BAMBOOZLED, DUPED, AND HOODWINKED

KEYS TO ESCAPING THE TRICKS, DECEPTIONS, AND HALF-TRUTHS OF THE MEDICAL INDUSTRY

BAMBOOZLED, DUPED, AND HOODWINKED

KEYS TO ESCAPING THE TRICKS, DECEPTIONS, AND HALF-TRUTHS OF THE MEDICAL INDUSTRY

JOSEPH G. JACKO, MD

ethos
collective

Printed in the United States of America

Published by Igniting Souls
PO Box 43, Powell, OH 43065
IgnitingSouls.com

LCCN: 2024920478
Paperback ISBN: 978-1-63680-401-9
Hardcover ISBN: 978-1-63680-402-6
e-book ISBN: 978-1-63680-403-3

Available in paperback, hardcover, e-book, and audiobook.

Dedication

This book is dedicated to independent thinkers,
those with the courage to challenge conventional thought.

Table of Contents

Part IV

Part V

Part VI

Conclusion

Appendices

About This Book

As I gathered the information for this book, I divided it into six sections. In the first section, I develop the concept of the half-truth by reviewing why it is so common, dangerous, and under-recognized. I review the psychology of those who have mastered the art of the half-truth and how they employ it in medicine. (The discussion on the half-truth has applications outside of medicine and will help you recognize the half-truths of politicians and the media tell.)

Evil exists in medicine. You may find my discussion on evil over the top, and some of my language too harsh or unfair to specific individuals at the center of COVID-19 management. However, I am confident such views will change by the end of the book.

Though I cite some examples of half-truths in these early chapters, the first section largely sets the stage for the remainder of the book.

In the second section, I'll examine how Big Pharma has gained control of the medical profession using bribes, kickbacks, threats, and blackmail while showing how it spreads its wings with its money far and wide into the medical infrastructure. You will also see how pharmaceutical companies manipulate and fabricate medical evidence, the foundation on which medicine is built. You will come to realize that science and evidence-based medicine are significantly flawed.

The third section debunks commonly held myths regarding medicine's contribution to longevity, shows the limitations of science in its ability to get to the truth, and discusses the detrimental effects of removing the art of medicine from the profession. You will see how little benefit medicine provides from our chronic disease management, and that there are less costly and more efficient ways to improve the quality and quantity of life.

The fourth section uncovers the incestuous relationship between the FDA and Big Pharma and why drug companies manufacture drugs the way they do. This process has more to do with obtaining patents and making money than improving health.

In the fifth section, I discuss my awakening to the corruption in medicine, the cancer therapy business, and the media's role and how it actively participates in bamboozling, duping, and hoodwinking us. I offer tips to patients and physicians on protecting themselves from future deception permeating the halls of the medical establishment.

Finally, the sixth section addresses the COVID-19 pandemic and how the half-truths were fully implemented with the aid of the media to deceive us about the pandemic's severity. The media misrepresented the safety and efficacy of the mRNA COVID-19 vaccines and fomented fear. I expose the decades-old criminal activity of a corporate entity at the center of the pandemic.

This Book's Goal

I want to be clear that I speak for myself but provide convincing evidence based on extensive research and expressed and viewed as thoughtful and persuasive arguments when I share my opinion. My goal is not to claim I am right. My goal is to find something increasingly absent in medicine—*the truth*.

One of this book's goals is to prompt you to do your own thinking and research and then propel yourself into action. You have access to the same information physicians do. You no longer need doctors or the media for health information. At some point, you must decide to educate yourself, take ownership of your health, and refuse to be bamboozled, duped, or hoodwinked. Sooner or later, you must say, "Enough is enough."

No one wants to hear that they have been fooled—bamboozled, duped, and hoodwinked. One ongoing challenge I encountered was striking a balance in my attempt to inoffensively educate and even wake up some of you. I apologize in advance if I am not always successful in that endeavor.

Remember that I, too, have been bamboozled, duped, and hoodwinked. We are all in this together. We need to look closely at ourselves to understand how we allow ourselves to be misled.

At some point, you must decide to educate yourself, take ownership of your health, and refuse to be bamboozled, duped, or hoodwinked.

For medicine to change, patients and awakened physicians will have to generate a grassroots movement. Physicians must have a strong desire, coupled with action, to wrest back control of their profession from the blue suits steering it off a cliff.

What You Need to Know About Me

Fortunately, I've had a unique and diverse career in medicine in comparison to most physicians, which perhaps gave me a broader view of medicine with different perspectives based on many experiences. We tend to see things or problems only as they relate to ourselves, and then, only from a narrow prism. My prism is broader than most physicians' and, perhaps, it makes me uniquely positioned to write this book.

I have been blessed to have learned from and worked with some of the best physicians and surgeons in the country, many of whom have been pioneers in their fields. I try to see where the future of medicine is heading and then get there as quickly as possible. I like to be on the cutting edge.

My medical career began with a formal primary care sports medicine fellowship at the Hughston Orthopaedic Clinic (now the Hughston Clinic), following up at the Cooper Clinic and Institute for Aerobic Research in Dallas.

I spent the bulk of my career with Southwest Orthopedic Institute (since merged with the Texas Orthopaedic Association), treating elite high school athletes. There, I worked with some of the best sports medicine surgeons in the country and the finest athletic trainers you can find. Two of my partners served as head physicians for the United States Olympic Team, the only practice in the country that can make that claim.

Later, I joined the Steadman-Hawkins Clinic of the Carolinas and trained and practiced Age Management Medicine with Cenegenics Medical Institute—a pioneer in hormone optimization that also focused on exercise, nutrition, and lifestyle medicine as the essentials to health and longevity.

Finally, in December 2022, I departed a large physician-owned primary care practice on the forefront of population- and value-based medicine.

Along the way, I completed a fellowship in regenerative medicine and certifications in the use of peptides and as a personal trainer. I now have a small concierge practice implementing everything I have learned and providing my patients with a wide selection of treatment options. Our practice includes dieticians, exercise physiologists, personal trainers, massage therapists, athletic coaches, and three fitness centers with the latest technology in sports performance recovery.

Breakthroughs in any field occur when there is a breakthrough in thought. For that to occur, you must abandon conventional thought, which becomes a stagnant pool over time. But you may find it difficult to swim upstream. I have a selective contrarian mindset and do not fear going against the current. Truth be told, I've learned that being in the majority is not always the best place to be.

My situation is also unique—I can speak more freely than many physicians because I am not employed, nor do I accept insurance for my services. Thus, I am less constrained by the medical establishment, and that freedom allows me to write what you are about to read.

Broad View of Medicine

Throughout my years as a physician, having learned from leaders in the field, I have seen how medicine is practiced across the spectrum. Mostly, I've called myself a sports medicine physician, but I never really considered sports medicine a distinct specialty as much as a philosophy for caring for patients and helping them achieve optimal health and function. I apply the sports medicine approach to all patients regardless of age and occupation.

Surprisingly, achieving optimal health and function has never been the goal of medicine, and we cannot achieve it with a pharmaceutical-driven approach that is the mainstay of today's medicine. Medicine is like all other professions in that it has become self-serving. It wants illness. It needs you to *not* be well.

Some of what you will read is not new. Others have reached similar conclusions, but I hope to package and present it in an easy-to-understand style. My goal is to connect the dots to show you the interplay of our complicated healthcare system and how it doesn't benefit you as much as you think or as much as it should.

Introduction: What You Will Learn from This Book

You probably bought this book because you sense something is wrong in medicine and cannot pinpoint exactly what or why.

If you feel that way, you have a good reason. Non-medical people hijacked medicine and now control it with the inside help of some physicians. Today, medicine's primary purpose is to maximize profit while patient care takes a back seat.

Medicine has a dark side, and this book reveals what goes on behind the scenes.

Like much of society, medicine has become increasingly corrupt. We expect some corruption within society, but not in medicine. Yet, medicine *is* fertile ground for corruption because it is the last place one would think it could occur. The deceptions baked into half-truths go primarily unnoticed in medicine.

Medicine is run by the blue suits: the CEOs of pharmaceutical companies, insurance companies, hospital systems, large group practices, directors of federal health agencies, and patient advocacy groups. They have the inside help of medical journals and their editors, as well as medical societies and organizations.

They conspire to maximize profit, protect each other, and control physicians while providing marginal patient benefits. Physicians are the conduits through which most money flows. By controlling what physicians are taught, coupled with strong micromanagement, physicians have become unknowing pawns in a system designed to enrich the medical establishment.

The book emphasizes that much of medicine is based on half-truths and that the science on which much of medicine is built is tainted, invalid, and in some cases, completely fabricated. There is a strong intent to mislead patients and physicians with "science."

Though I had talking points and topics in mind, I had no idea how or where to start. But just starting somewhere is 90 percent of anything. Unknowingly, I followed the advice of William Cobbett, an English journalist, politician, and pamphleteer from the 1700s:

> *Sit down to write what you have thought,*
> *and not to think about what you shall write.*

I found myself intuitively doing that—simply writing what I thought. The biggest challenge was knowing when to stop writing. Most of this book was written by mid-July 2024, but as I was revising it, I kept coming across pertinent new information and tried to weave it into the text. But I found this later information most helpful in tying topics together, reinforcing what I already wrote, and bringing better clarity.

I delved into one topic more than I had planned. Outside of the COVID-19 vaccines, I had no intention of discussing vaccines, but one last-minute discovery was hard to ignore and necessitated changes to two or three chapters.

Some of what you are about to read is shocking. Some of it is also shocking to me, even though I had an inkling before embarking on this project. But the half-truths and deception of medicine are far worse than I thought.

"Having Light, We Pass It Onto Others" is the motto of Wittenberg University, where I completed my undergraduate studies. What I have uncovered about the half-truths of medicine has enlightened me, and I believe my calling is to pass that light and knowledge onto others.

The book's take-home message will make many readers uncomfortable:

The people who control medicine are willing to risk your health in their quest for money, power, and control.[IP]

What You Will Learn

- Medicine does not always have your best interest in mind.
- Some medical misinformation comes from within the medical establishment and is hidden in half-truths.
- The corrupt nature of medicine.
- The nature and the seductive power of the half-truth and why we fall prey to it.
- The psychology of those who perpetrate half-truths and why we fall for them.

- Who controls medicine and the tactics used to gain and maintain a grasp on the medical system.
- The shortcomings of science and evidence-based medicine, the false security they provide to patients and physicians, and the fact that these entities are the source of most of the half-truths in medicine.
- When it comes to chronic disease management, we spend a significant amount of money to get only slightly better results than if we did nothing at all.
- Medicine adds little to longevity.
- The downside of taking a profession that is an art and a science and turning it into a pure science. Science does not address human interaction. Medicine is based on it.
- Medications and vaccines are overutilized and are not adequate substitutes for a healthy lifestyle. They do not provide as many benefits as they promote.
- The mRNA vaccines for COVID-19 are not as "safe and effective" as stated because "safe and effective" does not mean what you think it means.
- The media's role in bamboozling, duping, and hoodwinking you when it comes to your health.
- When it comes to medical information, your physician is essentially a middleman. You have access to the same information they do.
- Tips so you can become less dependent on the healthcare system, making it less likely that you will be bamboozled, duped, and hoodwinked by the profession.

- How half-truths and fear were masterfully used during the COVID-19 pandemic by those you trust, those you believe are credible, and those you think hold your best interest in mind.
- The Top 40 Not-So-Wacko Jacko Rules of Medicine.

The Top 40 Not-So-Wacko Jacko Rules of Medicine

Over the years, I've developed forty rules of medicine. I've peppered these rules throughout the book, some more than once. These rules will help you understand much of this book.

1. The people who control medicine are willing to risk your health in their quest for money, power, and control.
2. Medicine needs more scientific integrity as it is partially built on tainted science.
3. Medicine has become a big business, more than a profession caring for patients.
4. Patients and physicians are pawns in the health-care system created to make money for others.
5. Medicine is fertile ground for deception because it is the last place you would expect such acts to happen.
6. Abandon the thought that those supposed to help you in medicine have your best interest in mind. Their primary purpose is to help themselves; any benefit you receive is subordinate to it.

7. The first characteristic of a successful half-truth is that it emanates from a trusted source, which includes your trusted doctor, your trusted news source, and your trusted government and its agencies.
8. Financial gain and control are the endpoints of the half-truth. That is its second characteristic.
9. Your trust in the medical system makes you an easy target for deception and makes medicine an unexpected venue for others to take advantage of you.
10. For medical decisions to succeed, they must go through physicians without their knowing or recognizing that they are being used.
11. When you receive conflicting health recommendations, consider more strongly the advice from those who have little to gain from that advice and have the most practical experience.
12. Big Pharma makes money on drugs that are still on patent. It manipulates the medical system to ensure these drugs become the first line of treatment.
13. We emphasize drugs so much that we consider nature the "alternative." We have it backward. Nature was here first.
14. Half-truths, fear, and micromanagement power today's medicine.

15. If you are intent on deceiving and controlling as many people as possible and getting away with it, then politics and medicine are where you want to be, hiding in the open and functioning under the guise of helping people.
16. If you control the physicians' minds, you control medicine since physicians are the gateway to medical care. Big Pharma owns those minds.
17. Medical education, science, and published research are devices used to manipulate and control physicians and the practice of medicine.
18. The need for medical science is frequently heavily promoted by those who know how to manipulate it.
19. Evidence-based medicine only delivers when all the evidence is made available and is untainted.
20. Not all medical evidence is made available. Some is suppressed. Much is tainted.
21. If medical research is tainted, then the authenticity of medicine as a profession is questionable.
22. Science is always at least partially wrong until it gets it right, which may never be.
23. Science changes, but truth does not.
24. We get the most significant gains in life expectancy from the least expensive interventions.
25. The numbers do not tell the story. The numbers *behind* the numbers tell the real story.

26. We test what we can measure and think it is relevant because we can measure it. That is not always true.
27. Data on an individual is more valuable than the results of a study of a few thousand.
28. Big Pharma has made itself indispensable, not because of its drugs, but because of its money.
29. Keeping you alive as long as possible and as sick as possible while extracting as much money from you as possible has become the outcome of today's healthcare system.
30. Science doesn't happen overnight, but common sense does.
31. Medicine or healthcare does matter. It matters much to a few but little to many, and it's detrimental to some. It follows Pareto's Principle.
32. Taking a drug long-term alters your biochemistry in ways we do not always fully understand.
33. Just because a drug may work doesn't mean it's the only thing that works or it's the best thing that works.
34. Regarding health data, data from an insurance company is likely more accurate than that from a government health agency. Insurance companies go out of business if they have poor data; health agencies do not.

35. Medicine is not the pure science we are making it out to be. There is a reason it is called the "practice of medicine." Science does not address human interaction, while medicine is based on it.
36. Regarding research, especially medical, follow the money.
37. You are more likely to become financially healthier by buying stock in pharmaceutical companies than you are to become physically healthier by buying their drugs.
38. Avoid mainstream media for your health news.
39. Many people have a plan for their life, including their health. Some people want to control you and will attempt to do so, whatever the cost. It would be wise for you to have a plan of your own. You are the only one who has your best interests in mind.
40. Bonus Rule for Life: Stop being a coincidental believer. Few things happen by chance.

Some of what you will read is not new. Others have reached similar conclusions, but I hope to package and present it in an easy-to-understand style. I'll try to connect the dots to show you the interplay of our complicated healthcare system and how you are not benefiting from it as much as you should.

If we ask *why* long enough, eventually, we get to the heart of the matter. Frequently, we stop short of that in medicine, which prevents us from getting to the root of many problems. But it is when we find ourselves asking *why not* that the Eureka moment is close and the solutions are about to be discovered.

When I look at medicine and ask why, I conclude that much of what we do in medicine makes little sense because much of medicine is built on half-truths. Some of it is based on faulty precepts and hidden agendas.

The key to getting the right answers is to ask the right questions. The answer to every question or problem already exists. We just need to find it. We cannot discover the answers without the right questions. Unfortunately, I have not reached the Eureka moment to ask why not and provide meaningful solutions to the medical system. Instead, I will offer a few suggestions that will enable you to become less dependent on it.

A quote from John F. Kennedy's commencement address at Yale applies to this book's message:

> *The great enemy of the truth is very often*
> *not the lie—deliberate, contrived and dishonest—*
> *but the myth—persistent, persuasive and unrealistic.*[1]

The other half of the truth is both a lie and a myth. Let's begin to uncover the truth.

PART I

Medicine Is Built on Half-Truths

Be a free thinker and don't accept everything you hear as truth.
Be critical and evaluate what you believe in.
—Aristotle

You are being bamboozled, duped, and hoodwinked by the medical establishment. You are not alone. So is your doctor and many others. The only ones not being bamboozled, duped, and hoodwinked are those who run and control medicine.

The purpose of this book is to provide insight and information on how the medical profession operates behind the scenes. What will be discussed will be shocking to many, including those we call physicians.

Much of what we do in medicine is built on half-truth; some truth and just enough truth that the deception behind the half-truth goes unnoticed.

The word "medicine" has different definitions depending on the context. One definition, according to the *Merriam-Webster Dictionary*, is the "science and art dealing with the maintenance of health and the prevention, alleviation, or cure of a disease." A second definition is a "substance or preparation used in treating disease."[2]

When addressing the first definition, I am focusing on the non-surgical fields of medicine, specifically those specialties that rely heavily on medications for chronic disease management. This then leads us to the second definition.

Medicine as a Scam

Not-So-Wacko Jacko Rule of Medicine:

Medicine needs more scientific integrity as it is partially built on tainted science.

Part of medicine is a scam built on tricks, deceptions, and half-truths. The challenge for patients and physicians alike is knowing where the scams hide. My experience tells me patients do a better job identifying the scams and deceptions than physicians. Many physicians are oblivious to the deception to which they are exposed.

What is a scam?

Merriam-Webster defines scam as "a fraudulent or deceptive act or operation.[3] *Oxford Learner's Dictionary* defines scam as a "clever and dishonest plan to make money."[4] I use the word to mean both definitions.

In medicine, this scam isn't being perpetrated intentionally by a vast majority of the physicians. Most physicians truly believe they are helping patients and have their best interests in mind.

But physicians are being used, and many are unaware of it. The medical establishment controls what physicians know. The scam is perpetrated by the real powers behind medicine—those who sit behind desks wearing blue suits.

Misinformation circulates, and much of it comes from within the halls of medicine.

A Bad Taste of the Taste to Come

How bad are the half-truths that come from within the walls of the medical establishment? I will give you a look at how corrupt medicine is, but what follows is the tip of the iceberg.

Let's look at what former editors of two of the more prestigious medical journals, *The Lancet* and *The New England Journal of Medicine*, say about my profession.

Richard Horton, editor in chief of *The Lancet,* wrote, in 2015, "The case against science is straightforward: much of the scientific literature, perhaps half, may simply be untrue."[5]

In 2004, Dr. Horton said, "Journals had devolved into information laundering operations for the pharmaceutical industry."[6]

In 2009, former editor of *The New England Journal of Medicine*, Dr. Marcia Angell, said,

> It is simply no longer possible to believe much of the clinical research that is published, or to rely on the judgment of trusted physicians or authoritative medical guidelines. I take no pleasure in this conclusion, which I reached slowly and reluctantly over my two decades as an editor.[7]

And in 2002, former editor-in-chief of *The New England Journal of Medicine*, Dr. Arnold S Relman, said that

> the medical profession is being bought by the pharmaceutical industry, not only in terms of the practice of medicine,

> but also in terms of teaching and research. The academic institutions of this country are allowing themselves to be the paid agents of the pharmaceutical industry. I think it's disgraceful.[8]

I trust I now have your attention, but let's not stop there.

Former FDA Commissioner, Herbert L. Ley Jr., who served as FDA Commissioner from 1968 to 1969, stated that

> The FDA protects the big drug companies, and is subsequently rewarded, and using the government's police powers, they attack those who threaten the big drug companies. People think that the FDA is protecting them. It isn't. What the FDA is doing and what the public thinks it is doing are as different as night and day.[9]

And finally, here are the words from John Abramson, MD, Harvard Medical School.

> The first step is to give up the illusion that the primary purpose of modern medical research is to improve America's health most effectively and efficiently. In our opinion, the primary purpose of commercially funded clinical research is to maximize financial return on investment, not health.[10]

There you have the truth from four highly esteemed physicians and a former FDA Commissioner. I have given you just a taste of the bad taste to come. I will spend much of the book demonstrating and explaining why these individuals said what they said.

Medicine is about making money, even if it means misleading you with "scientific" research.

Doctors do not realize that they are being bamboozled, duped, and hoodwinked by questionable science, and patients, in turn, are bamboozled, duped, and hoodwinked because their physicians believe what they read in the medical literature.

The Powers That Control Medicine

The greatest evils in the world will not be carried out by men with guns, But by men in suits sitting behind desks.
—C. S. Lewis

What is evil? The word has many definitions. One is "morally wrong." Another is "arising from imputed bad character." Another is "causing harm." And then, we have "corrupt."

I use a definition that embodies all of the above. For the purposes of this book, I define evil as the "intentional act of deceiving or misleading others, or the strong desire to control people through deceptive acts, many times, carried out under the guise of helping them."

And that is what we have in medicine today. Medicine is full of such evil and deception masquerading as good intentions, and much of it is spewed from the desks of the suits who run medicine.

The blue suits function in the background. I refer to the blue suits as the medical establishment, which includes CEOs of pharmaceutical companies, insurance companies, hospital systems, and large physician practices, as well as directors of federal health agencies, medical societies, and medical journals. Combined, they control medicine because they control physicians.

Medicine goes through physicians, and if you want to control medicine, you must control physicians. You must regulate what they learn and shape how they think, so you can constrain their actions. Some might call that conditioning, brainwashing, indoctrination, or even grooming. You can decide what you might call it.

The health outcomes we get in medicine are dismal for the money we spend. The financial outcomes are great for the powers of medicine. Financial outcomes are more important than health outcomes to the blue suits. Patients and physicians exist for them to make money. Physicians and patients are pawns in a system rigged to make money for others who have little interest in your health.

I am sixty-four years old. I've been in medicine since I started medical school in 1982. Medicine has many wonderful aspects, but there is a dark side that is unrecognized. However, when it is recognized, it is not discussed.

A good part of medicine is built on half-truths and is driven by money to earn more money. The medical profession has become increasingly corrupt in my years in the field. I find it hard to imagine any profession being more corrupt than medicine right now, other than government and mainstream media, which goes without saying.

The Corruption of Medicine

What is corruption? Transparency International defines corruption as the "abuse of entrusted power for private gain."[11] I would broaden the definition to include "corporate gain" as well. The medical profession revolves around trust, and that trust in the system makes it a profession ripe for deception. It is easier to deceive those who have blind trust or near blind trust in something or someone.

Medicine is a microcosm of today's society. It is corrupt. It has become unethical. It is led by those motivated by greed and a lust for power and control. Corruption in our society is so rampant that it has reached a point where little attempt is made to even hide it, except, perhaps, in medicine.

Medicine is big business, representing 18–20 percent of our nation's GDP, a result of the focus on business and increasing profits rather than patient care.[12] Profits keep the doors open and provide for an increasingly better quality of care. But the profit-driven mentality is leading to unethical actions and tactics that hurt patients, even though patients may perceive that they are being helped.

Not-So-Wacko Jacko Rules of Medicine:

Patients and physicians are pawns in the healthcare system created to make money for others.

The Goal of the Half-Truth

That is one goal of the half-truth: to provide a benefit, or perceived benefit, to limit any questioning of ulterior agendas. We are less likely to question anything from which we derive some benefit.

Not much happens in medicine without the doctor-patient relationship, yet an increasing number of barriers serve to hinder and disrupt that relationship. Physicians are the gatekeepers of the system. Nearly everything in medicine runs through physicians. Here is why it is important to recognize this.

Not-So-Wacko Jacko Rule of Medicine:

To be successful, the medical deceptions must go through physicians without them knowing it and recognizing they are being used.

And the real powers of medicine have managed to pull that off.

In the process of using physicians, the blue suits have created a system that appeals to neither physicians nor patients. Both ends of that relationship are afterthoughts and merely a reason for an unnecessarily complex system.

An outgrowth of World War II was the military-industrial complex. In medicine, we have the Pharmaceutical-Medical Complex. The pharmaceutical companies are the main force behind medicine, with their hands involved in medical training and education, medical research, medical publishing, medical societies and organizations, dissemination of information through the media, and government and healthcare policy.

Many consider the military-industrial complex a necessary evil. We cannot live safely in America without it, but such a complex situation comes with risks of becoming too powerful and serving its own interests rather than those of the public.

The Pharmaceutical-Medical Complex

Much the same can be said about the pharmaceutical-medical complex. It largely serves its own interest in throwing dog bones to patients and physicians. A major difference between these two complexes is that the pharmaceutical industry is less necessary for our survival. Its "miracle drugs" are reported to be safe and effective, but that is based

If we took better care of ourselves and looked for better alternatives than medications, we would have less need for pharmaceutical companies, and, in turn, the pharmaceutical companies would have less influence on medicine.

on half-truths and, in fact, may be perpetuating chronic illness.

The military-industrial complex is a necessary evil due to the evil in the world. The Pharmaceutical-Medical Complex is a less necessary evil but largely exists due to the evil we do to our own health. Some of that harm, however, is inflicted upon us by the medical system itself.

If we took better care of ourselves and looked for better alternatives than medications, we would have less need for pharmaceutical companies, and, in turn, the pharmaceutical companies would have less influence on medicine.

And that is where medicine needs to put more focus—on getting out from under the control of pharmaceutical companies.

Sick-Care Medical System

The foundations of health—nutrition, exercise, and other lifestyle habits—are poorly taught in medical schools and residency training programs. We largely overlook the foundations of health and then wonder why we are so sick as a population. We are sick because the system wants us to be sick.

We have a sick-care model that benefits when sickness prevails. The medical system thrives on sickness. You and your doctor may want you to be well. But the system does not want you to be well. And the system, not your doctor, now calls the shots.

As you are about to learn, there is no money to be made in healthy people. At the same time, there is no money in dead people. Money is earned from those with illnesses, especially those with chronic diseases. Thus, the system is incentivized to promote a sick society or *at least give people the impression they are sick.* To some degree, we fabricate illness to justify treatments, some of which are unnecessary, and at best, many times, of marginal value.

As the medical system is currently structured, patients have little medical freedom. They are given limited options by physicians whose education is carefully scripted and crafted to serve the pharmaceutical-medical complex. The focus is on medications, medications, medications, with a sprinkling of surgery.

And, many times, the information you receive from your doctor is incomplete, limiting your ability to make the best decision for yourself.

Unnecessarily Complex Healthcare System

Managing sickness has become extremely complicated due to the unnecessarily complex healthcare system. Below is a schematic of our healthcare system that has evolved from the Affordable Care Act. Our healthcare system is so complex, I doubt anyone can get his or her arms around it well enough to explain it.

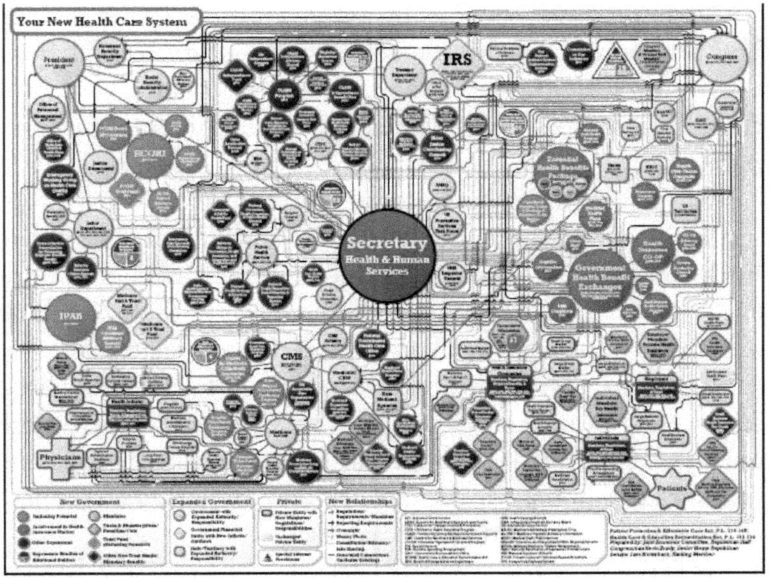

Healthcare Chart from the Joint Economic Committee, August 2, 2010.

At one point in history, this schematic would have only included patients and doctors. Now, you cannot even find them on the chart. Patients used to have direct access to doctors. Not anymore. Now, patients must leap, climb, jump, crawl, serpentine, sashay, and beg to see a doctor. Why so many middlemen? Do they benefit patients? No, the system benefits all the middlemen. The system is a big money-grabbing scheme with everybody trying to find ways to insert themselves into the flow of money.

From 1975 to 2010, the number of physicians in the US increased by 150 percent, keeping up with population growth. In that same 35-year span, the number of healthcare administrators grew 3,200 percent.[13] Considering that administrators do not improve our health, why do we need so many? We've made the system unnecessarily complex.

Patients have become insignificant under this system. You are represented by the star-shaped figure second from the bottom right. Shouldn't patients be at the center of this diagram? Nothing else exists on the diagram without patients.

Physicians have also become insignificant. We are represented by the cross symbol on the far bottom left. The entire healthcare system revolves around two entities that are not even next to each other. About 160 entities in that schematic are either supported by the doctor-patient relationship or profiting from it. Both doctors and patients are being used to generate profit and create jobs. Nearly every one of these entities has your private information too. Medicine is a convenient instrument for the government and others to collect data on you and invade your privacy.

It is not only the medical establishment that is bamboozling, duping, and hoodwinking you, however. The media plays a major role too.

The Media

You are also being bamboozled, duped, and hoodwinked if you rely on mainstream media for your health news. I will go into this in more detail in "Where You Get Your Information Matters," but beware that the mainstream media intentionally misleads you on some health matters.

The media have their own agenda, which is to help the ruling class control you by instilling unfounded fear. Fear is paralyzing and allows for conditioning. Also, the media receive significant amounts of ad money from the pharmaceutical companies, which I will discuss in "Big Pharma and Its Pursuit of Power."

Not-So-Wacko Jacko Rule:

Avoid mainstream media for your health news.

Just as physicians are unknowing pawns in the medical system, some in the media are also unknowing pawns spreading misinformation. The medical establishment, the government, and the media are masters of the half-truth. The half-truth is powerful. Let's find out how powerful it is.

The Power of the Half-Truth

A lie that is half the truth is ever the blackest of lies.
—Alfred Lord Tennyson

You have been bamboozled, duped, and hoodwinked by the medical establishment. Don't feel bad, though, as your doctor is equally bamboozled, duped, and hoodwinked.

Why is this? We easily fall prey to the most deceptive lie. That lie is called the half-truth, and it masquerades in the wide open, so much so that we don't see it.

Our tendency to fall prey to the half-truth dates to the Garden of Eden when Eve, then Adam, took a bite of the apple. The half-truth is the devil's invention and is the main device used today to fool others. When coupled with fear, it can motivate one to do almost anything. We witnessed that during the peak of the COVID-19 pandemic.

Pervasiveness of the Half-Truth

NASCAR cars sport so many sponsors that you don't even notice them. The half-truth is much the same. It is so commonplace today that it barely tickles our consciousness.

We perceive the half-truth as the whole truth, with the consequences of the outright lie, which makes it so dangerous. Unlike the outright lie, the half-truth goes undetected until it is detected, and that may never happen.

Medical misinformation and disinformation from unreliable and illegitimate sources abound. There is also medical misinformation and disinformation from perceived credible and legitimate sources. Yet, the misinformation and disinformation that are most dangerous are the ones you listen to and act on.

Who you listen to matters.

Would you follow advice from someone or something you don't trust? Likely not. The misinformation you don't listen to won't harm you; instead, it is the misinformation you listen to that will.

Thus, half-truths are most effective when they come from a source, either an individual or organization, that you perceive as credible, trustworthy, and caring, such as your trusted doctor, news source, or government and its agencies.

Not-So-Wacko Jacko Rule to Live By[IP]:

The first characteristic of the successful half-truth is that it emanates from a trusted source.[IP]

The people you trust most are most apt to misguide and deceive you. Not all of them, but a few will, and they may be your accountant, lawyer, financial planner, family, or, if you are Shohei Ohtani, your interpreter.

Not-So-Wacko Jacko Rule:

Medicine is fertile ground for deception because it is the last place you would expect such acts to happen.

Medicine is the last place you would think such deception would occur. But remember: The love of money is the root of all evil, and that applies to medicine too.

"Certainly, no one is going to put money above my health, would they?" Yes, they would, and they do every day. "Certainly, the recommendations I am receiving for my health are in my best interest." Maybe, but not always.

You need to adjust your thinking about medicine. Many times, what is best for you and your health is not always what happens.

While healthcare providers are essentially benevolent, those who control them are not.

Unlike your physician, the blue suits behind medicine do not know you. They do not know your name, do not know where you live, do not know what you do for a living. Everything they don't know makes it easy for them not to care about you. You are merely an entry on a spreadsheet.

Not-So-Wacko Jacko Rules of Medicine:

The blue suits are willing to risk your health in the quest for money, power, and control.

Your trust in the medical system makes you an easy target for deception and makes medicine an unexpected venue for others to take advantage of you.

The problem is that most physicians have been bamboozled, duped, and hoodwinked themselves. They are being taken advantage of and used without realizing it.

Everyone Can Be Bamboozled, Duped, and Hoodwinked

Let's look at Bernie Madoff, the mastermind behind the largest Ponzi scheme in the United States. He was intelligent, driven, charismatic, and he built trust and credibility with his clients so much so that extremely wealthy individuals gave him their fortunes to invest. In return, he bamboozled, duped, and hoodwinked them. These investors were intelligent, did their due diligence, were the least likely to be fooled, and yet, they were.

The half-truth is effective when tied to fear, but more so when it is also tied to greed. Fear and greed lead to emotional decision-making. Perhaps the desire (emotion) for greater riches blinded them to Bernie's half-truths. Regardless, he fooled his clients.

And you can be fooled, too, and you *are* being fooled.

Some of medicine is a scam. When I speak of medicine, I primarily talk of chronic disease management and those specialties heavily dependent on pharmaceutical solutions (little in this book applies to surgical fields). Within the system, physicians are primarily the pawns. The real powers behind medicine—the suits behind the desks—are the perpetrators.

If you are a physician, do not think for a minute that our profession has not deceived us. We have been lied to during our entire careers. It began with what we were taught.

If you are a patient, do not believe for one second that you are not being deceived by those with whom you trust your health.

The half-truth is the instrument of those who are looking to gain something, very commonly money or control over you.

Not-So-Wacko Jacko Rule:

Financial gain and control are the endpoints of the half-truth.
That is its second characteristic.[IP]

Do we find Bernie Madoffs in our government? Most certainly. Do we find Bernie Madoffs in our federal health agencies? You bet. Do we find Bernie Madoffs in pharmaceutical companies, health insurance companies, and hospital administration? Naturally. Do we find Bernie Madoffs on the boards of directors of medical societies and patient advocacy groups? Of course, we do.

Everyone probably has told a half-truth at some point. My questions are "Why did you do it? Did you have something to gain by doing so?" Most likely. That makes the half-truth so familiar and so enticing—the answer, frequently, is what benefits you more than the whole truth.

A group of people has mastered the art of the half-truth. They have perfected it. Telling half-truths is a daily routine for them. It is part of who they are. They are frequently charismatic and smooth talkers.

We call them sociopaths. Bernie Madoff had sociopathic features, and medicine is replete with such individuals too. Why should medicine be any different than the rest of society?

> **Disclaimer:** As a physician, I must be careful **not to make** a clinical diagnosis on someone I have not examined. Thus, I will describe individuals as having "features" or "characteristics" of a clinical diagnosis.

If a *sociopath* seems like too strong a word, you may not know what a sociopath entirely is. One need not be a sociopath to engage in half-truth telling, but the sociopath has perfected the craft and has taken it to another level.

In the next chapter, I will take a deeper dive into the psychological profile of the sociopath. Sociopaths are everywhere. Chances are, you cross paths with them every day and don't even realize it. They are the snakes of society, motivated by their self-interest to your detriment. Some are the powers behind medicine and government.

Not-So-Wacko Jacko Rule:

Abandon the thought that those supposed to help you in medicine have your best interest in mind. Their primary purpose is to help themselves; any benefit you receive is subordinate to it.

Half-truths and fear frequently co-exist. Create enough fear, and you can get people to do almost anything. You can get people to believe an outright lie with enough fear. And with enough fear, you can get people to give up their freedoms willingly. We witnessed that with COVID-19.

If the half-truth alone is not enough to get you to act a certain way in medicine, we add fear to the picture. "Well, if you don't want to die of a heart attack, you better take this pill." Or "You don't want your mother in the nursing home to die of COVID-19, do you? Get the vaccine, then."

Half-Truths Are Disinformation

Half-truths are a form of disinformation, and a majority come from the hallways of the medical establishment. Patients are given just enough information to act in a preferred way, being spared the whole truth.

The public perceives information coming from trusted and credible sources like doctors, medical societies, patient advocacy organizations, federal healthcare agencies, and other authorities to be whole, pure, definitive, and reliable, but frequently it is not. I suggest you start thinking otherwise.

You have already learned from medical editors that you cannot trust much in the medical literature, nor can you rely on the judgment of trusted physicians or authoritative medical guidelines. But worse than a half-truth is no truth or an outright lie coming from medical journals.

Half-Truths to No Truth

The Lancet and *The New England Journal of Medicine* are two of the most prestigious journals in the medical field. Thousands of physicians flock to them each week for the "best medical information," not knowing that, in some cases, they are being misled and, perhaps, intentionally misled.

During the height of the COVID-19 pandemic, both journals published articles, later retracted, related to the treatment of COVID-19. *The Lancet* article lambasted the use of hydroxychloroquine, but the study was based on unverifiable data (the authors eventually admitted), as was *The New England Journal of Medicine*'s article. Ultimately, the articles were found to be based on a non-existent or fictitious database—**a database that did not reflect science but rather science fiction.**[14]

Somehow, that escaped the editors and peer reviewers of these prominent journals. If two of the most prestigious journals publish articles based on a fictitious database, how much content of any medical publication can we trust? It casts a black eye on the entire profession.

Are these articles isolated events? Were the publications intentionally using the fictitious database, or were the editors incompetent? Either way, such occurrences now discredit or should discredit these "credible" publications and the veracity of all past, present, and future studies they publish, including Pfizer's studies on the Pfizer-BioNTech mRNA vaccines published subsequently in *The New England Journal of Medicine*.[15] Should we trust the results of those studies?

Physicians should be angry that two prominent journals published what is, in essence, science fiction, but there appears to be no meaningful negative reaction to it.

For the mRNA vaccines to be *tested* under Emergency Use Authorization (EUA), that meant no other safe and effective treatments already existed that were FDA-approved. Thus, treatments like ivermectin and hydroxychloroquine, both of which are FDA-approved, needed to look ineffective and dangerous. They manipulated science to do just that.

Medicine vs. the Law

The medical profession is now about money, and nearly everyone is on the take. That is how low the profession has sunk. Medicine is an increasingly corrupt profession, falling just below the government and mainstream media, and tied with the legal and justice systems. Go to PubMed.com and search "medicine and corruption." As I wrote this book, I found 1,277 results, and the number increases monthly.

The difference between corruption in the law and corruption in medicine is that corruption in the legal and justice systems is somewhat visible and expected. Corruption in medicine is hidden and unexpected, which makes it fertile ground for deception.[IP]

Another difference between medicine and the law is that medicine is a more significant part of your life. Some people may never have a meaningful encounter with the legal system. We encounter medical half-truths nearly daily. They are hard to escape, even when you know they exist. Like landmines, it's hard to know you stepped on one until it's too late.

Corruption in medicine is hidden and unexpected, which makes it fertile ground for deception.

Medicine is about making money, even if it means misleading you with "scientific" research.

Medicine has gone from a calling to a career and, today, for most physicians, simply a job. The blue suits have shifted the focus from patient care to pocketbook care while creating endless obstacles between doctors and patients. They shackle physicians who go against the grain in their attempt to do what is best for the patient.

Doctors and patients are being taken advantage of for the selfish purposes of those who now run the profession.

Half-truths Are Championed by Those Who Financially Gain from Them

In medicine, the half-truths will likely be championed by those who gain financially from spreading them. Invariably, half-truths lead to these individuals making more money.

The greater the potential for more money, the more likely they will use a half-truth. Those who genuinely have your best interests in mind are less likely to be motivated by money.

Of all the entities involved in medicine, those who deliver the care (providers, nurses, and ancillary support in patient care) are far more altruistic in their motivation than those who run the business entities. Physicians, generally, try to do what they think is best for patients. However, today, the medical establishment carefully manipulates their thinking, so what they think is best may not be.

People who give advice that they do not personally gain from are less likely to deceive you intentionally. Let's look at COVID-19 and the controversy regarding its treatment.

Physicians who recommended the use of ivermectin and hydroxychloroquine *did not profit* from that advice. If there were any financial profits, they were a mere pittance to the $63.2 billion Pfizer made in 2021 and 2022 from its COVID-19 vaccine.[16] Pfizer and Moderna profited the most, not individual physicians who recommended ivermectin or hydroxychloroquine.

The profiteers and barons of the medical establishment beat up those front-line doctors who challenged the medical establishment and tried to warn us. Yet, we have substantial evidence that physicians who opposed the medical establishment on COVID-19 management were right.

Practical Experience vs. Desk Experience

What did we do with COVID-19? Think about this for a minute. We turned our backs on those who had the most experience and were obtaining real-time information on what was working. We ignored those who rolled up their sleeves and got their hands dirty.

Instead, we took advice from those behind the desk, like Dr. Anthony Fauci, Dr. Rochelle Walensky, and Dr. Deborah Birx, none of whom treated *a single* COVID-19 patient. (Dr. Fauci, however, reports being part of a team that managed COVID-19 patients.) They did not propose any outpatient protocols beyond masking, distancing, and lockdowns (the World Health Organization stated lockdowns have "a profound negative impact"), all of which had a tremendous negative economic impact and did little to quiet the pandemic.

Those three individuals mentioned above misled the American public.

The Chinese had treatment protocols including the use of chloroquine as early as March 3, 2020, before most states in our country even had a case of COVID-19.[17] Death rates in countries using hydroxychloroquine (a cousin of chloroquine) were one-tenth the rate here in the United States. In Delhi, India, 97 percent of COVID-19 cases were successfully treated with ivermectin.[18]

While other countries were developing treatment protocols, our "health experts" were busy discussing lockdowns, masking, and distancing, and promoting "two weeks to flatten the curve" while passively waiting until monoclonal antibodies, antivirals, and vaccines were developed by and for the benefit of Big Pharma. Meanwhile, hundreds of thousands died unnecessarily.

For nine months, from March to December 2020, we watched *Seinfeld*, a show about nothing.

Common sense alone says we should have tried something, but we did not. We relied on passive measures. Our advice was, "Stay home until you get really sick, then go to the hospital." I'm not sure that a medical degree is required for such advice. The entire profession should be embarrassed, or at least that segment of the profession that discouraged trying something and promoted only passive measures.

Listening to our nation's "health experts" delivered this: The US represents 4.1 percent of the world's population, yet it was responsible for 15.9 percent of the COVID-19 cases and 17.4 percent of COVID-19 deaths worldwide.[19] Developing countries with living conditions more conducive to pandemics performed better than we did.

With the help of the mainstream media and widespread censorship, information was concealed from the public. We have heard from Mark Zuckerberg that the White House pressured Facebook (Meta) to censor information on COVID-19.[20]

From the beginning of the pandemic to May 2020, an estimated 500,000 preventable deaths occurred among our family, friends, and colleagues from COVID-19 due to our nation's poor leadership and passive approach.

[21]Why did we not do what was working elsewhere? What we witnessed was a stall tactic enabling Big Pharma to cash in on new drug development and vaccines. Who you listen to matters. You obtained limited and misleading information with respect to COVID-19 (and it likely trickles over to other topics). Clearly, our "experts" made poor decisions. Were those decisions their choices alone? Do those decisions represent intentionality or incompetency? (I will go into all of this in more detail in the COVID-19 chapters.)

Not-So-Wacko Jacko Rule:

When you receive conflicting health recommendations, consider more strongly the advice from those who have the most practical experience and the least to gain from that advice.[IP]

Physicians Fleeing the Profession

Half-truths have enticed people to go into medicine, but they are not always strong enough to keep them in practice. While many physicians may not see the half-truths, they do see a profession in increasing disarray, with many fleeing the profession.

Physicians may not agree with some of what I am stating, but they sense something is wrong with the medical profession. Physician Side Gigs is an online physician community boasting 185,000 members, including 110,000 members in its Facebook group. There are about one million to 1.1 million doctors in the United States. So, 15–20 percent of them are a part of the online community. Probably 90 percent of the remaining percentage would join the group if they knew of its existence.

A majority of the physicians in the Facebook group are frustrated and disgruntled with their career choices. Most of them refer to what they do as their "job," not position, opportunity, career, or profession, but *job*.

I don't post comments or reply to comments. I just read and "listen," and the posts are enlightening, entertaining, and discouraging. They provide a glimpse of the present and future of medicine from a provider perspective.

Nearly all those who post comments are looking for alternative ways to supplement their incomes so they can become less dependent on the practice of medicine and get away from patient care. Some have totally walked away from medicine in their late 40s or early 50s.

From its physicians' survey, *Physician Side Gigs* reported that 70 percent of its members would *not* recommend a medical career to their children. Forty percent of women physicians cut back or leave medicine entirely within their first six years, and 25–50 percent of physicians want to leave clinical practice in the next few years.[22] Though they may not see the half-truths, I believe the half-truths manifest in their opinions of medicine.

In other words, they feel the adverse effects of half-truths without seeing them.

The problem I see for these *Physician Side Gig* physicians is that they are job-hopping from one employment "job" to another. If a physician is employed, that physician is controlled, and it is hard to be professionally satisfied when controlled.

What a change from a couple of decades ago. During the early part of my career, it was not unusual for doctors to practice into their 70s or early 80s because they still loved practicing medicine and found it rewarding long after they were financially secure. Not anymore. Doctors are leaving the profession earlier and as soon as they can afford it.

That does not speak well to the system the blue suits have created. And it is not good for patients. Do you really want someone caring for you because it is a "job" or because they feel trapped in a profession due to the enormous debt they incurred in the educational process?

Seventy-four percent of doctors are now employed,[23] with many trapped by student loans. (The average debt is $200,000, with some up to $400,000.[24]) They wake up to the realization that they have become servants to their employers. The promises embedded in the half-truths that lured them into the profession have not been delivered upon, nor will they for most.

Employed physicians have little autonomy to do the right thing for their patients. They must do what the system tells them. They are micromanaged. Critical and independent thinking is no longer allowed.

I doubt the blue suits care that they are running off doctors. You might, but you don't matter in their system either. Patients should be front and center in any healthcare model.

The blue suits will replace doctors with less trained and less expensive physician assistants and nurse practitioners, which they are already doing, and patients will, ultimately, pay the price.

If the blue suits run off physicians, who make a decent salary, do they not think that they will eventually run off mid-level providers? These providers will be assuming more responsibility for patient care without the physician's salary. I predict that the mid-level providers will eventually flee the profession as well.

Patients should be front and center in any healthcare model.

Mid-Level Providers

What we once called mid-level providers are now referred to as "advanced practice providers" (APPs) and include physician assistants, nurse practitioners, certified registered nurse anesthetists, and certified midwives.

The change in the name to "advanced" is an attempt to bamboozle, dupe, and hoodwink you into thinking you are getting elite care. "Advanced" as compared to what? Physicians? Not likely. These "advanced" practice providers have about half the training as physicians.

Many of these mid-level providers do a very good job for their limited level of training compared to physicians.

Controlling language is a key to controlling you. "Advanced" is not the same as "mid-level," and "equity" is not the same as "equality." You are being bamboozled, duped, and hoodwinked into thinking otherwise.

Micromanagement

Nearly everyone I meet these days dislikes their jobs, and not just in medicine. Why? I think a big part of it is that almost everyone is micromanaged to death, becoming human robots, and that includes physicians and other healthcare workers. Micromanagement is a control device of the self-proclaimed elite, including the medical establishment. The elite only want people educated enough to obey orders. The medical system is now based on conformity, compliance, and standardization. Physicians desire fulfillment and meaning, not drudgery, and certainly not a miserable, repetitive existence, which is what medicine has become. Blindly following clinical practice guidelines, some of which are based on bogus science, does not make for an uplifting career.

Medicine is on a self-destructive path. It just doesn't know it yet. Patients are becoming increasingly distrustful of the medical system. COVID-19 mismanagement escalated that distrust. The medical establishment does not recognize the growing silent majority unhappy with the system the establishment has built. The system is teetering and may be one black swan event away from collapse.

Not-So-Wacko Jacko Rule:

Half-truths, fear, and micromanagement power today's medicine.

Where the Half-Truth Hides

Where do we find these half-truths? In short, everywhere.

Half-truths hide

- In the medication you take
- In medical education
- In medical research
- In the clinical guidelines physicians must follow to treat you
- In position statements put forth by physician organizations
- In lab tests

I will review these one by one, focusing on the first point and providing a more detailed discussion of some of the others in later chapters.

Medications

One of the more prevalent places where half-truths hide is within the medications you take, especially those you take for chronic conditions.

Many commonly prescribed medications are not nearly as effective as advertised, nor as safe. The term "safe and effective" does not mean what you think. Clever marketing and statistical distraction or sleight of hand cloud the actual safety and efficacy of prescription medications.

When you hear a drug is effective, you likely assume it works in most patients. That is not what it means. It really means that it works better than a placebo, which isn't expected to work at all. A drug can surpass a placebo and be FDA-approved, working only in a small percentage of patients. This scenario is commonplace.

It is a half-truth that you take medication to lower your blood pressure, cholesterol, or blood sugar. The reason you take such medications is to prevent premature death and the complications of conditions like heart disease and stroke.

It is a subtle but essential distinction.

Drugs are effective in lowering blood pressure, cholesterol, and blood sugar. They are not nearly as effective when it comes to preventing stroke, heart attacks, and premature death—the outcomes you are trying to avoid. Modifying a risk factor doesn't always alter the risk of getting a disease. We can show you that your blood pressure is lower, but it is much harder to prove that lowering it is doing you any good. That mindset presupposes that no other options exist that might be safer.

Treating a risk factor does not necessarily reduce the risk of a disease, at least not very well. For example, depending on the class of blood pressure medication, 86 to 140 patients have to take said medication for five years to prevent one heart attack or stroke.[25] The 86–140 are the "numbers needed to treat" (NNT) to prevent one cardiovascular incident.

Does that sound effective to you? Considering that such drugs would have performed better than a placebo and that performance meets statistical significance, those numbers meet the satisfaction of the FDA to approve. However, statistical significance is not the same as clinical relevance, which is what patients need to know and weigh.

Statistical significance means that the results are real and are not likely to have occurred by chance alone, but it does not mean the results are relevant in a clinical setting (clinical relevance). Clinical relevance is more subjective and considers a patient's risk tolerance and overall risk profile.

Is an NNT of 86–140 relevant? That's up to you as a patient to decide. Some might find a one in 86 chance of benefiting from a drug worth the risks, but some will not. But to make that decision, you need to know those numbers, but such numbers are hidden from you. All you see and hear are the *relative risk reductions.*

For example, if you watched the 2024 Summer Olympics, you likely saw plenty of pharmaceutical commercials. A commercial for Repatha, which lowers LDL cholesterol, boasted a 63 percent reduction in LDL cholesterol and a 27 percent relative risk reduction in cardiovascular events. Sounds impressive. What the commercial did not disclose is that a monthly Repatha injection costs $600 and that 81 to 104 patients must receive it to prevent one excess cardiovascular event at the rate of one per year.[26]

You received only the half-truth.

Statistical significance means that the results are real and are not likely to have occurred by chance alone, but it does not mean the results are relevant in a clinical setting (clinical relevance). Clinical relevance is more subjective and considers a patient's risk tolerance and overall risk profile.

Individual vs. Society

Some of you probably do not consider 86 to 140 acceptable numbers, but many times, numbers in this range are still cost-effective, and that is what drives their use. Let me explain. Let's use an NNT of 100 for blood pressure medicine to prevent a cardiovascular event at five years. It may be less expensive to pay for such treatment on 100 patients, despite 99 patients not benefiting from it, than it is to pay for the one heart attack that will be avoided.

In essence, even though we are treating you, we do so with the interest of society or the entire population in mind, not what is in *your* best interests. We treat 99 to benefit one, but that one saves the system money. Plus, we don't know who that one person is who will benefit, but there is only a one-in-a-hundred chance it will be you. Thus, we tend to overtreat disease.

These actuarial equations remove the focus from what is best for you as an individual to what is best for the population and medical system. It is assumed, incorrectly, that if we treat you and you do not benefit, then we are not harming you. We likely are harming some people with that approach, and you are likely to be subjected to more frequent office visits and unnecessary blood work.

Improving fitness will reduce mortality more than treating heart disease, diabetes, obesity, hypertension, and other chronic diseases. Yet, we do the opposite. We prescribe medications and ignore fitness.

This is a fundamental problem when trying to extrapolate data from a study on a few thousand patients and apply it to an individual. Science breaks down when applied to the individual.

We now hear about "population health." There is a simple way to improve the general health of the population without overtreating individuals and *without any medication.* Simply improving fitness will reduce mortality more than treating heart disease, diabetes, obesity, hypertension, and other chronic diseases. Yet, we do the opposite. We prescribe medications and ignore fitness. I will cover this more in "You Are Not Likely to Die of Anything, But Will Die from Something."

I will again review statistical significance and clinical relevance in "The Pharmaceutical Funded FDA," so don't worry if you don't quite understand now.

My purpose is to illustrate how often you are not given all the information you need and likely want to make the best decision for you, not the healthcare system.

The Number Needed to Treat

Numbers needed to treat are incredibly challenging to find in any published study, probably because, many times, they are not terribly impressive. Rarely will a study provide that information. Instead, it will discuss relative risk reduction, which is misleading, but it is the metric that prompts doctors to write prescriptions. More on that later. But there is a tool that can help you. That tool is TheNNT.com site.

This website can be a useful tool for the numbers to treat for some of the more commonly prescribed classes of medications. The data is based on 5–10 years of drug use.

Assessments or drug evaluations on TheNNT.com are color-coded green, yellow, red, or black.

- Green: presents good evidence of essential patient benefits (but even then, some of the NNT are high).
- Yellow: more study is needed to assess the benefit/risk of a drug.
- Red: benefits and harms are equivocal or equal.
- Black: a drug or class of drugs has clear harms without recognizable benefit.

If you want to search the NNT for statins (cholesterol-lowering drugs), you can research the benefits/risks in four categories of patients:

- Statins in persons at low risk of cardiovascular disease
- Statins for heart disease prevention (without prior heart disease)
- Statins for prevention (with known heart disease)
- Statins for acute coronary syndrome

In patients at low risk for cardiovascular disease, you will see that after ten years of statin use, there is no mortality benefit. Two hundred seventeen people would have to take a statin for ten years to prevent one nonfatal heart attack, and one in 313 people will be spared a nonfatal stroke. But one in 204 will develop diabetes, and one in 21 will experience muscle pain/damage.

The data on statins for three categories are coded in red. "Statins for prevention with known heart disease" is coded in green, but the NNT is quite high even then. Based on five years of statin use, statins help one in 83, one in 39 is spared a non-fatal heart attack, and one in 125 is spared a stroke, but one in 50 develops diabetes, and one in 10 develops muscle issues. Statins are known to raise blood sugar.

Also, to achieve these numbers needed to treat, you will soon learn that many "tricks" are employed by researchers to make the numbers look "as good as they do," which are not all that good.

The numbers needed to treat come down (improve) the longer a medication is used, but that is offset by the side effects and adverse drug reactions going up.

Some people will buy every product's extended warranty. Some buy none. Neither decision is right nor wrong. The choice simply depends on how much risk they are willing to take or how much uncertainty they tolerate. If a drug or other treatment has even the slightest chance of helping, some will want the treatment regardless of a plethora of potential side effects.

Then, you must assess your risk tolerance and motivation level to change your lifestyle habits if you opt not to be treated for a condition. You will never go wrong by improving your lifestyle habits, but sometimes, that may not be enough. Also, a high number to treat is not necessarily "bad" if the drug costs pennies a day and has few side effects. In that case, it might be worth taking such a drug even if there is only a one-in-100 chance it might help.

In general, drugs that treat chronic problems resulting from poor lifestyle have high numbers needed to treat. Keep in mind that reducing a risk factor does not lead to a commensurate reduction in preventing a chronic disease.

COVID-19 Vaccines

You likely heard that the COVID-19 vaccines were 95 percent effective in preventing infection and 100 percent effective in preventing death. Those are relative risk reductions, and they sound impressive, but they are misleading. Let's examine this further.

Just *one* COVID-19 death is prevented for every 22,000 people who are vaccinated, per Pfizer's study. For every 22,000 **unvaccinated,** two died from COVID-19. For every 22,000 **vaccinated,** one died from the disease. That represents a 100 percent relative risk reduction in deaths. Going from 2 to 1 represents a 100 percent reduction, but 22,000 must be vaccinated to achieve that one less death. That 100 percent relative risk reduction is very misleading. It is a half-truth.

The **absolute risk reduction** in getting the coronavirus if vaccinated was only 0.84 percent, which represents a 95 percent vaccine efficacy or **relative risk reduction**. I will go into how scientists derived these numbers in "Pfizer's Deceptive COVID-19 Vaccine Trial."

Would you have received the vaccine if you knew it takes 22,000 people to be vaccinated to prevent one COVID-19 death? **That is not misinformation**. You'll find it in black and white in Pfizer's 6-month study of its mRNA vaccine.

You got the half-truth. You heard 100 percent efficacy in preventing death and 95 percent efficacy in preventing infection without any explanation of what those terms mean. The full weight of the medical establishment bamboozled, duped, and hoodwinked you.

Would you have received the vaccine if you knew it takes 22,000 people to be vaccinated to prevent one COVID-19 death?

Furthermore, some of that data was not even available until more than half the population had already been vaccinated. Some of you were ramrodded into the vaccines before much was known about their safety and efficacy. And some of you got vaccinated for the "benefit of society" before much was known about their safety and efficacy.

Only two months of data were available when the vaccines were rolled out to the general population. More complete data wasn't available until September 15, 2021, nearly nine months after the mass vaccinations began. Some of you were never fully informed because the information did not exist when you were vaccinated. You were part of an experiment—the largest experiment performed on mankind.

If you were vaccinated after that date, were you informed of those numbers or at least received an explanation as to what they meant? Likely not, but why not? I will review this again in "COVID-19: Chaos, Confusion, and Coercion."

Medical Education

Half-truths hide in medical education. Academic centers take money from Big Pharma, which influences what is taught and how it is taught.[27] As it relates to non-surgical fields, the emphasis is on prescription medications. The fundamentals of health, nutrition, and exercise are glossed over. I go over this more in "Big Pharma and Its Pursuit of Power."

Medical Research

Medical research is riddled with half-truths, especially when it comes to drug studies. I will devote more time to this in "How Pure Is the Evidence?" You will see why former editors of *The Lancet* and *The New England Journal of Medicine* said much medical research cannot be trusted. Some of the medical literature is better described as science fiction.

Clinical Practice Guidelines

Half-truths hide in the clinical guidelines used today. Clinical guidelines are based on medical evidence as well as expert opinion. Instead of being used to "guide" physicians, such guidelines have become the "rule of law" for physicians. You have already learned from the editors of medical journals that the science is tainted, including the science that shapes clinical guidelines.

And the experts? Many have financial ties to various industries, not limited to the pharmaceutical industry, and thus have conflicts of interest.[28]

If science is so clear-cut, why do clinical practice guidelines vary from country to country? How can people look at the same evidence and come to different conclusions, and who decides whose conclusions are correct?

Pharmaceutical companies strongly influence clinical guidelines and play a role in determining when treatment for a condition should start and the treatment's target goal.[29]

Position Statements

Half-truths hide in position statements of the physician organizations, societies, and certification boards. These statements are designed to sway the way doctors practice medicine. They are somewhat like clinical practice guidelines, but more subjective and opinion-driven. These professional societies set the standards of care for medicine. Deviate from them as a physician, and you are not practicing the standard of care. With half-truths embedded within them, the standards of care become a device to control doctors.

Lab Tests

The "normal ranges" of lab tests, the reference ranges, often have little to do with what is optimal or normal and, therefore, are half-truths. They are **statistical ranges** that typically encompass the middle 95 percent of the population. Calling them "normal ranges" is a misnomer.

Many doctors are content with a vitamin D level of 30 ng/dl, which is the low end of the reference range. If that is your level, congratulations, 97.5 percent of the population has higher levels than you. Some health benefits from vitamin D do not kick in until your level is 55 or higher.

You can have symptoms related to any number of medical conditions despite expected lab test results, but frequently, your provider dismisses such symptoms because of "normal" lab results. "Your lab results are normal. Your fatigue must be in your head." They may suggest that you feel fatigued because you are stressed or depressed, even though you don't think you are.

Half-truths are designed to deceive you and to get you and your doctor to act in a particular way.

What's the end game of half-truths?

Half-truths are designed to deceive you and to get you and your doctor to act in a particular way. They are propagated by those who benefit most, the blue suits of medicine.

Much of what I just mentioned are summaries. I will be discussing these topics more in the "Big Pharma and Its Pursuit of Power" and "How Pure Is the Evidence?" chapters.

Military-Industrial Complex

A significant outcome of World War II was the establishment of the military-industrial complex. Before this permanent armament industry was invented, civilian factories would convert to making military equipment in times of war.

Today, we have the pharmaceutical-medical complex.

In his farewell speech on January 17, 1961, President Dwight D. Eisenhower expressed concern that the military-industrial complex (that he helped build) could become too powerful. This sentiment came from the former

Chief of Staff of the Army and the First Supreme Allied Commander Europe.

He also voiced concern about the industry taking over **academic research**. I include much of his speech related to the military-industrial complex because the issues and concerns he expressed are relevant today as they relate to the pharmaceutical-medical complex.

> This conjunction of an immense military establishment and a large arms industry is new in the American experience. The total influence—economic, political, even spiritual—is felt in every city, every state house, every office of the Federal government. We recognize the imperative need for this development. Yet we must not fail to comprehend its grave implications. Our toil, resources and livelihood are all involved; so is the very structure of our society.
>
> In the councils of government, we must guard against the acquisition of unwarranted influence, whether sought or unsought, by the military-industrial complex. The potential for the disastrous rise of misplaced power exists and will persist....
>
> ...Akin to, and largely responsible for the sweeping changes in our industrial-military posture, has been the technological revolution during recent decades.
>
> In this revolution, research has become central; it also becomes more formalized, complex, and costly. A steadily increasing share is conducted for, by, or at the direction of the Federal government.

> Today, the solitary inventor, tinkering in his shop, has been overshadowed by task forces of scientists in laboratories and testing fields. In the same fashion, the free university, historically the fountainhead of free ideas and scientific discovery, has experienced a revolution in the conduct of research. Partly because of the huge costs involved, a government contract becomes virtually a substitute for intellectual curiosity. For every old blackboard, there are now hundreds of new electronic computers.
>
> The prospect of domination of the nation's scholars by Federal employment, project allocations, and the power of money is ever present and is gravely to be regarded.
>
> Yet, in holding scientific research and discovery in respect, as we should, we must also be alert to the equal and opposite danger that public policy could itself become the captive of a scientific-technological elite.[30]

Within the speech is an important point I will return to—the complexity of research that almost necessitates a relationship between academia and industry.

Pharmaceutical-Medical Complex

Just like we need a military, we do need a pharmaceutical industry. Ours does some good, but not as much as patients think, and not nearly as much as doctors, who have been conditioned by the pharmaceutical companies.

I could say the medical-pharmaceutical complex. Instead, I put "pharmaceutical" first because it is the blue suits of the pharmaceutical industry who control the medical industry. The tail is wagging the dog.

How does the pharmaceutical industry control medicine? By controlling and strongly influencing every aspect of medicine—education, research, medical publishing, healthcare policy, federal healthcare agencies, physician professional societies, patient advocacy groups, government/politics, and others.

Not-So-Wacko Jacko Rule:

Big Pharma uses its vast sum of money to wield its influence and force its will on everything it encounters.

Big Pharma vs. Illegal Drug Cartels

A half-truth is most effective when it comes from a trusted source, and it is more effective if there is some benefit or perceived benefit for the person the half-truth is trying to trap.

People are less likely to feel that they are being bamboozled if they believe they have obtained some benefit. This enables the half-truth to prosper longer. Many patients believe they benefit from the medications they take, and sometimes they do, but not to the extent they think.

Pablo Escobar

Colombian drug lord Pablo Escobar was one of the world's biggest criminals. He was also one of the world's most generous. He spent money building roads, schools, libraries, hospitals, low-income housing, stadiums, plus he gave cash to several thousand people. This secured his support and loyalty from the Colombians, and though they benefited from his generosity, Pablo Escobar benefited still more. Many people look the other way if they have something to gain, and so it is with medicine as well.[31]

Big Pharma does much the same. It spreads its wealth to buy loyalty. It donates to the FDA, academic centers, medical journals, physician organizations, patient advocacy groups, the media, and physicians. Despite giving away a good portion of its money, it gets more in return.

It is hard to see any daylight between the tactics of Big Pharma and illegal drug cartels.

If you or I had a cure for cancer that costs a few bucks a month, you can be sure Big Pharma would not allow it to get to market. That is how much they don't care about you if they are not the ones making money. The only way your "cure" may get to market is if you sell it to Big Pharma. However, they may buy it without marketing it if more profitable options are available.

Big Pharma is about money first, foremost, and only. Big Pharma only wants people to be helped if it is the one making money, preferably with expensive drugs or on an ongoing basis, which we see with chronic disease management. Big Pharma wants customers for life. Big Pharma uses the FDA as its police force anytime it feels threatened.

Not-So-Wacko Jacko Rule:

Big Pharma makes its money on drugs still on patent. It will manipulate the medical system to make sure drugs still on patent become the first line of treatment.[IP]

Big Pharma made sure its patented products, like monoclonal antibodies and antivirals, were used first, and it discredited off-patent drugs already in the market. It will even "trash" its own FDA-approved drugs off-patent if necessary. Merck did this with ivermectin to promote molnupiravir, its antiviral for the coronavirus.[32] You can compare how poorly molnupiravir performed compared to ivermectin at C19early.org (look for molnupiravir under the RdRP inhibitors category).

The C19early.org website collects data on everything that has been tried in the treatment of COVID-19, from prescription medication (some off-patent, some still on patent), supplements, and lifestyle habits. It shows how many studies have been done on each treatment intervention, how many patients were in the studies, how many researchers were involved, and how many countries were involved in the studies, and, most importantly, it shows the outcomes associated with each treatment. Some existing FDA-approved drugs off patent performed better, and, in some cases, far better, than the more recent patented ones that Dr. Fauci and others were promoting.

Again, medicine is about making money, not getting the best results.

Half-Truth Chain of Command

The successful half-truth must have the following:

- The inventor or originator of the half-truth who is perceived as credible.
- Spreaders of the half-truth who are perceived as credible.
- Receivers of the half-truth.

The medical establishment is the inventor of a half-truth and uses others in the medical establishment to knowingly spread it. Physicians are both receivers and spreaders of the half-truth. They receive the half-truth but perceive it as the whole truth and, thus, spread it onto patients. Physicians are unknowing spreaders of the half-truth.

Physicians are being used, and many don't know it. The medical establishment has carefully groomed them to be useful pawns in the system. Conditioning, indoctrination, brainwashing, and grooming are at play.

Most doctors believe they are acting in your best interests, not realizing they have fallen prey to the same half-truths they help spread. Many times, they are just as bamboozled, duped, and hoodwinked as patients, perhaps even more.

Preparing You to Be Bamboozled, Duped, and Hoodwinked

Historically, governments have used medicine as an instrument to control people and gather information. In 1961, long before he was president of the United States and before being governor of California, Ronald Reagan discussed this encroachment of government on private citizens through healthcare as a way "to get a foot in the door" of controlling people.[33]

We fail to recognize that because, in our country, the encroachment on privacy and data collection via healthcare has been gradual. Unlike other countries, we have not had a rapid descent towards socialism. The descent has been more gradual, but it is rapidly accelerating. For those of you old enough, compare today's healthcare to 20 years ago. You will see there have been significant changes in the lack of privacy and loss of freedoms, and not only in medicine.

Now, for the preparation process.

Rapidly at the onset but slowly over time, the medical profession prepares you to be duped. It may not have been done intentionally, but it is a natural byproduct of how medicine is practiced.

What follows is an oversimplified explanation of this preparation. I will go over some of it in more detail when we get to the appropriate chapters.

System Dependency

First, society makes you a medical dependent. It does this quickly. You are groomed to be a medical dependent shortly after you are conceived. While still *in utero,* you are exposed to the medical profession and, subsequently, you have frequent visits to doctors during the first few years of life.

Seeing doctors becomes a routine part of your life. You think nothing of it, yet each medical encounter builds on the next. You become comfortable. The frequent medical visits are like eating sugar. Exposed to sugar when you are young, you don't realize you are addicted to an extremely addictive substance.

Just like sugar rewires your brain, repeated doctor visits condition you to become medically dependent with repeated doctor visits.

Note: This is not to suggest medical visits have no value.

As you age, you cannot escape seeing a doctor even if you don't have a problem. You might need a wellness exam, a sports physical, or an exam for employment. If you want to travel, you may need a doctor's note saying you are free of infectious diseases and up to date on your immunizations. If you are sick, you are required to see a doctor. If you are ill and want to go to work or school, you can't unless you see a doctor and get a note.

At some point, you may tire of seeing doctors, but the medical profession won't let you escape. Each medical encounter is an opportunity to "sell" you on a treatment. The doctor frequently discusses the need for prevention, not much in terms of lifestyle habits, but in the form of vaccines, ensuring you receive most of the ones available for your age.

You may be shown how you are sick or in poor health, even though you may feel fine. The doctor cites data from studies from leading medical journals showing how you may benefit from a drug, using misrepresented data with little discussion on addressing the problem at its root cause.

Trust Your Doctor

While you are being converted to a medical dependent, you are told to trust your doctors. Your doctors will proudly tell you that they are the only qualified healthcare professionals. They know what is best for you, so much so that even though you have access to all the same medical information, you have no reason to research anything, as that is the doctors' job.

Stroke Doctors' Egos

The medical education system strokes doctors' egos. They are told they are the best and brightest. They are trained, conditioned, and brainwashed to believe that they, and only they, have the answers to patients' health problems.

Doctors become convinced that they are superior to all other healthcare professionals and that treatments from other medical professionals are antiquated and inadequate. They believe other treatments are not based on "science," yet have little knowledge of these treatments to speak about them intelligently. In the end, you follow their advice, though much of what your doctor is doing is not working for you. If you express concern, you may find yourself terminated from the practice.

Conditioned Physicians

Just like you are told to trust your doctors, doctors trust their education, not realizing that what they learned is carefully scripted and crafted to serve the interests of the pharmaceutical-medical complex rather than those of patients. Doctors are conditioned to believe that they are receiving the best, up-to-date, and complete education, and the only one that can lead to true health because it is scientifically based, not realizing that some of science is misrepresented, and in some cases, completely fabricated.

They are conditioned to believe that the only acceptable form of therapy for most non-surgical problems is an FDA-approved pharmaceutical medication. Unfortunately, this medication often does not address the problem's root cause. They are so convinced of the medications' value that if you were to take the prescription pad away from many general internal and family practitioners, they would have no other tool in their toolbox to treat you. They have one skill—writing prescriptions. They're a hammer and see everything as a nail.

Drug Sales Pitch

Clever marketing and sales pitches misrepresent, through statistical sleight of hand, drug safety and efficacy data to physicians who may not be savvy enough to see through the deception. Such misrepresented information is replicated and reinforced when published in medical journals. Big

Pharma financially supports those journals through ad buys and article reprint purchases.

Consequently, doctors prescribe medications, sometimes bombarding patients with drugs that have marginal benefits and a plethora of side effects. Most patients are likely to suffer from a side effect rather than the drug's intended benefit.

What's the first characteristic of the half-truth? Trust in credible sources. You trust your doctor, and he or she trusts their training. Both of you are being bamboozled, duped, and hoodwinked in the process.

Medical Journals

Medical journals suppress articles potentially damaging to Big Pharma by not publishing unfavorable articles or publishing them in the least damaging way. Not only that, but researchers self-censor themselves by rarely submitting negative studies, so we never know about them.

When an article is published, pharmaceutical companies purchase thousands and thousands of reprints, dispensing them to pharmaceutical reps who deliver the reprints into the hands of physicians. Those reprints are not inexpensive and can account for as much as 50 percent of a journal's revenue.[34] This motivates medical journals to publish articles, even those of dubious value.

You can see how one entity scratches the back of the other. However, journals are not the only ones protecting Big Pharma.

TV Ads

Those pharmaceutical television ads serve a purpose other than being marketing aides. Big Pharma uses them to curry favor with television networks. The television networks receive about one-tenth of their television ad revenue from drug companies[35] and don't want to lose it.

Thus, they eagerly promote Big Pharma's drugs and help protect the drug companies against negative publicity, not unlike the FDA and medical journals do. The media and medical journals have knowingly become spreaders of half-truths.

The media strongly controls what health information consumers read or hear by steering them to certain sources to control the narrative Big Pharma and the medical establishment desire. They masterfully play on emotions while misrepresenting health information and creating fear.

The Game Within the Game

We have a game of cat and mouse playing out between pharmaceutical companies and the FDA, as well as the pharmaceutical companies and medical journals.

FDA and Medical Journals

Would you include damaging information about yourself on your résumé when you apply for a job? Probably not.

Pharmaceutical companies do the same when they submit their data to the FDA for approval or to a medical journal for publication. As much as possible, they present only favorable data; that is, they do not present all their clinical data. The FDA, medical journals, and peer reviewers base their decisions solely on the information provided.

For instance, if a drug company conducts a study on three thousand patients at four different centers, it may submit data on only two thousand patients at three of the centers because the fourth center's data may show negative results. There is no way for the FDA or medical journals to know about the patients at the fourth location if the pharmaceutical company does not disclose it.

The FDA and medical journals are sometimes bamboozled, duped, and hoodwinked too. But, at least, they know that they could be misled. They are aware of this game but are powerless to do anything about it. They don't have the authority or legal standing to force pharmaceutical companies to turn over all their evidence, which is considered proprietary information. This is part of the reason the medical editors at *The New England Journal of Medicine* and *The Lancet* said what they did.

Researchers use other tricks when submitting studies for medical publication, which will be discussed later.

Peer Review

The concept of a "peer review" may sound ethical and provide a level of confidence and reassurance to patients and doctors alike. Unfortunately, a peer review does not serve its intended purpose because it is working in a rigged system. Like the FDA and medical journals, peer reviewers make decisions based on the material they are given.

Some studies show the peer-review process is biased.[36] Peer reviews did not pick up non-existent data in the cases of the retracted articles published in *The Lancet* and *The New England Journal of Medicine* because the peer-review process is not designed to pick up on such deception.

And so, patients and most doctors play the pawns in this big money-grabbing game. Worse yet, some doctors are in on the game, taking money from the drug companies in any number of ways.

How Much of the System Can You Trust?

Physicians will not want to believe, and in some cases, will refuse to believe, their profession is tainted. I suggest they do their own research on PubMed, search "corruption and medicine," and read some of the 1,200-plus results.

Half-truths in medicine are so common that once you recognize their omnipresence, they present a real challenge. Who or what do you believe? Who do you trust?

Most of us want to trust those we perceive as authorities, those in positions of influence, those who inform us, and those who are supposed to be on our side as citizens of this country. Yet, they are more likely to be successful in misleading you.

I recommend you become more skeptical. Do your own research on anything related to your health. And when you conduct your research, look into how other countries, less influenced by Big Pharma's forces, diagnose and treat medical conditions.

In the US, we think we are more advanced when it comes to healthcare. You may be surprised how poorly we stack up against Australia, Austria, Belgium, Canada, France, Germany, Japan, the Netherlands, Sweden, Switzerland, and the UK. Despite spending more money per capita on healthcare, the United States has a lower life expectancy and worse health outcomes since the onset of the COVID-19 pandemic.[37]

Don't be afraid to ask questions. Start with *why* or *how*. After all, it is your health and your life. If you sense something is not adding up, it probably does not add up. Trust your instincts.

Many times, physicians are blinded by their proximity to a situation and are unable to step back to view the issue from a bigger perspective. That ability to detach from a situation is a rare but necessary trait for seeing something as it truly is.

Sometimes, you need outsiders to shed light on a problem. Speaking of outsiders, let's move on to the next two chapters. I will use their observations of medicine and science as talking points throughout the remainder of this book.

Observations of a Rapper

Nothing strengthens authority so much as silence.
—Leonardo da Vinci

The greater the power, the more dangerous the abuse.
—Edmund Burke

Until July 5, 2021, I had never heard British rapper Zuby. That day, he posted on social media 20 things he'd learned about humanity during the pandemic. He provided a twenty-first bonus thought, which I think is the key to understanding many of his previous observations.

I am reposting some of his observations that apply to this book, though I feel most of his observations are relevant to medicine. As we progress through the chapters, keep in mind most of these observations. Many have some application to medicine even before COVID-19.

You may disagree with some of his observations (some of which may seem outrageous) at this stage in the book, but I am confident your views will change by the end. To measure how your views may have changed, you may want to use the following scale to indicate how much you agree or disagree with each statement, and then repeat that exercise when you finish the book.

1. Strongly disagree
2. Somewhat disagree
3. Neither agree nor disagree
4. Somewhat agree
5. Strongly agree

His bonus thought is critical and largely explains why medicine is ripe for deception and corruption, and why we are easily bamboozled when we follow those we trust. I am going to focus on that observation in this chapter.

As they relate to this book, below are Zuby's words, as posted in order on Twitter (now X):

> ***20 Things I've Learned (Or Had Confirmed) About Humanity During The "Pandemic" (THREAD):***
>
> 4. Propaganda is just as effective in the modern day as it was one hundred years ago. Access to limitless information has not made the average person any wiser.
>
> 5. Anything and everything can and will be politicized by the media, government, and those who trust them.
>
> 6. Many politicians and large corporations will gladly sacrifice human lives if it is conducive to their political and financial aspirations.

11. People who are dismissed as conspiracy theorists are often well-researched and simply ahead of the mainstream narrative.

12. Most people value safety and security more than freedom and liberty, even if said safety is merely an illusion.

15. Science has evolved into a secular pseudo-religion for millions of people in the West. This religion has little to do with science itself.

17. Politics, the media, science, and the healthcare industries are all corrupt, to varying degrees. Scientists and doctors can be bought as easily as politicians.

19. Modern people are overly complacent and lack vigilance when it comes to defending their own freedoms from government overreach.

Bonus thought:

21. Most people are fairly compassionate and have good intentions (this is good). As a result, most people deeply struggle to understand that some people, including our leaders, CAN have malicious or perverse intentions (this is bad).[38]

The Sociopathic Nature of Those Who Have Corrupted Medicine

We want to trust the government and its agencies. We want to trust the leaders of the education system. We want to trust religious and business leaders. We want to trust the leaders of science and technology. **And that is what they are counting on.** That trust makes it easier to deceive you for those set on deceiving you. Not all want to deceive you, but a small number do, and it only takes a small number to succeed.

We want to believe that our leaders have our best interests in mind. The reality is that many times, such leaders have only their best interests in mind.

Blind belief in authority is the greatest enemy of truth.
—Albert Einstein

We don't want to believe that there are people who intentionally inflict harm on us or have ill intentions, especially when it comes to our health, or who only have their best intentions in mind. Even by the time we get to the end of this book, some of you will still refuse to believe that there are people in medicine with bad intentions. We have such strong innate desires to trust authority figures that we don't want to believe otherwise, even when it can be demonstrated otherwise.

Our failure to believe that there are leaders with ill intentions is why we are repeatedly hoodwinked. It is no more complicated than that. The medical profession is built on trust. We trust the system and the authorities behind it implicitly, yet unwisely, and, consequently, are misled or harmed as a result, some of the time.

Some of the people who have corrupted medicine are malicious and perverse, and you need to understand their psychology. They tend to have certain personality traits. The person with malicious and perverse intentions that Zuby speaks of is, frequently, a sociopath or has sociopathic features. And we find sociopaths throughout society.

These individuals possess some very desirable qualities that make it challenging to identify them. They have leadership qualities; thus, we find many sociopaths in the upper levels of organizations of all stripes.

Sociopaths perpetrate evil. Their defining quality is that they have little or no remorse for their actions and little conscience. The concept of "good and bad" does not register for them.

As long as they get what they want (money, power, fame), they do not care what happens to others. They will use whatever means necessary to get what they want.

A patient of mine is a clinical psychologist. He shared with me that the psychological profile of a criminal, a criminal defense attorney, and a career politician is the same: the profile of a sociopath.

When I asked him for a reference, he steered me to *The Sociopath Next Door* by Martha Stout, PhD, a clinical psychologist who had served on the faculty of Harvard Medical School's Department of Psychiatry.

Dr. Stout reports that one in 25 individuals is a sociopath.[39] They are crossing your path every day. You just don't see them because sociopaths are so deceptive and clever. Her book helps you identify the sociopath.

Dr. Stout describes sociopaths as persons who

- are frequently intelligent, charismatic, and persuasive;
- learn early to show sham emotions but live only to dominate others and win.
- have a charisma that makes them more charming or interesting than people around them. They are more spontaneous, intense, complex, or sexier than everyone else;
- crave stimulation and excitement, often showing brief, intense enthusiasms that they later drop;

- are seductive, encouraging others to take risks; and
- will tell you that you are just like them. Don't believe it.

Other sociopathic features include

- being fearless, sometimes to the point of being reckless;
- having a high sense of self-worth and can be narcissists;
- engaging in deviant behavior;
- being arrogant, selfish, and manipulative;
- attempting to control others with threats or acts of aggression;
- having calculating minds; and
- failing to accept responsibility for their actions.

Some of these traits are desirable and possessed by many who have climbed the ladder of their profession. This seems to suggest that the higher we ascend, the more likely we will encounter those with sociopathic features.

When asked, in a 2012 interview, if sociopathy was more prevalent among politicians, Dr. Stout responded that

> Politicians are more likely than people in the general population to be sociopaths. I think you would find no expert in the field of sociopathy/psychopathy/antisocial personality disorder who would dispute this… That a small minority of human beings literally have no conscience was and is a bitter pill for our society to swallow—but it does

explain a great many things, shamelessly deceitful political behavior being one.[40]

She went on to say

> As it turns out, the majority of sociopaths/psychopaths never kill anyone with their own hands, nor do they end up in prison.... A smart sociopath can avoid prison and find other, less conspicuous ways to satisfy his or her lust for dominating and controlling others, and what better way than through politics and big business.

Healthcare is a big business, and it is the biggest in our country. And within that big business of healthcare is the biggest one of all—Big Pharma. Big Pharma is the force behind medicine. It does some good but is the master of deception, cleverly enlisting the help of others, including physicians.

Though not elected officials, many government bureaucrats function like and have characteristics of politicians. Many are career bureaucrats who wield great power, sometimes more than politicians. For instance, for thirty-eight years, Dr. Anthony Fauci served as NIAID director from 1984 to 2022. He called the shots on COVID-19, at least, in front of the television cameras. For comparison, J. Edgar Hoover was director of the FBI for thirty-seven years, from 1935 to 1972.

Career bureaucrats in government agencies carry out much of the government's function. These non-elected people have garnered too much power and control over your life and your health.

John Whitehead, an attorney and noted author, says this about political sociopaths:

> Political sociopaths are all largely cut from the same pathological cloth, brimming with seemingly easy charm and boasting calculating minds. Such leaders eventually create pathocracies—totalitarian societies bent on power, control, and destruction of both freedom in general and those who exercise their freedoms.[41]

Evil

Evil does exist. We all recognize that. But we forget that it takes evil people to commit evil. Evil doesn't happen of its own accord. It needs a source. Liars lie, cheaters cheat, thieves steal, and evil people do evil things—it's part of their DNA.

What is evil? For the purposes of this book, it is the intentional act of **deceiving others or the strong desire to control them through deceptive acts** carried out under the guise of helping them. Does such evil exist in medicine? Unquestionably.

Make no mistake. Some people don't want you to succeed, and they will ensure you don't. Others don't want you to do better than they are. And then, some are only happy when you are miserable, and they will make your life miserable so that they can be happy.

Evil needs evil people to exist.

Some of these people occupy positions of power and influence, having infiltrated the ranks of our institutions and organizations, including the entities that run medicine (insurance companies, hospital systems, pharmaceutical companies, etc.) and the physicians who collaborate with such entities and no longer care for patients.

When physicians leave the patient care arena, their focus changes, usually away from what is best for the patient to what is best for themselves and the pharmaceutical-medical complex. Some of them become bought-and-paid-for agents of the medical establishment, primarily controlled by Big Pharma.

Harming People by Hiding in the Open

Dr. Stout's comments on sociopaths finding less conspicuous ways to satisfy their lust for domination and control through politics and business remind me of a quote from Gus Fring speaking to Walter White on *Breaking Bad,* who said, "I hide in plain sight, just like you."[42]

Politics and medicine, including government health agencies, are the perfect venues for domination, control, and committing deception in plain sight and behind the illusion that one is doing his/her job helping people.

Bad healthcare policy decisions will harm more people than a mass shooting. From 1982 to 2024, deaths from mass shootings in the US totaled 1,150.[43] That's not 1,150 mass shootings. That's the number of deaths from 150 mass shootings. Far more people died unnecessarily in the US from our nation's handling of the COVID-19 pandemic than from forty years of mass shootings. You don't need a gun to kill or harm people. The tragedy of 9/11 proves that. Bad healthcare policy is also proof.

As a profession, medicine failed in its COVID-19 management. Many patients died unnecessarily—five hundred thousand through May 2020 because of bad policy masquerading as an attempt to protect the public.[44] Masks, distancing, and semi-lockdowns were never going to serve the purpose sold to the American public due to little science to support them. Those measures gave the illusion that the appropriate measures were being taken, despite accomplishing very little.

The American public was bamboozled, duped, and hoodwinked by such folly. The medical system withheld effective and inexpensive treatments until preferred profit-making therapeutics could be developed. Our passive and disillusioned approach denied early treatments with repurposed drugs, allowing patients to die. The bigger question, which I will leave unanswered, is why. Why did we not do more?

Not-So-Wacko Jacko Rule of Medicine:

If you are intent on deceiving and controlling as many people as possible and getting away with it, then politics and medicine are where you want to be, hiding in the open and functioning under the guise of helping people.[IP]

Perhaps that is the evil to which C. S. Lewis referred when he said that the greatest evils in the world will not be carried out by men with guns, but by men in suits sitting behind desks.

Many of us believe that our federal health agencies, with Big Pharma's help, poorly managed COVID-19. They took advantage of people's trust in them using half-truths, fear, and coercion, and, consequently, harmed many individuals.

Medicine Attracts Warped Minds

For some reason, we think our society is immune to such evil. I am here to tell you that there is evil in medicine.

Medicine has a history of attracting persons with warped and twisted minds and those thirsting for control and power. We've all read about physicians and nurses intentionally killing patients or conducting harmful human experiments.

Let's look back at World War II. German physicians joined the Nazi Party at four times the rate as other professionals. In fact, over 50 percent of German physicians joined the Nazi Party and participated in the many atrocities that happened in that war.[45]

Zyklon B, the gas used in the concentration camps during World War 11, was originally developed as a pesticide, and later, they discovered it could kill humans. Two civilian scientists/businessmen whose company supplied Zyklon B to the Nazis were tried as war criminals, found complicit in the murder of civilians by means of poisonous gas, and hanged on May 16, 1946.[46]

Take a moment to review Zuby's sixth observation now and again at the end of the book and see if you think it applies today.

> **Note:** In a later chapter, I will address the Nuremberg Code regarding human experimentation, a result of atrocities occurring during World War II. Our handling of COVID-19, specifically as it relates to vaccines, can be argued to have violated that Code.

There is much evil in this world because there is an overabundance of evil people.

Scientific Totalitarianism

I end this chapter with a discussion on scientific totalitarianism. Robert F Kennedy Jr., in *The Real Anthony Fauci,* paints quite a different picture of Dr. Fauci than the one we saw on television. Mr. Kennedy provides a thorough shakedown of

Dr. Fauci's career and the totalitarian approach he used in his thirty-eight years as Director of the National Institute of Allergy and Infectious Diseases (NIAID).

Mr. Kennedy describes how Dr. Fauci transformed NIAID into a pharma subsidiary and implemented a two-decade strategy of promoting false pandemics as a means for promoting vaccines and drugs benefiting the pharmaceutical industry. He writes

> Tony Fauci does not do public health; he is a businessman who has used his office to enrich his pharmaceutical partners and expand the reach of influence that has made him the most powerful—and despotic—doctor in human history.[47]

Kennedy describes Fauci as someone with strong influence over the CDC, FDA, HHS, NIH, and other organizations; he has the power to destroy or enrich careers, manipulate scientific journals, dictate study protocols, and control the *outcome* of scientific studies globally.

However, he is not the only one who has such conclusions about Dr. Fauci. Charles Ortleb, who has followed Dr. Fauci's career since he took over as the Director of the NIAID in 1984, says, "Scientific totalitarianism is the background music of Anthony Fauci's brilliant and long-lasting Ponzi scheme."[48]

On April 9, 2024, Senator Rand Paul reported that as early as January 2018, fifteen federal agencies were informed of the intent of the DEFUSE project to create a virus very similar, if not identical to COVID-19.[49] EcoHealth Alliance and the Wuhan Institute of Virology were seeking federal funding for the project in 2018.

Not one agency alerted the public that the Chinese lab was ready to move on such a project. The NIAID, headed by Dr. Fauci, was listed as a participant in the initial DEFUSE pitch.

And in Dr. Fauci's own words, "…it's been proven that when you *make it difficult* for people in their lives, they lose their ideological bullshit, and they get vaccinated."[50] *Making it difficult for people* to live their lives is a totalitarian tactic.

Challenging Dr. Fauci's actions in his management of COVID-19 was not permitted. The truth should not mind being questioned, but a lie might. Dr. Fauci did not like being questioned or second-guessed. Anyone who challenged his and his colleagues' actions was quickly dismissed as a quack or a "conspiracy theorist." There was no room for discussion, yet medicine and science are all about discussion.

Andrew Huff states that Dr. Fauci is guilty of 25 million counts of negligent homicide.[51] If those numbers are accurate, Dr. Fauci is responsible for more deaths than Adolf Hitler and Joseph Stalin combined. If Mr. Huff is correct, we see a perfect illustration of the degree of evil and harm possible when someone hides in the open under the guise of helping people while sitting behind a desk.

We should not be surprised, then, that Dr. Fauci accepted President Joe Biden's pre-emptive pardon, one of the president's last acts in office.[52]

Totalitarianism exists when discussion ceases or is prevented. That is where we find ourselves today, and not solely in medicine. On any given topic, only one view is now allowed to exist. We are going down a path of no return if it continues.

Medicine is mutating into a totalitarian profession where only the desires of federal health agencies and the medical establishment are permitted to exist. Patients' and physicians' concerns, now, matter little.

You need to understand Zuby's 21st observation:

> Most people are fairly compassionate and have good intentions (this is good). As a result, most people deeply struggle to understand that some people, including our "leaders," CAN have malicious or perverse intentions (this is bad).

His observation is real; it is ever present in our country and has taken root in medicine.

A Comedian's Observations

The truth does not require your participation
in order to exist. Bullshit does.
—Terence McKenna

Let's move on to something a little lighter in tone. Outsiders sometimes see things better than insiders and frequently state the obvious. They see the elephant in the room. In this chapter, I share the observations of an outsider, a comedian, and television host.

Bill Maher's Anti-Pharma Rant

In Bill Maher's four-minute, ten-second rant against Big Pharma, he summed up much of what is wrong with medicine. Though his 2007 rant was meant to be humorous, he exposed many hidden truths.

Let me set the scene. It is September 2007, in the middle of the presidential primaries, and he is discussing the health plans of the three remaining Democratic Presidential candidates, Hillary Clinton, Barack Obama, and John Edwards.

Briefly, in an entertaining way, Mr. Maher said:

- The government subsidizes illness in America because of the money illness generates.
- We make ourselves sick.
- Medicine is a big business and needs sick people.
- We treat a patient's symptoms with drugs without curing them.
- We come up with new diagnoses to justify using more drugs (known as medicalization).[53]

Mr. Maher mentions several conditions that used to be rare but are now mainstream. The conditions he mentions are primarily chronic and often require ongoing management for a lifetime. He is not speaking of the flu, appendicitis, acute sinusitis, urinary tract infections, or poison ivy.

He mentioned that in Hillary Clinton's health plan, the words "nutrition and exercise" appeared once, but the word "drugs" appeared 14 times, "just as the pharmaceutical companies want it."

I agree with his views.

We do well in medicine with acute conditions. We don't manage chronic conditions with the same level of success, though. That's because chronic diseases are largely lifestyle-related, and we emphasize medications over lifestyle changes. We push drugs over lifestyle changes for chronic conditions. That's one of the points he was making—we throw drugs at problems and create new diagnoses.

My specialty in internal medicine is nothing more than the clinical practice of pharmacology, but with a pharmacology background far from commensurate with the number of prescriptions we write.

Pharmacists spend three to four years studying pharmacology. I recall sixty hours of pharmacology in medical school, if that. Yet, ads tell you to ask your doctor. You are better off asking your pharmacist. Ponder that for a minute. You would think that the people prescribing medications would be expected to have more training and knowledge than those dispensing the medications.

If you were to take the prescription pad away from primary care providers, many would have no other option left in their toolbox to treat you. Many physicians have been conditioned to disregard any treatment that is not an FDA-approved medication.

Not-So-Wacko Jacko Rule to Live By:

Just because a medication may work does not mean it is the only thing that works, nor does it mean that it is the best thing that works.[IP]

That concept is lost on many physicians due to their medical training.

Not-So-Wacko Jacko Rule to Live By:

If you control physicians' brains, you control medicine.

Big Pharma excels at doing this. Big Pharma recognizes that much of medicine goes through physicians, and it owns the brains of most physicians. It has acquired this ownership slowly, incrementally, subtly, and mostly unnoticed by the medical profession. If Big Pharma had its way, doctors would happily treat every sign and symptom with a branded FDA-approved drug.

Do you need all these medications?

A good personal trainer will do more to improve your health than a good doctor. The latter will keep you alive as long as possible, but in a poor-to-fair state of health by administering medications. The former will help you improve your state of health by focusing on typically free lifestyle changes. A good personal trainer will enable you to live longer and healthier.

Not all physicians believe it is their responsibility to make you healthier.

Sometimes the patient's view of their doctor's role differs from the doctor's view. Some physicians readily acknowledge that they treat sick people and have little interest in preventing disease. They do not see prevention as their role. They think, "If you want to be healthy, work with a personal trainer, dietitian, or health coach. I treat sickness, and I do that with drugs."

In my opinion, that view is short-sighted, but if a physician is upfront about it, then a patient can choose to see someone else. You, as a patient, want to ensure you and your doctor are in alignment with what his or her role in your health should be.

The net effect of our chronic disease management is that you live to about seventy-seven years of age, but your health span—those years lived in good health—is about sixty-six.[54] In general, lifespan has increased from 59.6 in 1922 to 77.5 in 2022.[55] I will discuss the factors most responsible in "Does Medicine Matter?" But those additional years are not very functional. Our treatments for chronic disease may add years to your life, but they are not frequently good years. Medicine's net effect helps you live more crappy years.

Not-So-Wacko Jacko Rule to Live By:

Keeping you alive as long as possible, as sick as possible, while extracting as much money from you as possible has become the outcome of today's healthcare system.[IP]

Our nation has had to keep the military-industrial complex relevant and operational. (Could that be the reason for periodic wars?) Wars are expensive but lucrative.

Likewise, medicine and the government must keep the pharmaceutical industry financially healthy. Big Pharma makes its big money from drugs still on patent. They need an ongoing pipeline of new drugs as older drugs come off patent. It also helps if there are new diagnoses that create demand for new drugs.

Big Pharma has an expensive lifestyle, and it needs to keep generating higher and higher profits. It has two ways to induce physicians to write more prescriptions. First, new drugs for new diagnoses should be created, and second, "guide" physicians to use drugs earlier and earlier in the disease process by setting target goals for treatment requiring drugs.

Pharmaceutical companies sometimes have one to three generations of drugs for a condition like hypertension or diabetes. However, that leads to diminishing financial returns because the generations compete against themselves, and it becomes more difficult to make drugs better than what already exists. (Tidbit: New drugs are not necessarily more effective than older ones.)

Big Pharma is having a harder time creating patentable drugs for existing medical problems or diagnoses. One way to combat that problem is to make new diagnoses. As Bill

Maher suggested, Big Pharma periodically needs new conditions to treat, enabling them to patent new drugs as existing drugs come off patent.

We are beginning to label many symptoms as diseases. Some may be legitimate, but not all. Pharmaceutical companies like this idea because they can create new drugs. Patients like it, too, because they cling to a diagnosis. "I have such and such…." Or "My such and such is acting up. I can't come to work today." In some cases, having this symptom/diagnosis frees them from taking any responsibility for their health.

Another strategy to boost pharmaceutical profits is to increase the use of existing drugs by expanding the boundaries of problems like hypertension, diabetes, and cholesterol problems. This encourages drug use at earlier stages to get even lower blood pressures, blood sugar levels, and cholesterol levels. The target goals of treatment are also lowered in these conditions.

Medicalization

The process of adding new diagnoses and expanding the boundaries of a diagnosis is called "medicalization," and pharmaceutical companies play an active role in that process.[56] These companies want you to believe that every physical, social, or personal illness you have is the result of a molecular disease for which they can provide a molecular solution.

The medicalization and expansion of diagnostic boundaries raises concern among some in the medical profession; it gives Big Pharma too much influence in defining disease and expanding treatment guidelines to promote the use of more medication and at earlier stages.[57]

Patients use medications as a substitute for making lifestyle changes. "I took my diabetes medication, so I can eat this piece of chocolate cake." Thus, reliance on medications only perpetuates chronic disease.

When you exercise or improve your diet, the physiological changes benefit every organ system in your body. Medications will not give you the same universal benefits.

Medications typically block a natural biochemical process that is somewhat out of balance rather than improve or facilitate normal function.

We have SSRIs (serotonin reuptake inhibitors). We have ACE (angiotensin-converting enzyme) inhibitors. We have ARBs (angiotensin II receptor blockers). We have PPIs (proton pump inhibitors). We have PDE5 inhibitors (phosphodiesterase 5). We have HMG CoA reductase inhibitors (statins). We have COX-2 inhibitors (nonsteroidals). I will discuss this further in "Patented Drugs: Where the Money Is."

One thing we fail to recognize is that when we use a drug to block something from happening, we are also interfering with the production of downstream metabolites of whatever molecule we are blocking. Many downstream metabolites provide health benefits, and when they become deficient, side effects and other diseases occur.

Not So-Wacko Jacko Rule of Medicine:

Taking a drug long-term alters your biochemistry in ways we do not always fully understand.

Pharmaceutical companies make inhibitors and blockers for a reason. It is easier to get a patent to make them. Pharmaceutical companies cannot get patents on naturally occurring compounds. They must find a backdoor or workaround to get patents. Thus, drugs do not replicate or facilitate normal biochemical or physiological functions. To some degree, they are fighting against normal functions. Unless they are bioidentical, all drugs are toxins, at some level.

In the short term, many of the drugs in these classes are safe, but we do not know what the long-term consequences are of using a drug over several years and its possible impact on your body's physiology.

Medications do not give you the overall benefit to your health as lifestyle changes do. Yet, much of the practice of medicine relies on medications.

Pandemics and Vaccines

Not everyone needs a blood pressure medicine, for example, which limits the value of medicalization. But is there a pharmaceutical intervention that could be applied to the masses on a repeated basis? Is there another way to create new diagnoses beyond merely labeling symptoms as diseases?

A third way for pharmaceutical companies to generate more profit falls into the category of "conspiracy theory" for many people. Mr. Kennedy touched upon this in his description of Dr. Fauci. This way promotes false pandemics that require vaccinations. Vaccines are highly profitable. Scientists can now make viruses, in case you did not know.

COVID-19 is a new disease that has never been previously described, and Big Pharma needed to "discover" solutions that were subsequently found in monoclonal antibodies, vaccines, and antiviral medication, even though simpler solutions already existed.

The World Economic Forum shows five pandemics occurring between 2003 and 2019, which overlap with the gain-of-function research era. Five pandemics in sixteen years! The five pandemics before 2003 ranged from occurring in 1889 (H2N2) to 1981 (HIV/AIDS), or 92 years.[58]

Keep in mind that the living conditions in the late 1800s to the early to mid-1900s were far more conducive to pandemics worldwide and here in the US than we are now. I cover more on the importance of water purification and sanitation in limiting infectious disease in "Does Medicine Matter?" but will leave you with this thought for now.

It is not strange that health improves when the population gives up using diluted sewage as the principal beverage.
—Dr. Thurman Rice, 1932

Gain-of-function research was coined in 2011 but has existed longer than that. Gain-of-function involves making a pathogen more virulent than found in nature. There is also loss-of-function research, which consists of weakening a pathogen. This is what Louis Pasteur used in the late 1800s to develop vaccines for cholera, anthrax, and rabies.[59]

I found it difficult to find a date when gain-of-function research started (probably because it had no name before 2011). Still, I did learn that Georgetown researchers looked at scientific papers from 2000 to 2022 and reviewed 488 studies that involved the manipulation of pathogens.

Fifty-four percent of the studies involved gain-of-function research and 46 percent loss-of-function research only (some studies involved both gain- and loss-of-function). More than half the publications, 53 percent, involved US-affiliated researchers, and 21 percent involved China-related researchers. Twenty-four percent of the studies were related to vaccine development, and the most studied pathogens are those that cause high global health burdens. Less than 1 percent of the pathogens studied involved pathogens that the CDC recommended be studied under the highest levels of biosafety.

Pandemics are more likely to occur in the gain-of-function era, even with the best security measures in position (which may not have been the case in the Wuhan lab). And it is easy to bamboozle, dupe, and hoodwink the public into making a "pandemic" look worse than it is while providing the solutions to the problem.[60]

Big Pharma's Appetite

Big Pharma is a big beast that must be fed to fulfill its insatiable appetite. Remember, Big Pharma helps support much of healthcare, whether it be medical education and research, or financially by supporting advocacy groups and physician organizations, and, of course, politicians.

If the Big Pharma well dried up, many groups in the system would struggle financially. Big Pharma "subsidizes" much of medicine, thus giving it the "right" to control the practice of medicine.

Not-So-Wacko Jacko Rule to Live By:

Big Pharma has made itself indispensable, not because of its drugs, but because of its money.[IP]

In a way, you must congratulate Big Pharma for being savvy and positioning itself as well as it has. Big Pharma's primary goal is to make money, not to improve your health, though some of its drugs are beneficial. Its CEOs are responsible to their shareholders, not you or me.

How does Big Pharma do it? How does it spread its wings? How does it buy influence? I will discuss that in "Big Pharma and Its Pursuit of Power."

PART II

Big Pharma and Its Pursuit of Power

It's not that a handful of evil men can do evil things.
It's that a handful of evil men can convince a large majority
of ordinary men to help them do evil things.
—Devin Pendas, PhD

Devin Pendas, a professor at Boston College, teaches the history of war and genocide, war crime trials, and human rights. His quote is in response to the atrocities committed by the Nazi Party during World War II.

Keep in mind my definition of evil. I am not talking about Holocaust-type evil, but some of the tactics used then are used today to spread half-truths. Simply substitute *deceptive* for *evil* in the above quote so it reads:

It's not that a handful of deceptive men can do deceptive things. It's that a handful of deceptive men can convince a large majority of ordinary men to help them do deceptive things.

That is what Big Pharma does. It has mastered and used deceptive tactics to convince ordinary men to cede control of medicine without some of them knowing it.

All our institutions are corrupt. It does not take many evil or deceptive people to corrupt an institution or society. Sociopaths or those with evil intentions are good at enlisting help from ordinary people, many of whom have good intentions. Some of those ordinary people are physicians. As I stated previously, most physicians are unknowingly useful pawns in the medical system.

How do you convince ordinary and even good people to help you in your quest for domination and spread deception? They will offer financial rewards, bribes, and kickbacks, or use blackmail, threats, and coercion.

Big Pharma has been guilty of all those acts, some of which will be discussed in this chapter and some in later chapters. Financial rewards are the most common way Big Pharma garners control of medicine. It has bribed doctors and provided kickbacks.[61] It has even resorted to blackmail to cover up its misdeeds. While ignoring at least eighteen fines and lawsuits levied against his company since 1992, Dr. Albert Bourlas, CEO of Pfizer, labeled those resistant to receiving the mRNA COVID-19 vaccines as "criminals" by spreading "misinformation."[62]

Big Pharma does some good, but not nearly as much good as patients and physicians believe. Remember, a key to the successful half-truth is to provide some benefit.

We act as if their pharmaceutical solutions are the only solutions to our health problems. *We act as if the benefit of its drugs cannot be obtained in some other way.* But that is not true. No drug or group of drugs can bring the health benefits that exercise and diet can.

We speak of "natural alternatives," but we should refer to medications as "drug alternatives." We have it backward. We emphasize drugs so much that we now consider what we find in nature as the alternative. That is not to say that natural alternatives are the answer either. They tend to be less harmful; they may not be as effective as sometimes touted but can be effective.

Sometimes, we fail to see the forest for the trees. We get distracted or lose focus. The key to health is found neither in a pill nor a supplement; it is in your lifestyle.

Not-So-Wacko Jacko Rule of Medicine:

We emphasize drugs so much that we consider nature as the "alternative." We have it backwards. Nature was here first.[IP]

Big Pharma controls medicine by spreading its money far and deep into the medical infrastructure. As a result, much of the entire medical system is partially dependent on the financial health of the drug companies.

It's no different than a state becoming increasingly dependent on federal money, which is the carrot to compel the state to do what the federal government wants. The same is true with the pharmaceutical-medical complex.

Not-So-Wacko Jacko Rule of Medicine:

Big Pharma has made itself indispensable, not because of its drugs, but because of its money.

The remainder of this chapter may not be the most exciting to read but will perhaps be the most eye-opening. I will be throwing out many numbers to show how Big Pharma uses vast sums of money to control medicine.

I will use *Big Pharma* and *pharmaceutical companies* interchangeably, though more strictly speaking, Big Pharma refers to the world's largest publicly traded pharmaceutical companies.

There are two factors to consider when we discuss Big Pharma's control of medicine.

1. CEOs of pharmaceutical companies, health insurance companies, hospital systems, and large medical practices are beholden to their shareholders or stakeholders, not to patients or providers. That is an unsettling thought. They run their companies to optimize profits, and *profits are more important than health outcomes*.
2. The other important feature to recognize, as President Eisenhower discussed in his farewell speech, is that research is increasingly complex and expensive and requires vast intellectual and physical resources. This makes a "partnership" between industry and medicine nearly unavoidable. Frequently, the partnership tilts in favor of industry, in this case, Big Pharma. When it partners, even with academic centers, Big Pharma runs the show.[63]

Often, Big Pharma funds the missing dollars that government and academic centers cannot provide for research. In exchange for that money, academic and research centers invariably give up control of the research and how it is used.

If we were CEOs of any of these entities, we might make similar decisions to enhance our bottom lines. Personally, I would hope that there would be ethical barriers past which I would not venture. Yet, a problem is that those who run pharmaceutical companies, insurance companies, and hospital systems frequently cross ethical barriers.

Let's follow the money. Big Pharma donates to:

- political campaigns
- the Food and Drug Administration (FDA)
- patient advocacy groups
- academic and research centers
- medical journals and their editors
- physicians
- the media
- medical societies
- itself

Whether discussing medicine, politics, religion, or any other institution, one only must corrupt/compromise/bribe/payoff the head of an organization (and, perhaps, a few key underlings) to corrupt the entire organization and compromise its original mission. Big Pharma uses that tactic to gain control of medicine.

Big Pharma could not get away with some of what it does without physician participation, but many physicians view that as a good thing. Many physicians believe the pharmaceutical-medical complex benefits patients, Big Pharma, and themselves. But they do not know many of the behind-the-scenes tactics used by Big Pharma, which you are about to learn. They don't realize they are sometimes being duped by the industry.

I doubt much of what you are about to read is well-known to physicians.

Political Campaigns

It is always nice to have politicians promoting your interests, and Big Pharma spends more money on lobbying lawmakers than any other industry. According to STAT analysis, more than two-thirds of Congress cashed campaign checks in 2020 from pharmaceutical companies.[64] This included 72 senators and 302 members of the House of Representatives receiving $14 million from pharmaceutical political action committees or PACs. Pfizer's PAC donated money to 228 lawmakers, and Amgen donated to 216. Pfizer also donated to 1,048 individuals running in state legislative races.

From 1999 to 2018, the pharmaceutical and health product industry spent $4.7 billion—$233 million a year—in lobbying expenditures at the federal level.[65] This is more than any other industry.

This total includes $414 million in contributions to candidates in presidential and congressional races, national party committees, and other outside spending groups. Of the senators and the House members who received the most contributions, 39 belonged to committees with jurisdiction over health-related legislative matters.

[66]Some of these contributions bought influence when key referenda on drug pricing and regulation were presented. Campaign contributions and lobbying have been shown to influence elections and legislative outcomes.

Pharmaceutical donations go beyond the federal level. The industry showers campaign cash at the state level as well. *STAT News* shows that 25 percent of state lawmakers nationwide have accepted money from the pharmaceutical industry since 2019.[67] In Illinois, 79 percent of its 177 lawmakers cashed pharmaceutical checks. In California, 85 percent accepted checks from the pharmaceutical industry.

In 2019-20, nearly two thousand state legislators received campaign contributions from major pharmaceutical companies. Keep in mind, it is typically the governor's office that appoints those who serve on the state medical boards.

Here is a peek at what specific pharmaceutical companies and their lobbying arm, Pharmaceutical Research and Manufacturers of America (PhRMA), spent on campaign contributions at the state level in 2019. Keep in mind that PhRMA is the pharmaceutical industry's most powerful trade group.

- Pfizer sent $777,695 to 994 candidates or lawmakers.
- PhRMA sent $769,321 to 545 candidates or lawmakers.
- Lilly sent $493,440 to 454 candidates or lawmakers.
- Merck sent $407,900 to 491 candidates or lawmakers.
- Novartis sent $304,450 to 222 candidates or lawmakers.[68]

Pharmaceutical companies would not spend this money at the federal and state levels if it were not effective in influencing healthcare policy and legislative action.

To learn more about contributions possibly made to *your* representatives, go to KFFHealthnews.org and search for individual legislators to see whether they received any contributions, the amount, and from which pharmaceutical companies.

FDA

The FDA is not fully supported by tax dollars. Many people, including physicians, do not know this. Some of its funding derives from user fees from the various industries it regulates, which are more than just pharmaceutical companies.

Sixty-five percent of funding for drug approval by the FDA comes directly from the drug companies.

The FDA receives 45 percent of its total funding from user fees[69] but user fees make up 65 percent of its budget for the drug review and approval.[70] In other words, 65 percent of funding for its drug review and approval processes comes directly from the drug companies themselves. That seems like a recipe for conflicts of interest and leads to regulatory capture, where the industry controls the regulators.

We have a situation where the inmates run the asylum.

Now you better understand Mr. Ley's words, which I quoted earlier in the book.

> The FDA protects the big drug companies, and is subsequently rewarded, and using the government's police powers, they attack those who threaten the big drug companies. People think that the FDA is protecting them. It isn't. What the FDA is doing and what the public thinks it is doing are as different as night and day.

Patient Advocacy Groups

You may think that a patient advocacy group website from the American Diabetes Association or the American Cancer Society provides unbiased medical advice. You may want to rethink that belief as millions of dollars flow from Big Pharma to patient advocacy groups.[71]

Some of these patient advocacy groups, like the American Diabetes Association, take money from the food industry as well.

The New England Journal of Medicine (NEJM) reported that 83 percent of 104 patient advocacy groups received drug company support with widespread conflicts of interest.[72]

Thirty-seven percent of the advocacy groups in the *NEJM* focused on cancer. Of the 18 groups that did not report industry support, thirteen provide no list of any donors (obviously, they must have donors). Only 59 advocacy groups listed the amounts of their donations. Of those groups, 23 received at least $1 million from industry. Only 12 of the 104 advocacy groups had policies addressing institutional conflicts of interest.

Public Citizen is a consumer advocacy nonprofit. It reported that, between 2010 and 2022, the lobbying groups of pharmaceutical companies provided $6 billion in grants to more than 20 thousand organizations, including patient advocacy groups.[73] Public Citizen also uncovered:

- More than $720 million in grants were given out in 2021. And close to $600 million in grants were given out on average each year from 2018 through 2022.[74]
- More than 460 organizations received money from five or more PhRMA Network entities. More than 70 organizations received money from 10 or more PhRMA Network entities.
- Thirteen of the nation's largest and most powerful patient advocacy organizations received more than

$10 million from the PhRMA Network. In total, they received $266 million.

Now for some specifics.

- Over the 12-year period, the American Heart Association received $64.1 million, including $8.3 million from Pfizer and $29 million from AstraZeneca, two major drug companies.
- The American Cancer Society and its affiliate, the American Cancer Society Cancer Action Network, received $23.1 million, including $6 million from AstraZeneca, $4.7 million from Merck, and $3.4 million from Pfizer.
- The American Diabetes Association received $26.4 million, with more than $11 million from Sanofi and more than $7 million from Eli Lilly, both drug companies.

That kind of money always raises conflicts of interest, and due to the money these groups receive from pharmaceutical companies, the information on those websites may be biased.

Academic and Research Centers

This discussion primarily relates to industry-funded and independently funded research. Industry-funded research is just that—research funded by interested industries. In the case of medicine, this would include the pharmaceutical industry as well as the medical device industry. We should note that many pharmaceutical companies have medical device divisions or subsidiaries. This type of research has a vested interest in the outcomes of studies.

Independently funded research is funded by groups without a vested interest in the outcome of a study. This would include the government through agencies like the NIH, independent research groups, and charitable organizations. Thus, independently funded research is less likely to be biased.

Since 1982, industry-funded research has exceeded independently funded research, and now, industry funds over 50 percent of research conducted at academic centers.

For industry-funded research, not only does industry fund the research, but the pharmaceutical company usually designs, organizes, audits, analyzes the data, and writes up the findings with the help of their subcontractors. Often, pharmaceutical companies use contract research organizations (CROs) to do their work for them. About 70–75 percent of the industry's expenditures on clinical trials go to CROs, which had an estimated revenue of $50 billion in 2020.

It is not uncommon for ghostwriters to draft manuscripts even when an academic center led the industry-sponsored trial. Sergio Sismondo coined the term "ghost management," referring to the behind-the-scenes tactics used by pharmaceutical companies to get trial findings published.[75]

Since 1982, industry-funded research has exceeded independently funded research, and now, industry funds over 50 percent of research conducted at academic centers.[76]

Pharmaceutical companies spend more money on research than the National Institutes of Health.[77] Most contracts between industry and academic centers give ownership of the data to the industry (pharmaceutical company). The pharmaceutical company decides which data is used, how it is used, if it will be published, and how it will be published. The industry uses "intellectual property" and "proprietary information" as reasons to control what and how information is disseminated.

A 2018 study found that among 127 academic institutions in the US, only one-third required their faculty to submit research consulting agreements for institutional review. Only 35 percent of academic institutions thought it was necessary to review the agreements. When agreements were reviewed, only 23 percent of the institutions reviewed the publication rights.[78]

Here are some interesting findings:

- Industry-funded research is published at a lower rate compared to independently funded research. Big Pharma-funded studies are five times more likely to go unpublished, most likely because it does not want to publish negative results.[79] That seems to suggest they conduct a lot of negative studies. (I will go into this in "How Pure Is the Medical Evidence," but thirty-seven of thirty-eight studies that showed favorable outcomes of antidepressants were published, but only three of thirty-six negative studies on antidepressants were published.)[80]
- Industry-funded published research is more likely to show favorable results. Trials run by industry are 70 percent more likely than government-funded trials to show a positive result.
- *The New England Journal of Medicine* published seventy-three studies on new drugs. Pharmaceutical companies funded sixty of those studies, fifty featured

drug-company employees among the authors, and thirty-seven of the lead researchers received money from a drug company.[81]

- In 2014, pharmaceutical companies funded 6,550 trials, and the NIH funded 1,048.[82]

We can conclude that industry-funded research weeds out its bad outcomes, and because such outcomes are not published, no one knows about that research. This results in a publication bias in scientific research, making drugs look more effective than they are.

Industry interests can drive research agendas away from relevant questions that need to be asked. As I stated before, sometimes we are not asking the right questions. Some of that is due to industry influences that serve the industry and not public health. And questions are being asked that will lead to more prescription drug use.

Be careful how much you trust science. Remember my Not-So-Wacko Jacko Rule: Evidence-based medicine only meets its objectives when all evidence is available in untainted form.

The cozy relationship between Big Pharma and academic centers extends to boardrooms. Since 2012, every major US-based pharmaceutical company has had at least one board member in a leadership position at a US academic medical center. Such board members received an average compensation of $312,564 from the pharmaceutical companies.[83]

Big Pharma and academic centers should have competing interests. The pharmaceutical industry wants to protect its discoveries and intellectual property. Its focus is on profit, and it will suppress negative information when possible.

Academia should strive for the discovery of truth and the dissemination of *all* information. Unfortunately, academia frequently succumbs to pressure due to the money it receives from Big Pharma.

Medical Journals

Through legal proceedings and with the help of whistleblowers, expert witnesses, and investigative reporters, we have learned that pharmaceutical companies have rigged clinical trials, suppressed or hidden unfavorable results, used ghostwriters, paid kickbacks to physicians, produced fake medical journals, and manipulated treatment guidelines.[84]

Funding for medical journals stems from several resources. As previously mentioned, they receive money from advertisements from drug companies and medical device companies. A big source of income that patients and physicians may have never considered comes from article reprints. The industry uses these reprints touting the safety and efficacy of their drugs and devices and disseminates them to physicians, hospital groups, and other potential customers.

Revenue from reprints can represent 23–53 percent of a journal's revenue.[85] This revenue is so important that medical journals may even publish articles with questionable data.

Payments to Medical Journal Editors

You might say that some medical publications are based on a pay-to-play model.

Medical journal editors play a significant role in determining which scientific studies are published, thus controlling what is read and influencing the overall practice of medicine. Medical journal editors' influence goes beyond that, though.

Indirectly, with their decisions to publish, medical editors shape the financial health of companies in the pharmaceutical and medical device industries. They also decide who will peer-review their publication. They can become powerbrokers if they so choose.

In light of the above, would you be surprised to learn that some medical journal editors receive direct payments from pharmaceutical and medical device companies?

A study published in *The British Medical Journal* looked at payments by US pharmaceutical and medical device companies to US medical journal editors. The study looked at high-impact-factor US medical journals across 26 specialties involving 713 journal editors.[86] High-impact journals are those that are highly reputable, have a large reading audience, and their published articles are frequently referenced in other studies.

Using the Open Payment database, the researchers checked to see which editors received money from industrial sources (pharmaceutical companies and medical device companies), and if so, how much.

In 2014, of the eligible editors, 361 or 50.6 percent received some type of payment from industry sources. Editors may receive one of two types of payments, general and research. Journal editors in subspecialty areas like cardiology received the highest median general payments. Below are the median payments to a select group of journals.

Journal	General Payment	Research Payment
JAMA	$6,331	$84,516
JACC (cardiology)	$475,072	$119,407
J Clinical Oncology	$5,957	$160,304
J Infectious Disease	$44,140	$17,526F

Diabetes Care	$96,688	$212,426
Internal Medicine	$9	$122,712

Derived from "Payments by US Pharmaceutical Companies and Medical Device Manufacturers to US Medical Journal editors: A Retrospective Observational Study." October 26, 2017. https://doi.org/10.1136/bmj.j4619.

Some of these journals have several publications and editors. For instance, the *Journal of the American College of Cardiology* has at least ten publications with up to 20 or more editors per publication.

These general payments are not bribes but payments in exchange for work that a physician may do on behalf of a pharmaceutical company or other industry source, including consulting work, educational programs, speaker fees/honoraria, and more. We tend to look favorably upon entities that pay us, which may create certain biases.

The results provided by scientific methods through publication are only as good as the gatekeeper medical editors.

Not So-Wacko Jacko Rule of Medicine:

Regarding research, especially medical, follow the money.

Money to Physicians

Pharmaceutical companies give money and gifts to physicians, as well. Some of this giving is relatively benign in the form of providing lunches to physicians and their office staff in exchange for physicians meeting with pharmaceutical representatives to learn more about their medications, especially new ones being launched.

There are also dinner presentations at upscale restaurants that physicians are invited to attend. The speaker is a physician paid to give a talk or seminar. Physicians who speak at these events can earn revenue well into the six figures over the course of a year.

Physicians are paid to help conduct clinical trials. And they are paid as consultants to help develop medical devices, including surgical instrumentation, artificial joints, cardiac catheters, vascular stents, artificial valve replacements, and so on.

Many of us probably find payments to conduct clinical trials and for medical device development somewhat necessary and appropriate, and often, they are. I think many people would find it comforting to know that physicians use their expertise in clinical drug trials, but also in medical device development.

Such arrangements create an ethical dilemma for the physicians that they may have never considered. What if the drug they are studying has significant adverse effects, yet the drug company finds a way to manipulate the data to make it look safe? If a physician blows the whistle, he or she likely will have broken their contract with the drug company and will probably be blacklisted from participating in future clinical trials. If such an event were to occur, would they blow the whistle or stay quiet, knowing some patients would be harmed?

From a patient's perspective, you want to make sure you are getting a joint replacement or cardiac stent that is ideal for your circumstances and not one simply because your surgeon or cardiologist helped develop it.

How Much Money Did Industry Spend on Physicians?

From 2013 to 2022, the *Journal of the American Medical Association* (*JAMA*) found that industry made 85 million payments to more than 820,300 (57 percent) of eligible physicians across thirty-nine specialties.[87]

The mean amount paid to the top 0.1 percent of physicians ranged from $194,933 for hospitalists to $4.8 million for orthopedic surgeons. Payments to the median physicians ranged from $0 to $2,339.

The greatest sum of payments went to orthopedic surgeons and amounted to $1.4 billion, followed by $1.3 billion to neurologists and psychiatrists, $1.3 billion to cardiologists, and $825.8 million to hematologists/oncologists.

One study found that 139 US oncologists, representing 1 percent of them, were paid $24.2 million. Payments were a minimum of $100,000 with a median payment of $154,000.[88] Many of these doctors held leadership roles in hospitals, academia, national health institutes, and guideline-making, potentially creating conflicts of interest.

Physicians practicing preventive medicine received the least amount of payments. As Bill Maher said, "There is no money in healthy people."

I suspect many physicians see the collaboration between industry and the medical profession as a win-win-win for patients, physicians, and industry. However, they are not aware of the tactics the industry employs in publishing studies, and they may not see that they are being used.

The Media

Only two countries allow pharmaceutical ads on television: the United States and New Zealand.[89] The pharmaceutical ads you see on television have a secondary purpose other than simply informing consumers of pharmaceutical products. Those ads are just as critical to the financial health of the media companies as the ad revenue is to medical journals. Those ads keep the media on Big Pharma's side.

How much is that ad revenue worth?

In 2022, television ad revenue grew to $74.9 billion. Three years earlier, pharmaceutical ads amounted to $6.6 billion or nearly one-tenth of the TV ad revenue.[90] To put those numbers into perspective, that $6.6 billion nearly equals the FDA's $7.2 billion 2024 budget.[91]

In 2022, thirty-second commercial spots during the Academy Awards ran from $1.7 million to $2.4 million. Viewers saw ads from Pfizer, Novartis, Lilly, and Incyte.[92]

Pharmaceutical companies doubled their TV ad spending between 2012 and 2016. Big Pharma spends $19 on promotions and advertising for every dollar spent on basic research and development.[93]

Does that amount of revenue to the media protect pharmaceutical companies from negative publicity? Big Pharma has a tremendously long rap sheet of crimes it has committed. Have you heard of these offenses through the media?

Medical Societies

Pharmaceutical companies frequently sponsor medical conferences held by many medical societies. I have been a member of approximately twelve medical societies and organizations over the years. The only one that I have belonged to that does not accept any outside money is the Seeds Scientific Research & Performance Institute (SSRP Institute).

Let me share part of its mission and focus statement:

> We must emphasize that we do not solicit or accept funding from pharmaceutical companies, supplement manufacturers, or any entity selling health-related goods. Our commitment is solely to our patients, our profession, and the scientific truth...we strive to be transparent as possible in all our dealings, collaborations, and research findings.[94]

The statement infers that outside money corrupts and precludes getting to the truth, and science is all about truth. What the SSRP Institute is doing is an example of what medicine is sorely missing today. Outside forces, specifically pharmaceutical companies, have hijacked medicine.

Big Pharma's Spending on Itself

What I am about to share probably puts everything in perspective in terms of where Big Pharma's values and interests lie. Big Pharma spends more money on executives and stockholders than it does on research and development.

This came out in a hearing held by the Senate Committee on Health, Education, Labor, and Pensions on February 6, 2024, chaired by Senator Bernie Sanders.[95]

- In 2022, Johnson & Johnson made $17.9 billion in profits; its CEO received $27.6 million in compensation while the company spent $17.8 billion on stock buybacks, dividends, and executive compensation, and only $14.6 billion on research and development.
- In 2022, Bristol Myers Squibb made $6.3 billion in profits, and its former CEO made $41.4 million in compensation. The company spent $12.7 billion on

stock buybacks, dividends, and executive compensation, and $9.5 billion on research and development.

- In 2022, Merck made $14.5 billion in profits, and its CEO received $52.5 million in compensation. The company spent $7 billion on stock buybacks, dividends, and executive compensation, and spent $13.6 billion on research and development.

If Merck's cancer drug, Keytruda, were its own company, it would have sales that rival the annual revenue of McDonald's and exceed the revenue of Marriott's hotel chain. Keytruda can cost a patient about $191,000 a year in the United States.

That's a lot of money for an industry that produces many products that provide marginal benefits.

Big Pharma's High Crimes and Misdemeanors

In 2010, the pharmaceutical industry surpassed the defense industry as the leading defrauder of the federal government, paying over $19.8 billion in penalties over a 20-year period. The largest penalty is off-label promotion.[96]

Once a drug is approved by the FDA, pharmaceutical companies can market it only for the approved indication(s); however, physicians can prescribe it, in their better judgment, for any condition they think reasonable, with some exceptions. This is called off-label use. Pharmaceutical companies are not allowed to promote off-label use because the drug was not studied for these other conditions. Nonetheless, they use various tactics to encourage off-label use and, sometimes, they get caught.

I doubt many of you heard or read much of the following civil and criminal penalties levied against pharmaceutical companies from the news media:

- Public Citizen published its findings of pharmaceutical settlements from 1991 to 2017 in its study, "Twenty-Seven Years of Pharmaceutical Industry Criminal and Civil Penalties 1991 Through 2017."[97] During that period, pharmaceutical companies and federal and state governments reached 412 settlements for a total of $38.6 billion.
- The most common violation from 1991 to 2017 was overcharging government health insurance programs, mainly through drug pricing against state Medicaid programs.
- The single violation leading to the largest settlements was the unlawful promotion of drugs (off-label use).
- During that same period, GlaxoSmithKline (GSK) reached thirty-two settlements and Pfizer thirty-four. GSK paid the most financial penalties at $7.9 billion, followed by $4.7 billion by Pfizer.
- Johnson & Johnson, Merck, Abbott, Eli Lilly, Teva, Schering-Plough, Novartis, Mylan, and AstraZeneca each paid more than $1 billion in fines during that time frame.

Company*	Total Financial Penalties ($ millions)	Percent of Total**	Number of Settlements***
GlaxoSmithKline	$7,901	20.4%	32
Pfizer	$4,728	12.2%	34
Johnson & Johnson	$2,857	7.4%	20
Teva	$1,990	5.1%	16
Merck & Co.	$1,840	4.8%	22
Abbott	$1,840	4.8%	16
Eli Lilly	$1,742	4.5%	15
Schering-Plough	$1,339	3.5%	6
Novartis	$1,275	3.3%	21
Mylan	$1,180	3.1%	22
AstraZeneca	$1,035	2.7%	13
Amgen	$901	2.3%	12
TAP	$875	2.3%	1
Bristol-Myers Squibb	$815	2.1%	14
Serono	$704	1.8%	1
Purdue	$646	1.7%	5
Allergan	$601	1.6%	2
Daiichi Sankyo	$586	1.5%	8
Boehringer Ingelheim	$441	1.1%	16
Cephalon	$425	1.1%	1
Other****	$4,100	10.6%	196
Total	**$37,822**	**97.9%**	**473**

*Parent company at time of settlement. If company is non-existent now, name at time of most recent settlement was used.

**Percent of $38.647 billion in overall penalties.

From Public Citizen, "Twenty-Seven Years of Pharmaceutical Industry Criminal and Civil Penalties: 1991-2017."

https://www.citizen.org-work/hcalth-and-safcty/pharmaccutical-industry-penalities.

Violations included:

- overcharging government health programs;
- unlawful promotion (off-label uses);
- monopolistic practices;
- kickbacks (to physicians, providers, and hospitals);
- concealing data on company-sponsored studies, other data from the government, and falsifying data to the federal government;
- poor manufacturing practices;
- environmental violations (Clean Air Acts and Clean Water Acts);
- financial violations; and
- illegal distribution (unapproved products).

The penalties of $38.6 billion represent 5 percent of the $710 billion in net profits from the eleven largest global drug companies during just ten of those 27 years. We don't have one bad apple or rogue company within the pharmaceutical industry. We have a systemic problem involving the entire industry.

Large but Small Fines

Thus, while the fines paid by pharmaceutical companies may seem high, they represent pennies relative to profits and are not likely to deter repeated bad behavior in the future.

This may be one reason Big Pharma may have a penchant for pushing the envelope with activities that border on being unethical and illegal. Fines are simply the cost of doing business and are factored into the cost of drugs.

Though not quite as large as the pharmaceutical industry, the US market for medical devices was $182 billion in 2024.[98]

Certainly, the pharmaceutical companies' drugs provide some benefits, but **how much benefit depends on whether you think such benefits cannot be obtained elsewhere**. Physicians are conditioned to think medications are the only solution and must use them first, with little knowledge of alternative treatments.

We have been bamboozled, duped, and hoodwinked into thinking that the only solutions to our health problems are pharmaceutical ones.

Big Pharma Intimidation of John Buse, MD

In 1999, John Buse, MD, discovered that GlaxoSmith Kline's (GSK) diabetes drug, Avandia, was associated with a higher risk of heart disease than in patients not on Avandia. Subsequent studies showed a 43 percent increased risk of heart disease in those on Avandia. Dr. Buse reported his findings only to find himself being threatened and intimidated by GSK officials.[99]

It was discovered in a 2007 Senate Finance Committee Report that a GSK official emailed the company's chairman of research and development to write Dr. Buse with a warning that "punishment will be that we will complain up his academic line and to the CME granting bodies that accredit his activities." There were threats of suing him for the $4 billion drop in the company's stock valuation.

After feeling he had no choice, Dr. Buse caved and signed a letter walking back his scientific findings, which GSK characterized as a "retraction letter," though he continued to have concerns about the drug.

The Senate Committee concluded that

> Corporate intimidation, the silencing of scientific dissent, and the suppression of scientific views threaten both the public well-being and the financial health of the federal government, which pays for healthcare. The behavior of GSK during the time that Dr. Buse voiced his concerns regarding the cardiovascular risks he believed were associated with Avandia was less than stellar. Had Dr. Buse been able to continue to voice his concerns, without being characterized as a "renegade" and without the need to sign a "retraction letter," it appears that the public good would have been better served.[100]

In 2004, Dr. Gurkipral Singh of Stanford University testified at a committee hearing that he was threatened and intimidated by Merck for requesting information on Vioxx, which was also linked to an increase in heart attacks. Both Avandia and Vioxx have since been taken off the market due to increased risk of heart conditions related to their use.

History repeats itself. We continue to see the intimidation of those physicians who came out against the federal government's handling of COVID-19. We no longer live in a society where there can be a free exchange of ideas and thoughts in medicine. The healthcare system has been hijacked.

How to Increase the Number of Patients on a Drug

When it comes to business, Big Pharma is smart. Once a drug is on the market, Big Pharma will try to get it to be used for everything. It has already spent the money on research and development, so it may as well get the biggest bang for its buck.

But it uses the following tactics to cheat. It

- creates and financially supports patient support groups and patient compliance programs;
- works with medical organizations to define disease and treatment; and
- seeks regulatory approval to promote off-label use.[101]

Support Groups and Compliance Programs

Compliance programs are conducted by insurance companies, hospital systems, large practices, and independent companies. These programs have some value in that they ensure patients are taking their meds, but they also serve as a ploy to get physicians to prescribe more medications. I receive notices from such compliance programs that say, for example, "based on the guidelines, your patient may benefit from a statin."

Support groups enable patients going through a similar experience, like a cancer diagnosis, to share their story, including their treatment and any medications. Those stories have value, but when a pharmaceutical company financially supports them, obviously, another agenda is in play.

Define Disease and Treatment

I discussed medicalization in the previous chapter, that is, creating diagnoses and expanding the boundaries of a diagnosis. This is probably no truer than when it comes to mental health disorders.

The whole concept that psychiatric disorders represent a "chemical imbalance" is not supported by biological psychiatry and is largely a pharmaceutical marketing phrase. It does not necessarily mean psychiatric drugs do not work; "chemical imbalance" is an over-simplification and even misleading, but it has become an effective marketing term successfully used on both patients and physicians with SSRIs now among the most prescribed class of drugs.[102]

We are increasingly quick to label patients with a diagnosis for an emotional response that is part and parcel of daily life.

So much of our population is now on SSRIs, including little kids, because their parents are told their child suffers from a "chemical imbalance."

We are increasingly quick to label patients with a diagnosis for an emotional response that is part and parcel of daily life. You should be anxious if you must give a talk to two hundred people. You should be depressed if a loved one dies. You should feel abandoned if your spouse walks out on you. You should feel anger if someone sabotages or threatens you. Such patients need help, but none of that means they necessarily need a drug.

For example, a recent study published in the *British Medical Journal* showed that exercise (walking, jogging, yoga, and strength training) was moderately effective in treating depression. But depression isn't the only area where Big Pharma sets the agenda.[103]

We see a push to start patients on diabetes drugs earlier. We see patients taking cholesterol drugs when their cholesterol levels are historically normal. (A study on total cholesterol and all-cause mortality showed that the sweet spot for total cholesterol was 210 to 249 mg/dl.)

Big Pharma has done a good job convincing physicians and patients alike that nearly everything is due to a molecular mishap, and it has the molecular solution to address it.

Regulatory Approval for Off-Label Use

The practice for getting FDA-approved medications used off-label, therefore, for non-FDA-approved indications is called "evergreening." Regardless of the tactic, the strategy is to get drugs used for practically everything. One way for pharmaceutical companies to promote off-label use and be within the law is for drug companies to have medical journals publish articles that show a drug may have other benefits beyond the FDA-approved conditions. The FDA views published articles as protected commercial speech and does not regulate their content.[104]

Big Pharma does serve a beneficial role in medical education, charity, and patient advocacy, but such roles are not its reason for existing. It is a business first and foremost. Its benevolent acts serve as conduits to make more money.

Not-So-Wacko Jacko Rule of Medicine:

You are more likely to become financially healthier buying stock in pharmaceutical companies than you are to become physically healthier buying their drugs.

Medicine is heading down a destructive path. It just does not know it yet. More and more people are being turned off by today's medicine. But those who sit behind the desk are oblivious to the growing distrust in the system.

The single best thing the medical profession can do is to get out from under the pharmaceutical industry's control. It can work with it, but it should not be controlled by it.

Bottom Line: Much of the medical system relies on some funding from the pharmaceutical industry. He who pays the bills gets to control the system.

How Pure Is the Evidence?

Those who don't read the newspaper are better off than those who do insofar as those who know nothing are better off than those whose heads are filled with half-truths and lies.
—Thomas Jefferson

How pure is medical evidence, really? Much of the entire practice of medicine is based on published medical studies. How well can we trust such evidence, and if we cannot trust it, what does that say about the validity or authenticity of the entire medical profession?

In this chapter, I discuss the concept of evidence-based medicine and the business of medical publishing. This is a book about half-truths. Are there half-truths baked in the medical evidence? Let's find out. We will explore the original concept or goal of evidence-based medicine and how it has deviated from it. You will be shown the "tricks of the trade" in how researchers get the result they want by the way they design studies.

Evidence-based medicine sure sounds like a commendable concept, and it is. Certainly, we want to base medical decisions on evidence. But a couple of problems arise. We only see the published studies and data. We don't see the studies not published. We don't even know they exist.

And so much medical evidence contradicts itself. Why does science give us different answers to the same question? We gravitate or lean on science because we want the right answers to our questions, but science can make the search for the truth even more confusing.

Why is it that, in even years, fish oil supplements protect against heart disease, and in odd years, they increase the risk? Studies showing both outcomes are published, so the editors who published the studies must think the studies were well-designed and the results valid. Right? Maybe, maybe not.

Does the truth change?

Does the science change?

Does our understanding change?

Who decides which pieces of evidence are to be believed and published? And why aren't all studies published? A preponderance of positive outcomes studies dominates medical literature. Is negative evidence being suppressed from publication?

Here are the pivotal questions: Does evidence-based medicine really deliver what the name implies? Where is the evidence that evidence-based medicine works?

Like the science with which it is closely related, evidence-based medicine (EBM) has some shortcomings since part of evidence-based medicine is based on science, as we see in the quotations below.

The laudable goal of making clinical decisions based on evidence can be impaired by the restricted quality and scope of what is collected as "best available evidence." The authoritative aura given to the collection, however, may lead to major abuses that produce inappropriate guidelines or doctrinaire dogmas for clinical practice.

—Alvan R. Feinstein, MD

EBM does not represent the scientific approach to medicine: it is only a restrictive interpretation of the scientific approach to clinical practice... It is time to substitute the fashionable popularity of a strategy developed outside of clinical medicine with models and research based on the insights of clinical judgement and patient-doctor interaction, as Feinstein had outlined.

—Giovanni A. Fava

It would seem those gentlemen do not believe evidence-based medicine delivers what the name implies. Let's look at some of the shortcomings of evidence-based medicine.

Much of medicine is based on scientific evidence. There is an assumption that if something is published in medical journals, it is valid and that it has been properly vetted. You are about to find that that assumption is not always true. I believe this assumption is the major reason why physicians are bamboozled, duped, and hoodwinked.

You will find out why the medical editors at prestigious medical journals quoted earlier have said the medical "evidence" that your doctor relies upon may not be reliable. These editors are in the know. Why did they say what they said? You will soon find out.

Not-So-Wacko Jacko Rules of Medicine:

Evidence-based medicine only fulfills its goal if all the evidence that exists is made available and in an untainted state.

Not all medical evidence is made available. Some is suppressed. Much is tainted.

If medical research is bogus, then the authenticity of medicine as a profession is questionable.

Evidence-based medicine encompasses medical research and medical publication, but it also directs how that information is used and applied in the clinical setting.

In theory, evidence-based medicine is a worthy pursuit, but, like many concepts, it has been bastardized and co-opted by those with other agendas. This bastardization or hijacking of concepts is common. In the case of evidence-based medicine, pharmaceutical companies, medical journals and editors, and those who write clinical practice guidelines influence it. They have agendas not necessarily directed at reaching the truth. In the previous chapter, we saw the sway the pharmaceutical industry has on the entirety of medicine, including medical journals and information.

Much of evidence-based medicine is an illusion. Like many illusions, it makes us feel good but is deceptive. This illusion greatly affects the practice of medicine. As physicians, we pat ourselves on the back for being evidence-based in our approach to patient care, not realizing that in some cases, if not many, we have been bamboozled, duped, and hoodwinked by the "evidence."[105]

The opening statement of an opinion article published in the *British Medical Journal* sums up the situation: "Evidence-based medicine has been corrupted by corporate interests, failed regulation, and commercialization of academia, argue these authors."[106]

This leads us back to President Dwight D. Eisenhower's farewell address warning of the potential hijacking of academia by industry.

David Sackett and Evidence-Based Medicine

David Sackett, MD, is considered one of the fathers of evidence-based medicine. On several occasions, he had to clarify what he meant by evidence-based medicine. According to Sackett, evidence-based medicine (1) is not meant to be cookbook medicine, (2) is not meant to replace physician experience, (3) still gives patients a say in how they are treated regardless of the evidence, and (4) considers a **patient's experience as evidence** and, many times, the best evidence because it is evidence that pertains directly to them.[107]

Evidence-based medicine is more than scientific evidence. There are different levels of strength of medical evidence. The goal of evidence-based medicine is to apply the strongest level of evidence available for a particular problem without ignoring a physician's experience and judgment and a patient's values and desires.

The table below is one way to categorize the strength of medical evidence. Large randomized clinical trials providing definitive results are the strongest forms of evidence. Not all problems allow for such trials. Sometimes, the best you can do is the "expert" opinion.

Level	Type of Evidence
1	Large randomized controlled trials with definitive results
2	Small randomized controlled trials with unclear results
3	Cohort and case-control studies
4	Historical cohort or case-controlled studies
5	Case series or studies with no controls
6	Expert opinion

Going back to the four characteristics of evidence-based medicine that Dr. Sackett found necessary to qualify, none are employed today with any regularity.

Today's medicine is all about "cookbook" medicine. Physician experience has taken a back seat to the medical guidelines, especially for those physicians who are employed. They cannot deviate too often or far from clinical guidelines without risking their job. Evidence-based medicine through clinical guidelines is a way to control physician thought and behavior.

Physicians are increasingly judged by how well they follow the guidelines and less by outcomes, at least the outcomes that matter to patients. Thus, physicians tend to focus more on meeting and treating the guidelines rather than patients.

Many times, patients have been stripped of their voices about how they are treated. Frequently, doctors dismiss, downplay, or invalidate a patient's experience. If a patient does not do what a doctor says, they run the risk of being terminated from the practice. We saw this during the COVID-19 pandemic; doctors terminated patients from their practices if they had not been vaccinated.

Medicine is supposed to have evolved to the state of nirvana by providing personalized or individualized care. We hear slogans or ads like, "We provide personalized care." Or "We are here for you." Such concepts make for nice ad campaigns but rarely exist in practice. Instead, we plug everyone into the same guidelines regardless of their individual circumstances. Does that make sense?

Here is an example of some of the silliness that occurs in today's interpretation of evidence-based medicine.

There is a push to not prescribe antibiotics (and for good reason). However, if a patient says, "Despite sinus surgery, I still get three sinus infections a year. When I sense one coming on, I use a nasal spray, take an antihistamine and decongestant, and use my neti pot. But if I am not improving by day five, I need an antibiotic." **That is evidence**.

In that scenario, it should be perfectly acceptable to prescribe the antibiotic rather than follow clinical guidelines, rather than make the patient suffer for another week or two doing what they are already doing but isn't working. Yet many physicians will not do that because they are evaluated by how well they follow clinical guidelines. Often, these guidelines are based on "expert opinion" (the weakest form of evidence) and not rooted in any meaningful science. A doctor treating a patient becomes secondary to following the guidelines.

Evidence-based medicine is more than just scientific evidence, which is how it has become largely interpreted today. According to Dr. Sackett, evidence-based medicine can be thought of as the area in a Venn diagram where relevant scientific evidence, clinical judgment, and patients' values and preferences overlap. Evidence-based medicine is just not scientific evidence as so many believe today.

Evidence-Based Medicine

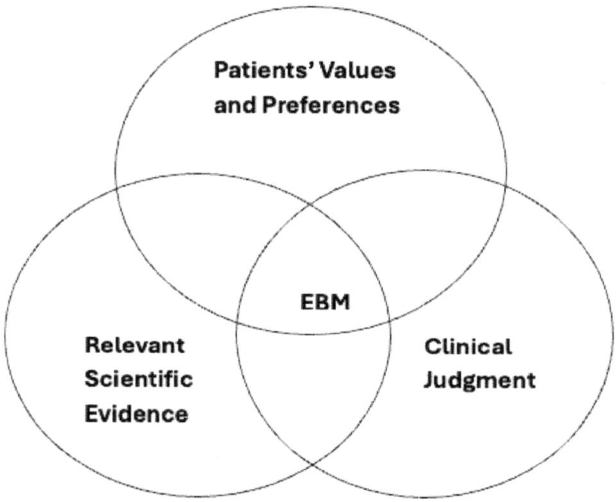

Adapted from Sackett DL, et al. BMJ. 1996;312(7023):71-72

For the most part today, clinical guidelines focus only on scientific evidence, ignoring a physician's clinical judgment and patients' experiences and treatment desires. Because of misunderstanding and misapplication, evidence-based medicine is bound to fall short of expectations.[108]

Misapplication of Evidence

Some guidelines are based on clinical studies. Frequently, we extrapolate a study's results and apply them to individuals outside the demographic that was studied. When doing so, we are not applying evidence-based medicine properly. For example, the results of a study on the management of sinus infection in people under age 65 do not necessarily hold true for those over age 65.

Pfizer's combined phases 1 and 2 trial on its mRNA vaccine for COVID was composed of only 45 healthy individuals under age 54. Before we knew the results of its 6-month phase 3 trial, which included people with cancer, heart disease, neurodegenerative disease, and pregnant women, we started to vaccinate individuals with those conditions without reliable safety data.

That was possible because the vaccine was being tested under Emergency Use Authorization (EUA), but it would have been nice to have data in patients with specific medical conditions ahead of vaccination. Strictly speaking, we abandoned evidence-based medicine during the time the EUA was in place.

Earlier, we discussed how editors at prestigious journals feel that much scientific evidence is unreliable, but the problem goes beyond that. Twenty years ago, *PLoS Medicine* published the article "Medical Journals Are an Extension of the Marketing Arm of Pharmaceutical Companies." The concerns expressed in that paper are likely more prevalent today, and much of what follows is from that article.[109]

How Researchers Get the Results They Want

If you want to obtain a certain result from your research, design the study to provide that result. Start with the end in mind and work backwards to prepare the study to yield the desired results. Researchers have several tactics to hide or misrepresent their data so that it is viewed in the best light possible. Most things come down to asking the right questions, either in honest pursuit of the truth, or the "right" questions to support an agenda or predetermined outcome. That is what well-seasoned researchers do.

Pharmaceutical companies get the results they want by asking the "right" questions of which there are several strategies. Here are some of those tricks:

- Conduct a trial of your drug against a treatment known to be inferior.
- Trial your drug against too low a dose of a competitor's drug.
- Conduct a trial of your drug against too high a dose of a competitor's drug, making your drug seem less toxic.
- Conduct trials that are too small to show differences from competing drugs.
- Use multiple endpoints in the trial and select those that give favorable results for publication.
- Conduct subgroup analyses and select those that are favorable for publication.
- Present results most likely to impress, for example, reduction in relative risk rather than absolute risk.
- Do not track down participants who have dropped out of the study.
- Conduct trials on subjects unrepresentative of the patient population.
- Publish only positive results and ignore negative results.

- Change the duration of the trial.
- Make lemonade out of lemons.
- Make stuff up.

Some of those tactics I believe are self-explanatory but let me explain them in more detail.

Trial a Drug Against One Known to Be Inferior

This tactic makes the study drug look more efficacious than it is, providing a halo effect, that is, the study drug is then perceived as superior to other drugs in its class.

For FDA approval, drugs are studied against a placebo—a treatment known to be inferior. Beating a placebo should not be hard to do and is a low bar to achieve for FDA approval. I go into this more in "The Pharmaceutical Funded FDA."

Sometimes, though, a drug is studied head-to-head against a competitor's drug to demonstrate its "superiority."

Trial a Drug Against a Low Dose of a Competitor's Drug

When comparing drugs, it is important to compare apples to apples and oranges to oranges. Ideally, the same dosage of the drugs would be studied (i.e., the lowest dose of the drug should be compared to the lowest dose of the competitor's).

However, studies are done where a larger dose of one drug, yet a dose not too high to cause additional side effects, is compared to a low dose of a competitor's drug.

They employ a similar tactic when studying supplements. Unknown to many, pharmaceutical companies have been quietly buying up supplement companies. It is common in studies on supplements to use too small a dose (likely intentionally in some cases) for a particular condition, thus making the supplement look ineffective and discouraging its use.

Many times, studies on vitamin D will use a dose of 400 to 800 IUs a day, which is barely enough to move the vitamin D level a few points. In those studies, vitamin D supplementation appears unhelpful.

I mentioned already that we don't always ask the right questions. Let's stick with vitamin D. Instead of focusing on the dose of vitamin D supplementation, we should focus on the vitamin D **level.**

Instead of asking whether 800 IUs of the vitamin reduces overall mortality or the risk of cancer or upper respiratory infections, a more appropriate question would be, is there a vitamin D level above which vitamin D supplementation improves mortality, reduces cancers, or reduces upper respiratory tract infections?

We know if you have a vitamin D level of 55 ng/dl, your odds of getting a hospital-acquired infection approach zero (about 60 percent of those hospitalized for COVID-19 had deficient vitamin D levels).[110] As a physician, you then determine how much vitamin D a patient should take to reach a target level, and the dose will vary greatly among patients. The level is important, yet studies are done on the doses, not the levels.

Conduct a Trial Against Too High a Dose of a Competitor's Drug

This probably is self-explanatory. The goal is to make the competitor's drug look dangerous or to dissuade use for a particular condition. This was done with hydroxychloroquine during the peak of COVID-19. Doses up to four to six times higher than recommended were given to COVID-19 patients, causing all sorts of side effects, including death, and providing ammunition against the use of hydroxychloroquine in the treatment of COVID-19.[111]

Conduct a Trial Too Small to Show a Difference with a Competitor's Drug

This tactic is used when a company has an inferior drug and tries to minimize the difference between its drug and a competitor's superior drug. Researchers purposefully design the study to minimize the difference between the inferior and superior drugs.

Use Multiple Endpoints and Select Those That Are Favorable

A clinical endpoint is an objective tool to measure how beneficial a medical intervention is. The primary endpoint is associated with the primary research question or hypothesis and is the main outcome of the study. It is well defined in advance and must be readily measurable with simple and easy-to-use tools.

For example, the number of cancer patients surviving one year following a particular intervention might be a primary endpoint. Another primary endpoint could be the number of people who avoid hospitalization following an intervention.

A study can have secondary endpoints as well. In the above example, several secondary endpoints might relate to quality-of-life issues. What percentage of cancer patients can function independently? What percentage can dress themselves and perform self-hygiene? What percentage can cook and eat without assistance?

In this example, some, and even many, of the primary and secondary endpoints may not have had favorable outcomes or results. What do you do as a researcher? If you start with several endpoints, one of them is likely to show favorable results, and that is the one you design your paper around for publication. However, if the results are unfavorable, you may not include or mention them in the paper you hope to publish. You ignore the bad outcomes.

Beginning in 2000, companies were required to register what they were measuring ahead of the study. Before then, 57 percent of trials showed positive results. After 2000, only 8 percent showed a positive result.[112]

A major flaw with Pfizer's 6-month mRNA COVID vaccine study was that death from *all causes* was not considered an endpoint. In Pfizer's study, more people died in the vaccine group than in the unvaccinated group, even though there was one less COVID-19 death per 22,000 cases of vaccination.[113]

Multicenter Trials and Picking Those with Favorable Results

Researchers, when submitting a drug trial for FDA approval or a paper to a journal, do not have to share all their findings. They can cherry-pick their data. The FDA and medical journals cannot compel them to turn over all their data, which is proprietary information.

For instance, at the beginning of a drug trial, researchers studied 3,000 individuals at six different centers (therefore 500 participants/location). The results at four of the centers were favorable, but the results at the other two were unfavorable. The researchers simply state that they studied the drug on 2,000 participants at four centers/locations. In essence, they weed out the bad results.

Select Favorable Subgroup Analyses for Publication

Subgroup analyses are a routine part of clinical trials to investigate whether treatment effects are homogeneous across the study population. Certain demographics may respond more favorably to an intervention than others. Let's say the study has 2,000 participants, comprising five subgroups of 400 participants.

Results are favorable in two subgroups of patients, but results for three subgroups involving 1,200 patients are not favorable. The results of the two favorable subgroups are submitted for publication. The medical journals have no way of knowing that 1,200 patients or 60 percent of the study participants did not respond to the intervention.

This tactic is similar to multicenter trials, where only favorable results from some of the centers are reported.

Present Results That Look Impressive but May Be Irrelevant

Perhaps the most common strategy used, especially by drug companies, is to report their findings in terms of relative risk reduction rather than absolute risk reduction.

Results reported in terms of relative risk look more impressive, and studies show that how information is presented to physicians influences whether they will prescribe a drug or not. They are more apt to prescribe a drug when the information is presented in terms of relative risk.[114]

Here is a real-life example.

If I proposed that you take drug X for forty months to reduce your risk of heart attack by 36 percent, would you be interested in that drug? The answer is most likely "yes," especially if you have a family history of heart disease and/or risk factors for it.

What if I suggested you take drug Y for forty months based on a one in one hundred chance to avoid a heart attack? Would you be interested in that drug? The answer is probably "no."

Now, if I told you that drug X and drug Y are the same drug, those two percentages would likely baffle you, but they are true. The drug I am speaking of is Lipitor (atorvastatin).

Pfizer makes Lipitor. In its study submitted to the FDA for drug approval, it reported in simplified terms: For every 100 participants who took Lipitor for forty months, two had a heart attack. For every 100 participants who received the placebo, three had a heart attack.[115]

The difference between three in the placebo group and two in the Lipitor group is one. One divided by three gives us 33 percent (36 percent when not rounding the numbers). That is the **relative risk reduction**. It measures the risk in the treated group relative to the placebo group. The difference of one between the two groups per 100 patients is the **absolute risk reduction**, in this case, 1 percent.

Yet, it takes 100 patients to take the drug for forty months for one patient to receive the intended benefit of the drug—avoidance of a heart attack. This provides us with a third number and perhaps the most important number. It is called the Number to Treat or NNT. The NNT and absolute risk reduction are similar ways to express the results.

The number of patients who need to take a drug for one patient to receive the intended benefit is the NNT, which is rarely reported in published trials. You may have enough information to calculate the NNT yourself, but that it is rarely visibly disclosed should speak volumes.

An NNT of 1 means that everyone who takes the drug benefits from it. No drug has an NNT of 1, but some approach it, like antibiotics, for certain infections. An NNT of 2 means that two patients must take the drug for one to benefit. That is akin to flipping a coin. An NNT of 3 means three patients must take a drug for one patient to benefit, and so on. An NNT of 50 or higher is worse than winning a minimal prize in the lottery.

Similar findings were found for AstraZeneca's Crestor (rosuvastatin), which is the most potent statin drug on the market. In its study, the relative risk reduction was 54 percent, but the absolute risk reduction was just 1 percent, and the NNT was 95.

The NNT is affected by the duration one takes the drug and comes down over time on a drug. It is estimated that the NNT for statin drugs approaches seven if patients stay on the statin for 30 years. This means that seven patients must take a statin for 30 years for one person to avoid a heart attack. For someone with a strong family history of heart disease and who has cardiovascular risk factors, an NNT of seven may be worth the risks. However, it's probably not beneficial to a reasonably healthy person who has elevated cholesterol.

The sad reality is that many commonly prescribed drugs have an NNT *well above* 20. A high NNT may not be significant if the drug costs pennies a day and has few and only minor side effects. This is not the case with statins, which have a litany of side effects, some of which are serious.

Keep in mind that those numbers are obtained with the help of statistical sleight of hand in some cases.

In my opinion, the NNT should be required to be specified in any drug study's first sentence, along with relative risk and absolute risk. For example, "In this study, the number to treat to achieve___ was____. The absolute risk reduction was ___ and the relative risk reduction was ___." That recommendation will never happen because it would lead to a decrease in prescription writing if physicians saw the NNT and absolute risk reductions prominently displayed.

Do Not Track Down Participants Who Have Dropped Out of the Study

Participants drop out of studies for any number of reasons, but statistically, they are more likely to drop out if they experience a side effect or have some other undesirable outcome. Therefore, for the purposes of results, pharmaceutical companies may not track them down, making their trial numbers look better. Researchers categorize such patients as "lost to follow-up."[116]

Conduct Trials on Subjects Unrepresentative of the Patient Population

Researchers did this with the Pfizer-BioNTech mRNA vaccine study for COVID-19. Phase 3 trial participants were healthier than the general population and far healthier than those who were dying of COVID-19, many of whom had multiple comorbidities.

Change the Duration of the Trial

Suppose a drug company plans a trial for six months and sees favorable results by four months. In that case, they may stop the trial prematurely because the results may become less favorable as the study progresses. Vice versa, they may extend the trial longer if, at six months, the results are approaching statistical significance but not quite there.

Initially, Pfizer's six-month trial on its COVID-19 vaccine was to be a three-year study, but they stopped it at six months, and its study showed waning efficacy as early as two months. I will examine this study more later in "Pfizer's Deceptive COVID-19 Vaccine Trial."[117]

Make Lemonade Out of Lemons

Drug studies are expensive. If a drug company does not get its anticipated results, it may attempt to salvage the study the best it can and find any positive correlation to build a paper around that result.

As a physician, there is no way to read every study, even just those within your field of expertise. It is not uncommon for physicians and others to read only the abstract and conclusions. Knowing this, another way researchers can salvage the study is to exaggerate or misrepresent the findings in the conclusion and abstract because many physicians will not read the entire study and discover the deception.[118]

Make Up Stuff

During COVID-19, both *The Lancet* and *The New England Journal of Medicine* published studies based on a non-existent database owned by the previously unknown company Surgisphere Corporation. This company claimed to have a global database with access to 96,000 patients from more than 600 hospitals over six continents.

Predicated on Surgisphere's database, *The Lancet's* study concluded hydroxychloroquine was ineffective and dangerous. In some instances, the data were unbelievable. In one Australian hospital, for instance, deaths attributed to hydroxychloroquine exceeded the total number of deaths for the entire country.

Nearly immediately, several scientists and clinicians across the globe questioned the authenticity of the data and results. Subsequently, we learned that the **database did not exist**. Eventually, three of the four co-authors of both studies requested to retract the papers because they "can no longer vouch for the veracity of the primary data sources." In the end, both journals retracted the articles.[119]

The Lancet and *The New England Journal of Medicine* are two of the most respected medical journals, and also home to two of the medical journal editors who, years earlier, stated the difficulty in trusting the science in the medical literature. Historically, these two have been among the most trusted medical publications. Unfortunately, those we trust most frequently deceive us.

We will see more issues with *The New England Journal of Medicine* when we get to "Pfizer's Deceptive COVID-19 Vaccine Trial." The journal's editor-in-chief also served concomitantly on the FDA Advisory Council, which approved the COVID-19 vaccines in the five-to-eleven-year-old population. At the same time, his journal published the primary studies on the Pfizer-BioNTech vaccines.

The Surgisphere case raises questions: Was this a one-time event? Are fraudulent studies published in medical literature a common occurrence? The Surgisphere case also highlights how an outright lie is easier to detect than a half-truth. The half-truth is powerful.

There are plenty of reasons we should be skeptical of medical research.[120] Fake articles and journals are more common than many might realize. Sometimes, we refer to fake journals as predatory journals.[121]

Retractions

Retraction of scientific papers is not new, but the number of retractions has quadrupled in the past 20 years, with 10,000 papers retracted in 2023 alone. Two-thirds of the papers were retracted for scientific misconduct rather than errors.

Unfortunately, retracted articles are continually cited in other studies even after retraction.[122]

Does Not Peer Review Help?

You might wonder whether the peer-review process helps to determine the credibility of the paper submitted for publication.

Peer reviewers are in the same boat as the editors of medical journals. They can only review what they are given. Editors will request authors submit related studies that they can then share with peer reviewers, but they have no way of knowing of any existing **unpublished** studies, perhaps unpublished due to disappointing results. Also, existing published studies may be using data from the same patient base, and editors and peer reviewers have no way of discovering that possibility.

The peer-review process itself has been shown to be ineffective, biased, and prone to abuse.[123] Peer review cannot detect anomalous data from inaccuracies, miscalculations, or outright fraud, as seen with the Surgisphere scandal. Journals do not require manuscripts to have accompanying data or analytical code, so reviewers do not evaluate manuscripts for analytical consistency.[124]

Properly conducting peer reviews is time-intensive, involving multiple rounds of communication with the manuscript's author(s) and working on revisions to strengthen and improve the manuscript. Peer reviewers may conduct several studies concurrently, and peer reviewing takes time away from their research. They are not paid, and they may not proceed with the diligence required because of time limitations.

When it comes to medical publications, we have mechanisms in place to ensure the process is legitimate and gives the appearance of integrity and credibility. But who regulates the regulators, who peer reviews the peer reviewers, and who edits the editors to verify there is no abuse, no fraud, no bias, and no corruption? And when it comes to disputes, who fact-checks the nebulous fact-checkers?

Not All Medical Evidence Is Available

Earlier, I mentioned that evidence-based medicine is worthy if all the existing evidence is available for review in an unbiased and untainted manner.

Not every study is published due to various reasons. Sometimes, editors won't publish a study because they found too many flaws in how the study was conducted. Such an instance is rare because seasoned researchers know how to conduct studies.

Sometimes, a well-conducted study may not add to the current knowledge base and is not considered valuable. At other times, should a study fail to show what the researchers were expecting, the researchers don't bother to submit it for publication.

As a result, studies showing an intervention's inefficacy or adverse effects are published at a much lower rate than positive outcome studies. Consequently, they are submitted for publication at a lower rate. Inadvertently or not, such studies are suppressed.[125]

You and I have no idea how many studies show negative results because they aren't reported. Have you ever seen a book titled *How I Screwed Up and Ruined My Life?* No, although such a book might be helpful to many. Negative outcomes are not published or discussed often.[126]

For example, the pharmaceutical company Sanofi completed 92 studies, but only 14 were published in 2008.[127] What happened to the other 78 studies? Negative studies can be valuable. Sometimes, knowing what doesn't work is just as important as knowing what does.

Why Negative Studies Matter

As I researched this book, I came across a paper published in *The New England Journal of Medicine.* The researchers of that study obtained reviews from the Food and Drug Administration for studies of 12 antidepressant agents involving 12,564 patients. Then, they conducted a systematic literature search to identify matching publications. The researchers were looking to see which and how many of the trials sent to the FDA had been published in medical journals. For trials reported in the literature, they compared the published outcomes with the FDA outcomes.[128]

Results

The math on this study is a little hard to follow, so I am going to break it down as simply as possible. The FDA determined that 38 of the 74 (51 percent) studies showed positive outcomes from antidepressants and 36 (49 percent) studies showed negative outcomes.

Of the 74 FDA-registered studies, 31 percent (23) were not published in the literature, leaving 51 (69 percent) studies that were published. The researchers then determined whether the published studies had positive or negative outcomes.

Thirty-seven studies viewed by the FDA as having positive results were published; one study viewed as positive was not published (one of the 23 unpublished). Therefore, in the eyes of the FDA, 38 studies (51 percent) showed a positive benefit to antidepressants, and 36 negative outcome studies (49 percent). What happened to those negative studies?

Only three studies viewed by the FDA as having negative or questionable results were published. We're down to 33 negative studies. What happened to them? Twenty-two of them were not published. Now, what about the remaining 11? Those studies were published in a way that, in the opinion of this study's researchers, conveys a positive outcome rather than the negative outcome as previously determined by the FDA.

Therefore, 48 of the 51 published studies (94 percent) showed positive outcomes to antidepressant use. In the eyes of the FDA, only 51 percent of the studies showed positive outcomes. Thus, if physicians read the literature and only see positive outcome studies on antidepressants, they might conclude that antidepressants are wonder drugs. The published studies have made antidepressants look more effective than they are in real life, which likely affects a physician's perception of antidepressants and subsequent prescribing habits.

Yet only 51 percent of the studies showed positive outcomes per the FDA, which lines up more with real-life experience. It is not unusual for a patient to try two or three antidepressants before finding one that works.

Other Ways to Suppress Medical Evidence

He who controls medical publishing indirectly controls medicine by controlling physicians. Medical publishing can suppress medical evidence, but it is not the only avenue by which this happens.

Hospital systems employ about 77 percent of physicians.[129] Hospital systems and other employers can control access to medical-related websites, permitting physicians to access some sites and blocking access to others.

The website C19early.org provides data on nearly every drug and supplement that has been tried in the treatment of COVID-19. Many physicians are unaware of the site; I strongly recommend you visit it. On the left side of the homepage, you will see the various interventions that have been studied for COVID-19. Most of the interventions are either existing drugs being repurposed for COVID-19 or common over-the-counter supplements.

As of this publication date, at least 5,349 studies on COVID-19 interventions have been entered into the C19.early.org database, as shown below.

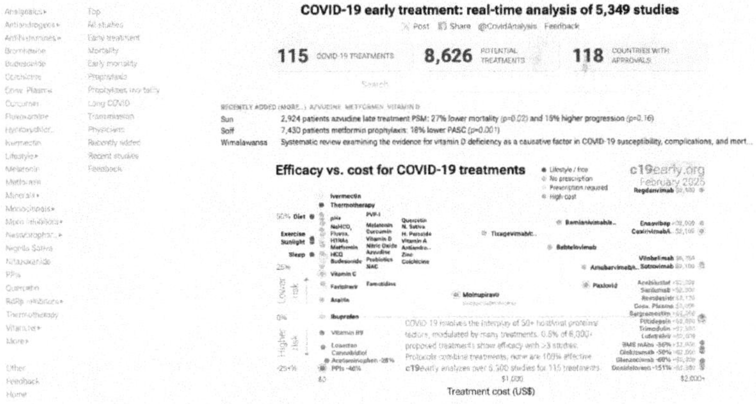

C19early.org home page as of March 3, 2025.

The C19early.org website provides a meta-analysis, pulling data from several studies showing the number of studies for that intervention, how many scientists were involved, how many patients participated, and the number of countries involved in the studies.

For each intervention, the results show the various outcomes or endpoints like mortality, recovery, hospitalization, prophylaxis, and so on. You do not want to see negative or red numbers. You want to see positive blue numbers; the higher, the better.

Plus, there is even a section on lifestyle, including diet, exercise, sleep, and sun. Look closely at these benefits. These lifestyle interventions are inexpensive (I believe sunlight is still free) and do not require a prescription.

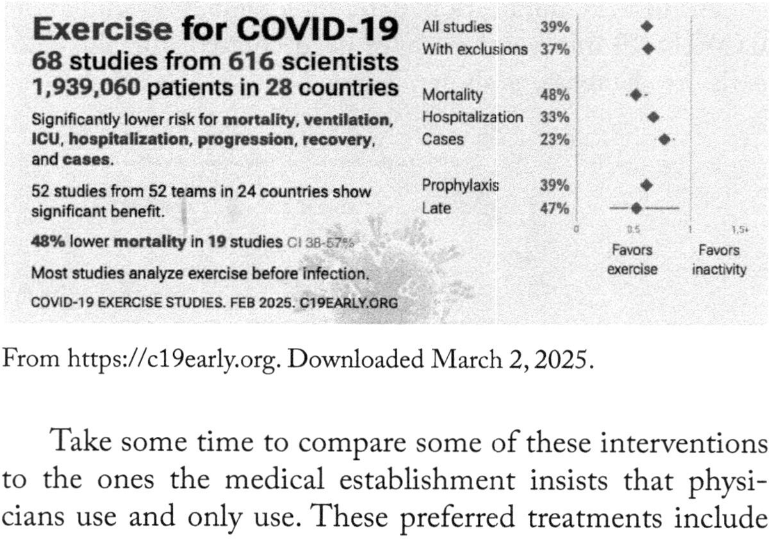

From https://c19early.org. Downloaded March 2, 2025.

Take some time to compare some of these interventions to the ones the medical establishment insists that physicians use and only use. These preferred treatments include Remdesivir, Paxlovid, molnupiravir, and monoclonal antibodies (which are rarely being used today since oral antivirals are available).

I am showing screenshots of some of the interventions, including ivermectin, hydroxychloroquine, quercetin (an over-the-counter supplement), and remdesivir (the medical establishment's preferred hospital treatment), which performed worse than other interventions I am showing.

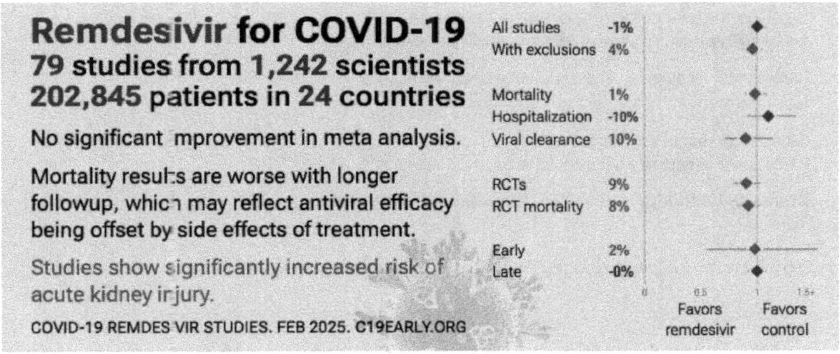
Remdesivir for COVID-19
79 studies from 1,242 scientists
202,845 patients in 24 countries
No significant improvement in meta analysis.
Mortality results are worse with longer followup, which may reflect antiviral efficacy being offset by side effects of treatment.
Studies show significantly increased risk of acute kidney injury.
COVID-19 REMDESIVIR STUDIES. FEB 2025. C19EARLY.ORG
All studies -1%
With exclusions 4%
Mortality 1%
Hospitalization -10%
Viral clearance 10%
RCTs 9%
RCT mortality 8%
Early 2%
Late -0%
Favors remdesivir
Favors control

From https://c19early.org. Downloaded March 2, 2025.

Many of these "non-approved" interventions perform better than the preferred and expensive interventions. Look at the results for ivermectin and hydroxychloroquine, the two drugs most discredited, and compare them to the preferred drugs, but especially Remdesivir.

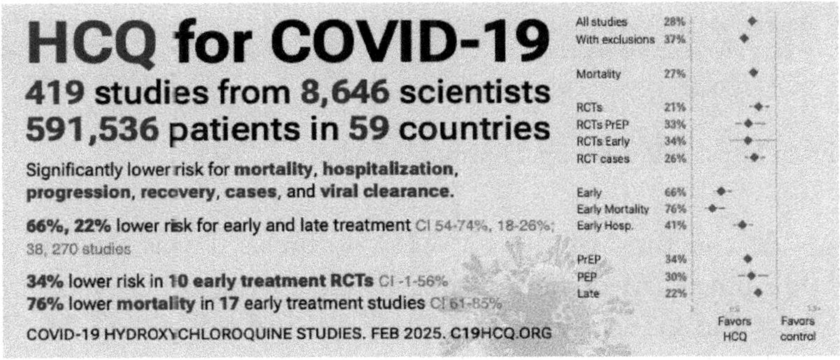
HCQ for COVID-19
419 studies from 8,646 scientists
591,536 patients in 59 countries
Significantly lower risk for mortality, hospitalization, progression, recovery, cases, and viral clearance.
66%, 22% lower risk for early and late treatment CI 54-74%, 18-26%; 38, 270 studies
34% lower risk in 10 early treatment RCTs CI -1-56%
76% lower mortality in 17 early treatment studies CI 61-85%
COVID-19 HYDROXYCHLOROQUINE STUDIES. FEB 2025. C19HCQ.ORG
All studies 28%
With exclusions 37%
Mortality 27%
RCTs 21%
RCTs PrEP 33%
RCTs Early 34%
RCT cases 26%
Early 66%
Early Mortality 76%
Early Hosp. 41%
PrEP 34%
PEP 30%
Late 22%
Favors HCQ
Favors control

From https://c19early.org. Downloaded March 2, 2025.

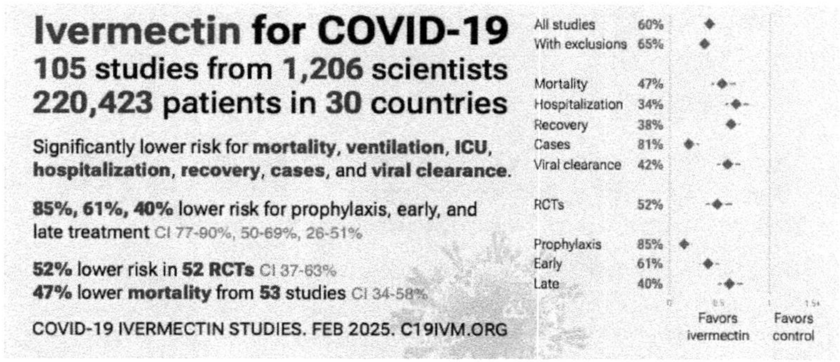

From https://c19early.org. Downloaded March 2, 2025.

The results of quercetin, which is easily obtained over the counter:

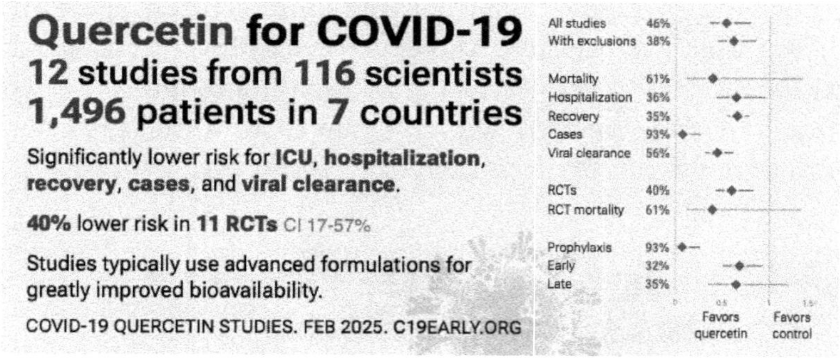

From https://c19early.org. Downloaded March 2, 2025.

At the time of the COVID outbreak, I was part of a 500+ physician-owned group. While in the office, I could access the C19early.org website from my cell phone, but I was blocked from accessing it from my work computer—another form of suppressing medical evidence. Coincidence?

Much of my research on the C19early.org site occurred after office hours from my home computer, and I had no issues accessing the website from home. Another coincidence?

How Medical Journals Survive Financially

Journals are incentivized to publish studies with a high impact factor (even if the reporting of results may be questionable). Yet, they must balance their content with their financial bottom line.

Medical journals receive income from several sources. Like many periodicals, some of it comes from subscription fees. Advertisements from pharmaceutical companies and medical device companies are another source. However, a suspect source provides a substantial part of their income—article reprints.

Articles read and then cited by other studies carry a high impact factor (IF). Many times, pharmaceutical companies supply such studies. To help get their "landmark" articles circulated, pharmaceutical companies buy reprints (sometimes several thousand) of an article and disperse them to their large sales staff, who then get them into the hands of physicians.[130]

Those reprints cost money. Lots of money.

The New England Journal of Medicine receives 23 percent of its income from reprints. *The Lancet* gets 41 percent of its revenue from reprints. JAMA receives 53 percent of its revenue from reprints. [131]

People who cast votes decide nothing. The people who count the votes decide everything.

—Joseph Stalin

He who controls medical publishing controls much of medicine. Who controls medical publishing? Follow the money to answer that question.

Payments to Editors of Medical Journals

In the previous chapter, I discussed payments made to editors of medical journals. While some payments may be appropriate, do such payments create biases for editors? We tend to look favorably on those from whom we receive payments. Why do some editors receive payments and others do not?

Sponsored Research

If pharmaceutical companies are not doing the research themselves, they frequently sponsor it. Frequently, pharmaceutical companies provide money for someone else to do the research, such as academic centers or independent research groups.

By involving an academic center, the pharmaceutical companies insulate themselves from criticism as they function in the background. Research performed by an academic center gives the results of any studies that might be published an air of credibility.

The academic center benefits by having an influx of funds, which enables it to maintain staff and facilities. The researchers benefit by meeting their "publish or perish" requirements as well as the prestige and honor that comes from being a prolific researcher and all the resulting secondary opportunities.

But here's the catch. The academic centers often do not own the research. They do the research, but they do not own the data.

Data ownership remains under the control of pharmaceutical companies. They determine what data is released, what is published, and how it is published. It is no different than if the pharmaceutical companies did the research with their staff.[132]

Not only do the companies outsource the research, but many employ ghostwriters to write the studies. The people conducting the research may not write the paper, though their names will be listed at the top of the study.

This type of outsourcing is not new. It happens in other industries too. Some well-known novelists now have ghostwriters pen their novels. The music of many hit songs from the '60s and '70s was outsourced to studio bands like the Wrecking Crew in Los Angeles, California, and the Muscle Shoals Rhythm Section in Muscle Shoals, Alabama. That might be one reason some musical groups do not sound as well when performing live. It is disappointing, though, to learn that the people getting credit for the music did not play it in the recording session.

Sponsored research is a tremendous win-win for pharmaceutical companies, academic centers, and the individual researchers involved. Perhaps we now better understand the words of Dr. Relman, former editor of *The New England Journal of Medicine,* when he said

> The medical profession is being bought by the pharmaceutical industry, not only in terms of the practice of medicine, but also in terms of teaching and research. The academic institutions of this country are allowing themselves to be the paid agents of the pharmaceutical industry. I think it's disgraceful.

Pharma-Funded Research Versus Independent Research

Drug studies can be funded by pharmaceutical companies, or they can be funded independently through government entities like the NIH or through academic centers or voluntary specialty groups (charities).

There is quite a difference in the outcomes of studies funded by Big Pharma and those funded by independent entities. Research shows a clear bias favoring products made by companies funding the research.[133]

In 2010, researchers from Harvard and Toronto examined 500 trials involving the five major classes of drugs and found 85 percent funded by pharmaceutical companies had positive results, whereas only 50 percent of government-funded studies were positive.[134]

In 2007, a review of 192 studies on statins found that pharmaceutical-funded studies were 20 times more likely to show favorable results for the test.[135]

In 2006, researchers looked at every trial on psychiatric drugs published in four academic journals over a ten-year period and found 542 trial outcomes. Pharmaceutical-funded studies showed favorable results 78 percent of the time versus 48 percent for independently funded trials.[136]

Ghostwriting in Action

In the previous section, I mentioned the practice of ghostwriting. Let me share a real case of this involving Wyeth and its combined estrogen/progestin drug Prempro.

A federal study linked Prempro to breast cancer in postmenopausal women. Wyeth commissioned a medical communication company, DesignWrite, to produce ghostwritten articles published under the names of leading physicians seeking to mitigate the perceived risks of breast cancer associated with Prempro. Ghostwritten articles defending Prempro were published in over 50 peer-reviewed journals.

The articles were designed to

- mitigate the perceived risks of breast cancer associated with Prempro;
- promote off-label and unproven uses of Prempro to prevent dementia, Parkinson's disease, and visual impairment;
- raise questions about the safety and efficacy of competing therapies; and
- promote Prempro's cardiovascular benefits despite the lack of benefit shown in randomized clinical trials.

This information came to light during litigation against Wyeth when over 14,000 women brought claims related to the development of breast cancer.[137]

When the FDA approves a drug, it is approved for specific indication(s) and drug companies are only legally able to promote a drug for the approved indication(s). However, physicians can prescribe a drug off-label for other conditions. One way for pharmaceutical companies to promote off-label use and be within the law is for drug companies to publish articles in medical journals showing a drug may have other benefits. The FDA views those published articles as protected commercial speech and does not regulate their content.[138]

Not-So-Wacko Jacko Rule of Medicine:

When it comes to research of any kind, but especially medical, follow the money.

Should All Medical Research Be Ignored?

Before I researched this book, I knew some things were shady with medical research, but I did not realize how bad, deceptive, and corrupt the research is. As a physician, I am now not sure I would trust any drug study sponsored by a pharmaceutical company unless there was also independent research to back up its results.

I think it might be wise to take a "guilty until proven innocent" approach with drug studies. This is most true of drugs still on patent. Studies by independent research groups studying a drug's repurposing are likely to be more honest.

My practice is less affected by potentially misleading results on drug studies, as I see drugs as a last resort and not the first option for many of my patients.

In addition to drug studies, any research involving medical devices or instrumentation that remains in the body, as is the case with some orthopedic and cardiology procedures involving joint replacements, cardiac stents, pacemakers, and instrumentation like plates and screws, should be viewed more carefully.

I know a neurosurgeon who feels one can get good results with cervical fusions using an autologous bone graft (one's own bone) at far less cost, but most of the published neurosurgical literature points to using plates and screws. Why? Because the medical device industry supports neurosurgical and spinal journals. No one makes money promoting the use of a patient's own bone.

Research on surgical and other invasive procedures can be heavily operator dependent (pun intended). Some surgeons and interventionalists are naturally more gifted than others and will get better results than other surgeons, despite doing the same procedure. Some surgeons have been known to keep procedures they developed as "trade secrets," only sharing them with their inner circle in fear the procedure may get a "bad name" if performed by those with lesser skill.

Insurance Companies

If I were the CEO of a health insurance company, I would be concerned knowing that a segment of the practice of medicine is based on less than honest research and misrepresented science.

Insurance companies base many of their decisions on what they will cover in their policies based on the published literature. The insurance industry needs to take a much closer look at the literature because it is likely making decisions on misrepresented science and may be covering therapies that are less effective.

Also, insurance companies often pay bonuses to physicians who meet specific performance goals and "important" metrics, typically based on clinical guidelines and published outcomes in the medical literature that may misrepresent a study's results.

In other words, the insurance industry may be getting ripped off by published literature. They, too, may be bamboozled, duped, and hoodwinked.

Not-So-Wacko Jacko Rules of Medicine.:

If medical research is bogus, then the authenticity of medicine as a profession is questionable.

Medicine suffers from a lack of scientific integrity and, thus, is partially built on science fiction.

PART III

Does Medicine Matter?

In the grand scheme of human longevity,
the contribution of modern medicine is minor.
—Jan Vijg, genetics professor,
Albert Einstein College of Medicine

Before we go much further, perhaps we should pause and ask a fundamental question. Does the field of medicine do any real good? Does it matter?

Is the whole field of medicine simply an exercise in futility? Maybe the entire profession is just one big lie because it is built on half-truths. Perhaps the profession is illegitimate in proportion to the illegitimate science that props it up.

After all, we are all going to die. We have a 100 percent mortality rate in medicine. Of all professions or industries, we have the worst results. What's the point in trying to be healthy and doing everything we can to stay healthy and treat illness?

We probably all know the person who spends every waking moment focused on staying healthy, making sure they eat well, get the right kind of exercise, get proper sleep, avoid unhealthy habits, keep unhealthy stress to a minimum, follow all the recommended guidelines for preventive care and vaccinations, and so on.

And that person will still die just like the person who totally neglects his or her health. This makes it hard to argue with the person who refuses to live a healthy lifestyle. But there is a way to respond to that person that I will mention later.

Again, I ask, "Does medicine matter?"

One way to answer that question is to ask another question: What is the impact of having no access to healthcare on premature death? You would think premature deaths would rise, possibly skyrocket, in the absence of healthcare. But do they?

Looking at data on life expectancy and premature death, and the impact of medicine on both, has led me to conclude that medicine is like many things we encounter in life. It follows the Pareto Principle, sometimes referred to as the 80/20 rule.

The Pareto Principle explains that 80 percent of the consequences or outcomes come from 20 percent of the causes. We can apply the principle to nearly everything, including the economy, investments, farming, crop yield, and coaching.

Many coaches will spend 80 percent of their time with the 20 percent of the athletes that will impact a team's success.

Typically, 80 percent of profits come from 20 percent of products. The McDonald brothers noticed this and trimmed their menu to a few items. Many individuals wear only 20 percent of their clothes 80 percent of the time. Most of the gains in your investment portfolio likely come from a handful of stocks.

Let me zero in on health. You do not need to do a thousand things daily to stay healthy. Five or six good habits, practiced daily, will take care of about 80 percent of your health needs.

Regardless of a physician's specialty, about 80 percent of care revolves around five diagnoses. The goal is to excel at managing those five diagnoses to provide excellent care to 80 percent or more of the patients.

About 21 percent of Medicare dollars are spent on 5 percent of the patients during their last year of life. That is not precisely 80/20, but it is still a 4 to 1 ratio.[139]

To improve health outcomes, we should zero in on the few things that make the most difference. We can do that without much healthcare.

The result of our efforts in medicine is this Not-So-Wacko Jacko Rule of Medicine:

We help a small number of patients a lot, we help many patients a little, but we also hurt some patients along the way.

How did I reach that conclusion?

The pathway to good health is determined more by behavior than interventions. We seem to want to credit healthcare anytime we see life expectancy rise or an improvement in quality of life. Still, many of these improvements are more behavior-driven or the result of public health measures.

Healthcare has much less impact on the extremely health-conscious person but will, potentially, have a greater impact on the person who is more neglectful of his or her health. Medicine has more opportunities to intervene with the neglectful person. In a system like the one we have in the US, where the emphasis is on treatment rather than prevention, it is the neglectful person on whom medicine feasts because it is more lucrative.

If the extremely health-conscious person lives to be one hundred, that improves life expectancy numbers, but that improvement is due to behavior and not healthcare.

Life Expectancy

Life expectancy in the US has improved since 1900, and our knee-jerk reaction is to thank modern medicine. I would say that praise for medicine may be overstated. The data below detail how life expectancy has changed since 1900. Life expectancy peaked in 2014, hovering in the 78–79 years range, and then dropped during COVID-19 by 1.9 years and slightly recovered in 2022.[140]

Year	Life Expectancy (Years)
1900	47.3
1922	59.6
2014	78.9
2022	77.5

That life expectancy has leveled off, despite medical advancement, means something. I am not sure what, but it means something. It might mean that we have squeezed the last little blood drop out of the turnip based on our current knowledge base and our drug-first approach, but some exciting advancements in cellular medicine might get us back on track. But for now, we have hit a plateau, despite advancements.

Or perhaps we have hit a plateau despite medical advancements because maybe, just maybe, medical advancements are not as significant as we think. That seems like a ridiculous comment or something a Wacko Jacko might say, but is it?

Life expectancy has nearly doubled compared to our hunter-gatherer ancestors,[141] and we attribute that increase to healthcare. But those numbers are misleading.

Many of our hunter-gatherer ancestors succumbed to an early death. If they lived past childhood, though, they lived to be 68–78 years old, not unlike what we do today, and they did it without any healthcare.[142] Anything that increases infant and childhood deaths considerably skews life expectancy numbers downward, which is why life expectancy numbers look better today than for our ancestors.

Without medical advancements, our hunter-gatherer ancestors lived about as long as we do today, if they reached adulthood. Basically, despite all our technology and all the billions we spend on healthcare, we are treading water. We must be overlooking something or some other factor at play that offsets our medical advancements.

It could be the toxic environment we live in that offsets the benefits of medical advancements. Toxins contaminate nearly everything we put into our bodies these days.

But for whatever reason, life expectancy has not improved in recent years despite ongoing advancements.

Much of the improvement in life expectancy over the past one hundred or so years centers around water/sanitation and reducing infant and childhood mortality.

It is not strange that health improves when the population gives up using diluted sewage as the principal beverage.

—Dr. Thurman Rice, 1932

Infant mortality skews life expectancy downward significantly. Anything that reduces infant and early childhood mortality has a more appreciable impact on life expectancy than something that reduces mortality in later years. For instance, treating a child for pneumonia will extend life expectancy more than treating pneumonia in the elderly because the latter are already closer to the peak of life expectancy.

The chart below shows how mortality rates have changed from 1900 to 1970 by age group. The line representing the big decline is for the under-one-year age group. Death rates for other age groups have remained stable during that seventy-year period, highlighting that the gain in life expectancy is due to reductions in childhood mortality. That questions the value or contribution of "medical advancements."

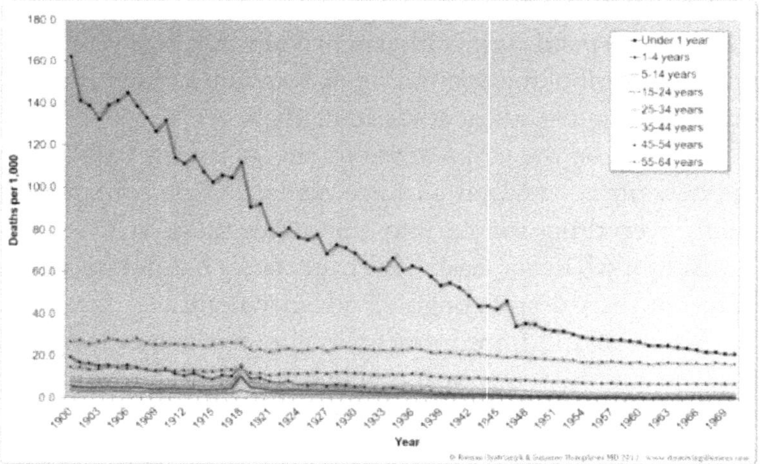

United States mortality rates for age groups from 1900 to 1970. (Historical Statistics of the United States—Colonial Times to 1970 Part 1, Bureau of the Census, p. 60)

From DissolvingIllusions.com.

The factors that most impact life expectancy center around sanitation and clean water, along with a reduction in childhood mortality from infection through antibiotics and, possibly, some contribution from vaccines.[143] Yet, frequently, we read how vaccines positively impact life expectancy and, thus, attribute improvement in life expectancy to childhood vaccines. We have accepted that as gospel, but that may not be true.

The graph below shows that death rates from infectious diseases had already reached a nadir by the time nationwide mass childhood vaccinations began in the early 1960s.

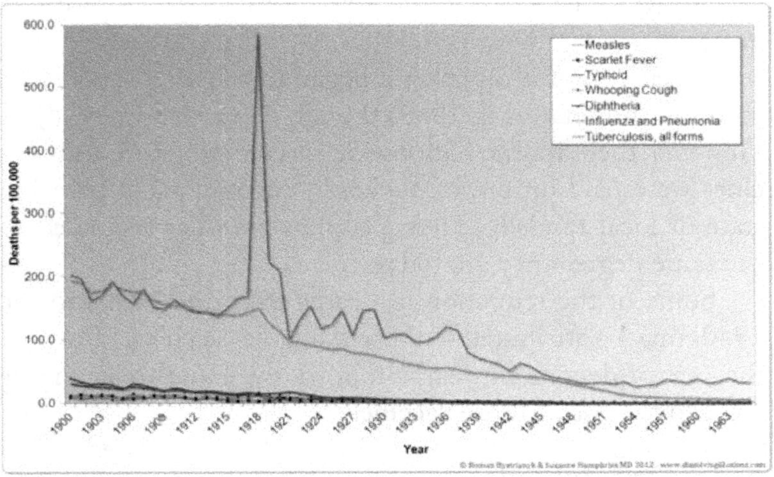

United States mortality rates from various infectious diseases from 1900 to 1965. (Vital Statistics of the United States 1937, 1938, 1943, 1944, 1949, 1960, 1967, 1976, 1987, 1992; Historical Statistics of the United States—Colonial Times to 1970 Part 1)

From DissolvingIllusions.com.

Before 1961, we vaccinated children for only five diseases: diphtheria, tetanus, pertussis, poliomyelitis, and smallpox.[144] We did not vaccinate children *en masse*.

Today, we vaccinate children for sixteen diseases: diphtheria, Haemophilus influenzae type b, hepatitis A, hepatitis B, human papillomavirus infection, influenza, measles, meningococcal disease, mumps, pertussis, pneumococcal disease, poliomyelitis, rotavirus infections, rubella, tetanus, and varicella.

Despite the increased number of vaccinations, we have not seen an appreciable decline in death rates from infectious diseases. But vaccines before 1961 may have played a role in getting to that nadir.

Let's review this graph and add some significant dates and events. The introduction of water filtration and chlorination in major US cities began between 1900 and 1940 and accounted for one-half of the 30 percent reduction in urban deaths.[145]

Vaccinating for diphtheria began in the 1920s, pertussis in 1926, and tetanus in 1938 (though developed in 1924).[146] However, there was no nationwide vaccine program, and vaccines were paid for out of pocket by individuals or by using state or local funds.[147] Thus, people were not vaccinated to the same degree they are today.

Some of the reduction in deaths from the 1920s to the 1940s may be attributed to those available vaccines. However, the rate of decline in deaths follows the same trajectory as prior to the use of those vaccines.

The spike in deaths from 1918 to 1920 is related to the Spanish Flu. Penicillin use started in 1942, with the subsequent development of other antibiotics. In 1955, we began vaccinating for polio after the Salk vaccine had been tested in about one million children in 1953–54. (For comparison, the Pfizer-BioNTech COVID-19 vaccine was tested on 22,000 participants in its phase 3 clinical trial.) Then Congress passed the Vaccine Assistance Act of 1962, which provided federal funds for vaccinations.

Note that even in 1900, some of these diseases had relatively low rates of death, even as low as 10 to 30 per 100,000 or 1 to 3 per 10,000, yet we vaccinate for them anyway. As you can see, mortality rates plummeted before the introduction of the Vaccine Assistance Act.

How Rare Is Rare?

Something with an incidence of 1 in 1,000 to 1 in 10,000 is considered rare in medicine. See the following table.

Term	Numerical rate	Percentage rate
Very common	More than 1 in 10	10% or higher
Common	1 in 10 – 1 in 100	10% – 1%
Uncommon	1 in 100 – 1 in 1000	0.1% to 1%
Rare	1 in 1000 – 1 in 10,000	0.01% to 0.1%
Very rare	Less than 1 in 10,000	Less than 0.01%

From HIV i-BASE. https://i-base.info/qa/812.

Even though the incidence of some of these infectious diseases was high in the early 1900s, the death rates for many of them were low enough to be considered rare by today's standards, despite the squalor in which many people lived during those times. Nonetheless, we still vaccinate for those infectious diseases with low death rates.

A Quick Look at Measles

Because measles is always a hot topic, let's zero in on this disease and look at the graph below showing the deaths from measles from 1900 to the introduction of the measles vaccine in 1963. In 1961, the death rate from measles was 0.237

per 100,000 population. Between 1900 and 1924, the annual death rate from measles was about 10 per 100,000 population. This decline from 10 per 100,000 to 0.237 per 100,000 represents a 98 percent decline in mortality before the introduction of the measles vaccine.

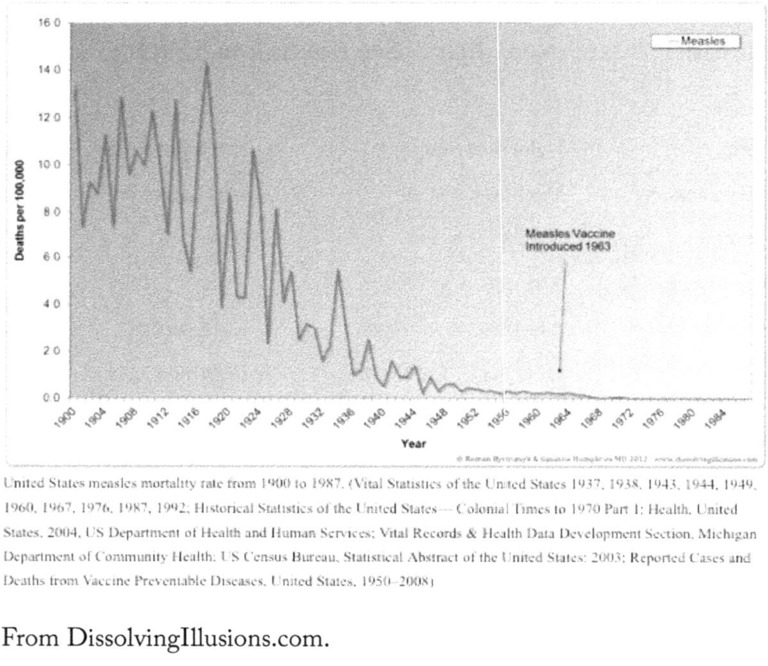

United States measles mortality rate from 1900 to 1987. (Vital Statistics of the United States 1937, 1938, 1943, 1944, 1949, 1960, 1967, 1976, 1987, 1992; Historical Statistics of the United States—Colonial Times to 1970 Part 1: Health, United States, 2004, US Department of Health and Human Services; Vital Records & Health Data Development Section, Michigan Department of Community Health; US Census Bureau, Statistical Abstract of the United States: 2003; Reported Cases and Deaths from Vaccine Preventable Diseases, United States, 1950–2008)

From DissolvingIllusions.com.

Let's look at the data on measles and its vaccine for 2024. Below is a screenshot from the CDC website. Notice three things. First, the 285 cases (not deaths) from measles are for all age groups. Second, some who contracted measles were vaccinated. Third, vaccine status for unvaccinated and unknown status is grouped together. This is a misleading way to present the data, which should be reported separately. Some of those individuals may have been vaccinated.

However, the way the data is presented makes it easy to conclude that 89 percent of the population was not vaccinated. Though not likely, it is possible that the entire 89 percent were vaccinated, but the status was unknown by the data collectors.

U.S. Cases in 2024

Total cases

285

Age
Under 5 years: **120 (42%)**
5-19 years: **88 (31%)**
20+ years: **77 (27%)**

Vaccination Status
Unvaccinated or Unknown: **89%**
One MMR dose: **7%**
Two MMR doses: **4%**

US Center for Disease Control and Prevention. "Measles Cases and Outbreak." https://www.cdc.gov/measles/data-research/index.html#cdc_data_surveillance_section_1-measles-cases-in-2024.

Let's look at the data for the under-five age group, which is the group we are usually concerned about when it comes to measles. In the under-five age group, there were 120 cases of measles in 2024. There are about 19,000,000 children under five in the US.[148]

Thus, the measles infection rate in the under-five population is 0.0006 percent (120/19,000,000 x 100). Few will die from measles. Plus, we don't know what comorbidities these children may have had or their living conditions.

Before the measles vaccine, 400–500 people contracted the disease annually.[149] Now, the number hovers around 300. Millions of vaccine doses are administered to lower cases of measles by 100–200 annually.

Thus, we can conclude that the measles vaccine contributes little to preventing measles cases and even less to improving life expectancy.

As a parent, you now have more data, and coupled with an understanding of your risk tolerance, you can make a more informed decision about the measles vaccine.

Moving forward, you do not need me or your physician to get such information. You can research other vaccines; it is all in the public domain. However, you must be curious enough to look for it. Curiosity is the key that stimulates critical thinking.

Vaccine Debate

This isn't a book about vaccines, but I wanted to explain how vaccines may not be as beneficial as we have been led to believe, especially when it comes to preventing childhood deaths. Parents have been more skeptical of vaccines than physicians, and it appears they have a legitimate concern.

Much of the vaccine controversy centers around vaccine safety. But perhaps that debate detracts from the bigger picture and overshadows a more fundamental question: Are some of these vaccines even needed, based on these charts?

I am not a proponent of either side in this vaccine debate; my only agenda is to try to explain these charts. So, let me share some food for thought.

Earlier, I shared some of the data for the COVID-19 vaccines and that, despite impressive "vaccine efficacy" numbers, those numbers do not translate into meaningful outcomes. What is more common: COVID-19, measles, mumps, or rubella? COVID-19, by far and away, is more common. If a 100 percent vaccine efficacy to prevent death from COVID-19 means 22,000 must be vaccinated to prevent one death, then the numbers to vaccinate to prevent deaths from measles, mumps, and rubella are likely to be even higher because the incidence of those infections are lower and not as deadly.

If a vaccine efficacy of 95 percent to prevent getting COVID-19 translates to an absolute risk reduction of 0.84 percent, then the absolute risk reduction to prevent an infection from vaccines for less common infectious diseases may be closer to zero. That could explain why we have not seen an appreciable lowering in deaths since the government introduced the Vaccine Act. When something already has a low incidence, any absolute risk reduction from an intervention will be low to the point of not being clinically relevant.

I suppose one can argue that, without the vaccines, the incidence of these diseases would increase, but the numbers had already plummeted before the Vaccine Act. The incidences would probably increase in the absence of sanitation and water purification, but that is not as much of a problem here in the US as it is in other countries where the incidence of childhood diseases is higher.

For readers interested in vaccines, I refer you to *Dissolving Illusions: Disease, Vaccines, and the Forgotten History* by Suzanne Humphries, MD, and Roman Bystrianyk. Dr. Humphries also has a lecture on vaccines on YouTube.[150]

I also recommend the websites Learn The Risk (LearnTheRisk.org/vaccines/diseases) and Vax Info Start Here (VaxInfoStartHere.com/did-vaccines-save-us). These sites feature more graphs showing the incidence of many infectious diseases declined before vaccinations, and you can learn about all the products used in making vaccines.

Physicians are poorly trained on vaccine history, that is, how vaccines are manufactured and how vaccine studies are conducted. We are taught only to recommend and persuade patients to receive them. In "The Pharmaceutical Funded FDA," I will discuss the approval of vaccines and the nebulous definition of vaccine safety.

In summary, water filtration, sanitation, and antibiotics are the main reasons for the increase in life expectancy, with some contribution from vaccines, but based on the above graphs, not as much as commonly believed. A close look at these graphs shows that the decline in deaths caused by infectious diseases that we vaccinate for corresponds to water and sanitation improvements. If we ever decide to go back to drinking diluted sewage, then vaccines would provide more value.

Impact of No Healthcare on Premature Deaths

Let me get back to the earlier question: How does no access to healthcare impact premature death? The answer is just 10 percent.[151] This would support Dr. Vijg's quote at the beginning of the chapter. Ninety percent of medicine adds very little and is built on half-truths.

In part, using previously published data from Mokdad,[152] Schroeder studied factors from five domains contributing to premature death. These included no access to healthcare, genetics, environmental exposure, social circumstances (socioeconomic factors), and behavioral patterns.

Genetics accounted for 30 percent of premature deaths, environmental exposures accounted for 5 percent, social circumstances accounted for 15 percent, and behavior patterns accounted for the principal cause of premature death at 40 percent. No access to healthcare accounted for the remaining 10 percent.

Behavior patterns caused 48.2 percent of all deaths.[153] These patterns included drug use, alcohol use, motor vehicle accidents, guns, sexual behavior, physical inactivity/obesity, and smoking. If we look at just the behavior pattern factors, smoking accounted for 18.1 percent of all deaths but 44 percent of premature deaths, inactivity/obesity accounted for 16.6 percent of all deaths and 37 percent of premature deaths, and alcohol 3.5 percent of all deaths and 8.6 percent of premature deaths.

Some Cold Hard Facts

Despite being one of the wealthiest nations and ranking first in healthcare expenditure, in 2022, the United States ranked 49th in the world for life expectancy at birth.[154] Our system has focused on new drug discovery and disease treatment rather than prevention. Consequently, we lag behind other industrialized nations when it comes to health outcomes.

A more recent meta-analysis of 15 studies on 17 countries estimates that 60 percent of premature deaths could be attributed to unhealthy lifestyle factors like smoking, excessive alcohol consumption, physical inactivity, poor diet, and obesity, with a healthy lifestyle increasing life expectancy from 7.4 years to 17.9 years (varied by country).[155]

How many drugs will add nearly 18 years to your life expectancy?

This seems to support the notion that medicine and healthcare follow Pareto's Principle of 80/20. That is, if our goal is to improve life expectancy, we should focus more on behavior (the 20 percent) than medical treatment (the 80 percent).

Improving fitness is far more critical than treating hypertension, heart disease, diabetes, and other chronic diseases in terms of reducing premature death. Exercise can be free.

Not-So-Wacko Jacko Rule of Medicine:

We get the biggest gains in life expectancy from the least expensive interventions.[IP]

We spend 18–20 percent of our nation's GDP on healthcare. It is the single biggest item we spend money on. It's debatable whether we get our money's worth when considering that behavioral changes are not expensive.

It seems such an obvious conclusion that we should spend more time on fitness, yet we don't. I think the fact that we focus more on medical treatments reflects the firm grasp Big Pharma has on healthcare and medical education/training.

There is no money to make when people are healthy, and little money to get people healthy via lifestyle changes.

The sad reality is that healthcare is more about money than health outcomes, but medicine must show that it produces some positive outcomes. It often does that through data manipulation, as we have learned from medical journal editors. Or we misrepresent the treatment goal, for example, by telling patients a drug treatment has successfully lowered their blood pressure even though that is not the actual goal.

Acute vs. Chronic Conditions

We need to make a distinction between acute and chronic conditions.

We do well when managing acute life-threatening emergencies, especially those involving severe infections requiring antibiotics and surgery. We also do well in managing acute trauma.

We have assumed that because we do well by applying interventions in acute care, the same would be true with chronic disease management. However, we do not deliver the same results because the underlying causes of chronic disease are largely lifestyle-related, and our system does not address them well. Remember, chronic disease management is more lucrative because it is ongoing.

Once you reach adulthood, and if you are then able to avoid life-threatening acute trauma and infections, the chance of you benefiting from healthcare is a flip of the coin. Some will benefit, some will not, and some will be harmed. We just don't know who.

Because antibiotics have helped treat acute infections, we have developed the mindset that medications are the answer to more chronic conditions.

As physicians, we think we have a greater influence on health than we do, and it's because we see a skewed population. We believe everybody is sick because we see sickness all day, every day.

When I did my pediatric rotation in medical school, I left with the impression that every young child has congenital heart disease, cancer, or a life-threatening infectious disease. But those children represent just a tiny fraction of the population.

Likewise, every patient that a cardiologist sees has heart disease. Thus, a cardiologist is prone to think more people die from heart disease than they do. Despite heart disease being the number one killer in the US, you need to know five hundred people to know one person who died of heart disease during the past twelve months. Many of you will not know one person who died of heart disease in the past year.

My Family Experience with Acute Trauma

During the pandemic lockdowns, my 20-year-old son had a bad motorcycle accident. He lost control while traveling at a high rate of speed, and he and his bike flew into a parked car. The bike was totaled. The car was totaled. And the left side of his body was totaled.

He is lucky to be alive and more fortunate not to have a spinal cord or traumatic brain injury. He avoided injury to other vital organs. His injuries were orthopedic, plus bad road rash that required a trip to the operating room.

Twelve surgeries over two years pieced him back together. His recovery has been remarkable. Despite some mild impairments, he manages to work as an auto mechanic.

He was lucky witnesses summoned an ambulance, and it was parked three blocks from the accident. He was lucky that the only level 1 trauma center in Columbus, Ohio, was no more than a mile-and-a-half from the accident.

He was lucky he got to the ER quickly, which is the key to improved outcomes for any acute trauma and medical emergency. He reached the ER before the police had arrived at the accident scene.

And he was lucky that the best trauma surgeon in the city was on call and performed his initial and subsequent surgeries with the help of a hand-and-plastics surgeon. He was lucky youth was on his side.

Changing any of those variables could have resulted in a very different outcome. Literally, he lost half his blood. A quick first emergency response coupled with timely and excellent care has helped to preserve his lifespan and health span. And thus, quality of life.

For my son, medicine mattered, and it mattered greatly. American medicine excels in acute trauma, emergencies, and managing acute infections. We do not excel at managing chronic problems.

We discussed the number needed to treat (NNT) some earlier. While the NNT for blood pressure medicine can be 86 to 140, the NNT for antibiotics can be as low as 1.1,[156] which means that for every 11 patients who receive an antibiotic, 10 will respond. That is quite a difference in results using a drug for a chronic problem like high blood pressure versus using an antibiotic for an acute infection.

Not-So-Wacko Jacko Rule of Medicine:

Anytime you take a drug long-term, your biochemistry is being altered in ways we do not always fully understand.

All drugs have side effects that, even if not serious, may still impact quality of life to one degree or another. Being nauseated, for example, is not fun and is usually the most common side effect of nearly all medications.

Thinking we are helping a vast majority with our chronic disease management with drugs is a half-truth. Plus…

We do some harm in medicine. Iatrogenic causes of death—those deaths caused by doctors and the healthcare system—have been the third leading cause of death behind heart disease and cancer. Only COVID-19 knocked it out of third place and down to the fourth leading cause of death.[157]

We do a less-than-stellar job with chronic disease management, but we also do a poor job with prevention. The two are linked because both rely more on behavior and lifestyle than medicine.

That can change, however, if we change our approach. About 70–80 percent of chronic diseases are related to lifestyle, so we have an opportunity to better affect those diseases if we alter our current approach of relying on medication.

The outcome of our chronic disease management is that we keep patients dying longer in a poor state of health. We help keep them alive past the time their health span has expired. Remember, your health span is the years you live in good health or, more specifically, the years you maintain full function. Our approach to chronic disease enables patients to die slowly and live more crappy years.

Not-So-Wacko Jacko Rule of Medicine:

We get the most significant gains in life expectancy from the least expensive interventions.

Drugs Help Some Chronic Diseases

I should make a distinction among chronic diseases because drugs can help certain chronic conditions, and I do not want to paint the picture that drugs cannot be effective.

We can break up chronic disease into asymptomatic and symptomatic categories. Asymptomatic diseases are typically lifestyle-related—high blood pressure, diabetes, and elevated cholesterol. Drugs are less effective in these conditions in preventing premature death and serious complications. As a patient, you cannot tell whether the drug is treating these conditions based on how you feel.

Symptomatic chronic diseases and autoimmune diseases, like rheumatoid arthritis and its cousins, may be effectively treated with drugs. Many of the biologics treating these conditions are life-changing. For these conditions, patients have proof that the drug is working—they feel less pain, have better mobility, and see their plaque psoriasis disappear.

Not-So-Wacko Jacko Rule of Medicine:

Medicine or healthcare does matter. It matters much to a few but little to many, and it's detrimental to some. It follows Pareto's Principle.

Let's go back to the extremely health-conscious person. What is that person looking for? What is the result of his or her effort to stay healthy?

The Goal of Medicine in One Word

What does an extremely health-conscious person want? What should be the ultimate goal of medicine?

I can distill that one goal into one word—ENERGY. That is what the person who is meticulous with his or her health habits is trying to do. Make and maintain a high level of energy.

When you have energy, you simply feel much better. When you have unlimited energy, you find yourself in an upward spiral. Living is much different when you have boundless energy. It is more enjoyable. You look forward to each day and the opportunity that it brings.

When you have energy, problems seem smaller; you brush off stress more easily and can do what brings you the most joy in life, longer and better. With energy, you have more time to make a difference, make an impact, and experience all that life offers.

Our thirty trillion-plus cells make energy in organelles called mitochondria. Nearly everything you put in your body either helps your cells produce energy or interferes with that life-giving process.

Medicine does not focus on improving energy production. We focus on treating symptoms and diseases, and many treatments fight the body's ability to make energy. In fact, numerous treatments drain us of energy.

For example, commonly used medications for diabetes, cardiovascular disease, and mood disorders interfere with coenzyme Q10 production, which is essential for energy production. Those classes include statins, beta blockers, ACE inhibitors, calcium channel blockers, diuretics, osteoporosis drugs, glimepiride, glyburide, glipizide, tricyclic antidepressants, and more.[158]

You may not recognize it, but what you want is ENERGY. Life stops the moment your body no longer produces energy.

Some patients, like those with heart failure, may take three to five of the above classes of medications, and their quality of life is not good. They are fatigued (some from heart failure but some from the medicine), but they put up with the side effects because it is better than the alternative. Nonetheless, their health span has come to an end. They are living crappy years.

The real key to health occurs at the cellular level—improving how the cell functions and improving the function of the basic unit of life. Improving cellular efficiency is where the future of medicine will be, and we are only now beginning to learn how to do that.

We would get better results if we emphasized lifestyle to prevent and treat disease. Let's look at lifestyle in action.

Lifestyle in Action: Blue Zones

If you hear of people being in Blue Zones, you might think they are depressed, but you would be wrong. A Blue Zone is not a mood. It is a place. A special place. We know of only five such places. Blue Zones are unique places where people tend to live longer than 90 years and even more than 100 years old. They are:

- Sardinia (Italy)
- Okinawa (Japan)
- Nicoya Peninsula (Costa Rica)
- Ikaria (Greece)
- Loma Linda (California)

We hear of athletes being in the zone—that rare intersection of peak performance, focused concentration, energy, and exhilaration. Blue Zones are like athletic zones. There we find individuals living long, productive, meaningful, and energetic lives.

Do Blue Zones have a secret?

The Secret of Blue Zones

Blue Zones are sometimes referred to as longevity hotspots. Michael Poulain originally developed the concept of Blue Zones in 2000.[159] Author Dan Buettner has written most extensively about Blue Zones, traveling the globe to study them and writing *The Blue Zones: 9 Lessons for Living Longer From the People Who Have Lived the Longest*.[160] (A documentary featuring Mr. Buettner's travels to the Blue Zones and his discussions of each is available on streaming services.)

What is the secret of these longevity hotspots? Is it a combination of modern medicine and technology? Is it nutritional supplements? Genes? That is what Mr. Buettner and others have been trying to answer. In a nutshell, the secret, if you can call it that, is lifestyle. So, not really a secret. And it's nothing you can package in a bottle. It is not a shortcut to good health either. The success of Blue Zones requires effort.

Members of Blue Zones share common traits, including

- an emphasis on family and social relationships;
- a plant-based diet with mild consumption of meat;
- daily physical activity;
- successful stress management, and
- incorporation of a spiritual or religious component.

Relationships and Roseto, Pennsylvania

Relationships are paramount in Blue Zones. Blue Zone members have both strong family and social relationships. They are active social participants in the community and life. The connection between longevity and social relationships has also been noted and reported in other populations.

Roseto, Pennsylvania, is not a Blue Zone but a case study in the importance of social connectedness. Roseto was settled by Italian immigrants from Roseto, Italy. In the 1950s, it was recognized that few people in Roseto died of heart attacks, which was nearly epidemic in those days.

Roseto's population had about a 35 percent lower mortality rate than the general US population. Heart attacks were virtually unheard of in Roseto in men under age 55. In men over 65, the rate of heart attacks was half that for men in Roseto compared to the rest of the US population.

Yet, their health habits were far from ideal. They prepared their Italian meals with lard rather than healthier olive oil. Forty-one percent of their calories came from fat. Many were heavy smokers, and many were overweight. Roseto was not a community of exercisers either.

Then, why so few heart attacks? Would they have had even fewer heart attacks if they had lived a cleaner lifestyle?

Many households contained three generations, and most individuals belonged to social clubs. This town of two thousand has 22 civic clubs and organizations. They treated the elderly with respect. There was essentially zero crime in Roseto. Eventually, researchers concluded that the town created a protective social structure that provided significant health benefits.[161]

When we feel connected, we feel wanted, and when we feel wanted, our outlook on life improves. We become more motivated and more confident. We come to know ourselves better and develop a sense of purpose. We are more peaceful, and peace is the opposite of stress.

Having a network of family and friends helps us dissipate and cope with stress when we go through tough times. Stress is a killer, figuratively and literally. Chronic stress shortens telomere length (telomeres are markers of aging), taking off eleven years of life span. That is more than smoking and obesity.

Plant-Based Diet

A plant-based diet is a low glycemic diet, that is, one that does not spike blood sugar. You will not go wrong if fruits and vegetables are your only sources of carbohydrates, but Blue Zone inhabitants do consume some starchy carbs.

Blue Zone inhabitants also eat some meat. Fish and poultry are healthy. Most evidence suggests limiting (not altogether avoiding) red meats, even if they are lean. In Blue Zones, fruits and vegetables are emphasized.

Daily Physical Activity

Inhabitants naturally incorporate physical activity into their daily lives. They work with their hands. They plant some of their food. They walk to the market and most everywhere. They live a slower-paced life yet are, paradoxically, more physically active than fast-paced Americans. Those of us not living in Blue Zones must work to be active because much of our day is sedentary. (I'm not exactly running as I write this.)

One does not have to go to the gym daily to be active though. Our non-exercise physical activity (all the calories we burn being active outside of formal exercise) may be a more important determinant of health than the amount of exercise we do. We tend to make being active more complicated than it is.

Stress and Spirituality

Inhabitants of Blue Zones tend to have a strong spiritual side. Given the geography of the five Blue Zones, it is likely that each population has differing spiritual beliefs. But having faith probably leads to similar health outcomes. Anything that reduces stress can help you live longer and healthier. Being religious or spiritual is one way to reduce stress. Faith is a way to find comfort in a world that often makes little sense. Faith is a way to put life in perspective.

Being religious gets us to look beyond ourselves and focus on the needs of others. That is healthy. Many have said that one of the best ways to help yourself is to help someone else. Religion encourages that. A belief in life after death makes it much easier to cope with practically everything we confront and must endure.

Lifestyle is more important than medications and medical interventions for improving longevity.[IP]

Amish Life Expectancy

Let's go back to life expectancy and examine it beyond water, sanitation, antibiotics, and vaccines, adding lifestyle into the mix. Earlier, we talked about Roseto, Pennsylvania. However, we have another example of how lifestyle affects life span.

To see the importance of lifestyle on life expectancy, and particularly water and sanitation, we can examine the Amish population in the US. In 1900, when the overall life expectancy was 47.3 years, for the Amish, it was 70.[162] In the early

1900s, the Amish did not live in crowded situations, so they would not have been subjected to the ill effects of poor-quality drinking water, unsanitary conditions, and air pollution. They ate food fresh from their fields, free from toxins, and they live a nearly identical lifestyle now.

Today, the Amish live slightly longer than the general population. Their lifestyle and life spans seem to support the premise that medical advancements and technology may not be as significant as we think. The Amish lifestyle is devoid of those things, and their life expectancy has remained relatively stable for over 120 years.

Lifestyle trumps medications.

Amish men take 18,425 steps daily, and Amish women take 14,196. Only 4 percent of the Amish population is obese compared to 41.9 percent of the general population. Rates of all cancers are 40 percent lower as well. Movement and healthy eating are essential—they are more important than medications.

Doctor Training Is Woefully Inadequate

We could increase the importance of medicine if we took a more comprehensive and integrative approach by removing our blinders.

Much of what I do in my practice I did not learn in medical school or residency training because it was not taught. It wasn't taught because no one had the experience to teach it.

When I was in middle school, more high schools in Ohio started playing soccer. Ohio is not exactly a soccer mecca, so few had ever played soccer. Consequently, even fewer knew enough to coach the sport. Some schools simply gave someone a whistle and said, "Congratulations! You are our soccer coach." Coaches learned to coach the game as they learned the game.

Something similar happens in medicine. That first wave of doctors must be willing to venture out and learn a new field by being in the field and learning from trial and error.

When I did my sports medicine fellowship in 1989–90, none of the dozen fellowship program directors across the country had ever completed a sports medicine fellowship themselves because such programs did not exist. They learned what they knew from doing it and then teaching it.

Traditional medicine does not embrace venturing out; it assumes that it provides all one needs to know. Conventional medicine has maintained a narrow focus on medication mixed in with surgery.

When some of the clinical faculty from my internal medicine residency program heard of my sports medicine fellowship, they said, "You know, that's not real medicine." Apparently, real medicine prescribes medication only.

If you look at all the ways that doctors can address a medical problem, conventional medicine addresses about a third to half, which is generous. Patients hear limited options when they see an MD or DO. Right out of the gate, patients get a half-truth, but not the half-truth I refer to in this book.

Physicians may have the least well-rounded education in medicine and health. Many physicians have never been exposed to other means of treatment. Frequently, they dismiss them due to this lack of knowledge about treatments such as acupuncture, chiropractic care, herbal medicine, electromagnetic therapy, biofeedback, and more.

Regardless of the longevity of alternative treatments, today's medical education system is primarily the result of the 1910 Flexner Report, which labeled complementary and alternative forms of medicine as quackery. It is not my intent to elevate alternative disciplines to the level of today's conventional medicine. However, some of those treatments are used increasingly and do have science to support them.

Magnets are used in diagnostic imaging, like MRI scans, to treat depression via transcranial magnetic stimulation and the treatment of soft tissue injuries. There are three different applications of magnets: Pulse electromagnetic therapy (PEMF) is FDA-approved and helps to heal tissues and ease pain. Electric current, in physical therapy, treats musculoskeletal problems, and implanted spinal stimulators aid those who suffer from chronic pain.

Dermatologists use phototherapy to treat skin problems. Light therapy treats depression and other mood disorders. Anything that helps with movement, like yoga and tai chi, is beneficial.

What I have observed is that patients abandon treatments that do not work. Acupuncture and chiropractic must work well enough in enough people that these treatments remain in demand.

Physician Gaps of Knowledge

Medicine would get better results by closing some gaps in physician knowledge.

Physicians have significant gaps in their knowledge. There are even areas where patients know more about a health topic than physicians, which is why many physicians frown on patients doing research. They close down the discussion to avoid being embarrassed about their inability to talk intelligently about a non-conventional option.

Do you know who knows the most about anabolic steroids, including testosterone? Not doctors. Not pharmacists. Not coaches. Athletes.

The average anabolic steroid user spends 268 hours studying the topic before they start taking anabolic steroids.[163] I recall something like 60 hours (if that) of pharmacology in medical school and none of that on anabolic steroids to put that in perspective.

Do you know who knows the most about nutrition? Not a registered dietician. Not a nutritionist or a sports nutritionist. Not a doctor. Bodybuilders.

Bodybuilders are looked down upon for any number of reasons and dismissed as dunces, but many are very intelligent. They have the rare ability to keep concepts simple, unlike doctors. They understand that food is fuel; if you want to power a Ferrari, you feed it high-octane fuel. You don't feed it the typical American diet of processed and sugary foods and drinks.

Do you know who knows the most about nutrition? Bodybuilders.

You eat certain foods before a workout and certain foods afterward. And some foods you never eat. Bodybuilders know how to lose fat and gain muscle without using anabolic steroids.

Bodybuilders have PhDs from the laboratory of experimentation but are also well-read on the topic, more so than 99 percent of physicians. They roll up their sleeves and get their hands dirty. They are on the field of play gathering real-time information. Real-time information—didn't I mention that earlier?

Practical experience matters more than desk knowledge. Bodybuilders learn, apply, refine their methods, and reapply. They rinse and repeat until they discover what works.

They are among the most disciplined people you will find. Most of them are more disciplined and meticulous with their eating than they are with their exercise. They know that "abs are made in the kitchen and refined in the gym." And without the right fuel, one cannot maximize the benefits of training. In essence, much of what they do is to improve cellular efficiency, though they may not think of it in those terms.

Our diets are at the core of many health problems. Unfortunately, in conventional medicine, we don't spend much time addressing nutrition. Much of our food supply is tainted with contaminants and toxins. There is a push for physicians to limit antibiotic use to curb the emergence of drug-resistant bacteria, but physicians are responsible for only about 30–35 percent of antibiotic use in the US. The remainder comes from the agricultural industry.[164]

We speak of "eating clean," which takes on two meanings. The first refers to avoiding unhealthy carbs and fats in our diet. The second refers to consuming meat and poultry that have *not* been fed hormones and antibiotics. Finding drug-free animals is a challenge these days.

Livestock are fed antibiotics and hormones, so the animals grow bigger and faster.[165] How this impacts our health is unclear, but it probably does not impact it positively.

Mixed Messaging

Medicine also sends out mixed messages that limit the results. Workers who smoke and are morbidly obese are plentiful in the healthcare industry. Many of them fall short when it comes to recommended exercise guidelines.

Hospital cafeterias feature some of the least healthy foods. The Cleveland Clinic, routinely ranked as the number one heart hospital in the world, had a McDonald's grace its food court for 20 years. Finally, in 2015, it severed ties with McDonald's.[166]

The Tip of the Iceberg

What we know, as physicians, is only the tip of the iceberg of everything there is to know. Unfortunately, physicians tend to see the tip as representing the entire iceberg. Like an iceberg, we know 20 percent of what there is to understand, and 80 percent sits below the water; however, more is within our reach if we take the time to look for it.

Our current approach to patient care enables us to help a few a lot, but most just a little bit, while hurting some in the process.

Science Is Always Wrong Until It Gets It Right

No science is immune to the infection of politics and the corruption of power.
—Jacob Bronowski

Science, science, science. We must have science. Science appeals to us because it seems so scientific, so legitimate. But is it?

Science is extraordinary when we use it to unveil the truth. But, as we have learned from former editors of prestigious medical journals, science is frequently tainted. Science can easily be used to deceive by inventing half-truths and manipulating data.

So, what good is tainted science? Do you want to be led by tainted science and put your trust in it?

Not-So-Wacko Jacko Rules of Medicine:

The need for medical science is frequently heavily promoted by those who know how to manipulate it.[IP]

Medicine needs more scientific integrity as it is partially built on tainted science.

If medical research is tainted, then the authenticity of medicine as a profession is questionable.

Should We Follow Science?

One mantra we have heard since the height of the COVID-19 pandemic is the need to "follow the science." Ironically, much of what was done during the height of the pandemic was not based on science or, at least, reputable science. To some degree, we followed science fiction.

I have found "following the science" to be misleading and, occasionally, poor advice, and I will present my case as to why throughout this chapter. To follow science, one better hope the science is correct.[IP]

One of the best discussions I have heard on the topic of "following the science" was given by Jordan Vaughan, MD, in testimony to Congress on June 26, 2024.

> The problem with following the science is that science does not lead anywhere. Science is an observer, measurer, and descriptor. Not a leader. Individuals lead. Pressing science to lead is a way decision makers avoid accountability for choices they make on the public's behalf. The leader is appealing to the authority of science to decide a course of action to conveniently sidestep accountability in the event

> of failure. I implore my fellow physicians and scientists to not follow the science but lead humbly with science.[167]

I think we should begin our quest for the truth with things for which there is universal agreement, things that have been proved, beyond doubt, to be true. The problem is that you will not find much universal agreement in medicine because **medicine is not a pure science** where one answer exists. We have eight billion people on the planet with eight billion different physiologies. A single-answer approach will not work.

However, "following the science" is a way for leaders to wash their hands when desired outcomes are not achieved. "Don't blame us, we followed the science" is an admission that science can be wrong. Also, the phrase "the science has changed" means science can be wrong.

Assuming honest science, following science is most appropriate when the science is pure, like physics or math. Medicine is not a pure science; often, there is more than one answer. I will go into this more later in the chapter.

Half the Stuff Is Outdated

In medical school, a movement began to get first-year medical students more clinical exposure. Part of that was meeting with a preceptor once a week.

My first preceptor was a general surgeon at the university. I arrived early on the first day, his secretary (a proper title in those days) shepherded me to his private office, and I waited for him to arrive. He had stacks of medical journals on his desk and the floor, some stacks three to four feet high.

When he arrived, he saw me looking at the journals and said, "Half the stuff in those journals will be outdated in five years. There is no way to know which half, though, so you must read it all."

We practice medicine five to ten years behind the existing base of knowledge, which means we are mostly wrong with our recommendations. But practicing medicine behind the times is the least of our concerns. Other issues are more concerning.

Those who fund medical research use science to promote half-truths for financial gain. As stated earlier, pharmaceutical companies frequently control the research questions. Some research is designed to justify the use of more medication.[168]

Half-truth science is a means to influence physicians and control how they practice medicine. Under the guise of science, research is conducted to support an agenda or prove a desired version of the truth. Typically, it is motivated with financial gain in the background, not the patient's best interest.

We practice medicine five to ten years behind the existing base of knowledge, which means we are mostly wrong with our recommendations.

What Is Science?

Science is a progressive method to discover the truth. The truth does not need our participation to exist. It just does. It does not require us to find it; it still exists. Even if we choose not to believe the truth, it exists.

Science is our human exercise to find the truth, not create or invent it. But create and invent it, we do. Science has value only when the research behind it is honest and unbiased, and in medicine, we have established that is no longer always the case.

When we discuss the importance and the legitimacy of science, we make a couple of assumptions. We assume we are embarking on an honest attempt to find the truth. We also assume we get closer to the truth with time and each subsequent study. But neither of those is necessarily true.

Because science is a method to get to the truth, let's ask some questions. How do we know when we are halfway to discovering the truth, finding the truth, or determining when "science is settled"? How do we know that we have reached a point where we are not helping patients but, at least, not hurting them?

Science is an ever-evolving process of finding the truth. Until it gets to the truth, which we frequently have no way of knowing, it is partially wrong.

Sometimes, being 1 percent wrong has devastating consequences. We can write entire books on all the times science and medicine have been wrong. Schools continually update their science books because of new "science."

Contradictions in Medical Literature

Have you noticed that medical research frequently contradicts itself and flip-flops on issues? Why should that happen if science is so pure that many individuals believe it to be the holy grail?

We've all heard about a link between caffeine and breast cancer, and that taking one baby aspirin every day is good. Then again, we've also heard that there is no link between caffeine and breast cancer, and taking a daily baby aspirin is risky.

Did the truth change? No, it did not. The problem is not the truth. The problem is not even science. The problem is us. Our understanding limits our comprehension.

How can flawed people (all of us) find something unflawed (the truth) given our biases, greed, ulterior motives, lust for power and control, and lack of intelligence? We are not nearly as bright as we think we are.

How Smart Are We?

We perceive ourselves as being smart because we build on the knowledge of previous generations, but we do so without *acquiring* that knowledge for ourselves. We seem to think that because our ancestors learned something, we don't have to.

I doubt anyone reading this book can accurately calculate the Earth's circumference using a makeshift sundial like Eratosthenes (who died in 194 BC) did. I doubt anyone reading this can go up and down the East Coast of the United States in a sailboat and accurately map out the coastline.

We can be smart—and dumb—at the same time.

I doubt any of us can construct buildings and roads that last two or three millennia like our ancestors. Our country is only 250 years old, and its infrastructure is falling apart in front of our very eyes. Some of that is planned obsolescence, as quality no longer matters in our country, but some stems from a lack of knowledge.

Our ancestors sailed to this country using stars and the sun as navigation guides. We get lost while using our car's GPS. There was a time we taught Latin in high school. We now teach remedial English in college.

Here is how smart and dumb we are. We put a man on the moon in 1969, but the United States Patent Office did not grant a patent for wheels on a suitcase until 1972.[169] That seems backward. Sometimes, we cannot see a need for something so obvious, and that applies to medicine too. People benefit every day from the wheels on a suitcase. Or how many years did we carry heavy trash cans down the driveway to the curb? We were smart enough to put handles on the cans but not smart enough to put wheels on them until recently. Going to the moon undoubtedly led to many discoveries and advancements, but it is hard to notice them in our everyday lives.

We overlook the simple for the complex. We tend to believe things are more complicated than they are, and consequently, we make them more complex than they are. A few simple habits will take care of most of your health needs—that's simple.

NASA completed 20 Mercury, Gemini, and Apollo missions before attempting to land a man on the moon. We barely tested COVID-19 vaccines before we embarked on the most consequential human experiment in history by vaccinating millions having little safety and efficacy data using a vaccine platform never used before.

Is that science? Is it ethical?

Yet, physicians, who supposedly embrace science, approved this mass vaccination program. Do you know why? They fell for half-truths and succumbed to fear, including fear for their own lives, evidenced by a good number of physicians shutting down their practices without adequate patient notification, leaving many patients in a lurch. They trusted the medical establishment and dutifully followed what they were told.

Is that science? Is it even common sense?

Trust in Leadership

We are supposed to trust those making these decisions without questioning them. During COVID-19, it was not permissible to disagree with Dr. Fauci. Though he became the face of the pandemic, I wonder how many of his decisions were his alone. Can someone as intelligent as him unintentionally make so many "wrong mistakes," as Yogi Berra might say?

COVID-19 was not Dr. Fauci's first rodeo. He reminded us of that and stated that he worked on HIV, Zika, Ebola, SARS, H1N1, and MERS. Two weeks to flatten the curve did not work. He was way off on projected COVID-19 deaths, and he kept changing the percentage needed for herd immunity and the duration of lockdowns. Eventually, he admitted the masking and six-foot distancing recommendations were not based on science. He hinged the success of COVID-19 management on vaccines using a new platform, even though he stated in May 2020 that there was no guarantee the vaccines would be effective. That is a lot of "wrong mistakes" made in less than a year.[170]

But he can wash his hands because he "followed the science," or at least one version of it, even though the version he followed was disastrous. Perhaps science bamboozled, duped, and hoodwinked him too. Why should "leaders" be immune to being fooled? Possibly, there were other reasons, but only he knows why he followed that "science."

Recall Albert Einstein's words: Blind belief in authority is the greatest enemy of truth.

Determining Intelligence

We are not that smart. We are certainly not nearly as intelligent as we believe. We are, however, arrogant, especially within the medical establishment.

It takes humility to recognize you don't know enough or that your understanding is lacking. It takes a certain amount of intelligence to know which questions to ask to get the correct answer or truth. It takes humility, integrity, and discipline to pursue the truth, rather than your handler's agenda.

If we were to take away computers and the internet, our stupidity would become much more apparent. Cashiers don't know how much change to return if someone gives them a $20 bill. It is no wonder some are easily bamboozled, duped, and hoodwinked.

I have two litmus tests to gauge how smart someone is without asking any questions.

- Do they ask good questions?
- Are they witty?

It takes a specific font of knowledge, interest, and curiosity for someone to formulate good questions that center around "why" that uncover the core of an issue. Anybody can look up answers using the internet. Giving answers tells little of someone's intelligence. The great differentiator is the quality of questions they ask.

Judge a man by his questions rather than by his answers.
—Voltaire

I know physicians who can quote medical literature forward, backward, upside down, downside up, and even inside out. They know all the information. They even know the dates studies were published and the names of the researchers.

But they do not take the time to question its validity. They never ask, "How true is this? Is this believable?" They assume that because it was published, it must be valid, which you now know is not necessarily true. They don't ask enough questions. Questions are the key to getting the answers.

The cardinal mistake most people make, especially physicians, is to believe that if something is published, it must be valid. Remember that journals stay in business by publishing articles. And to stay in business, they must regularly publish X amount of content regardless of quality or validity.

Here's an intriguing thought: Maybe it's the research not submitted for publication due to negative results that more closely approximates the truth than that which is published. But rarely do we learn from those studies.

I am not sure academia's "publish or perish" mentality is healthy, as it potentially leads to doing research with no meaningful purpose behind it. It also leads to the temptation of producing fake research to meet publication requirements. There is far more fake research than we know.[171] We would be better off with fewer but rigorously and honestly conducted studies.

When you look at all the evidence provided so far, you might conclude that the field of science provides a means and opportunity for "researchers" to report what they wish were true, for whatever reason they want to, and not what is true. Some of what is published is sophisticated storytelling cloaked in science.

Not-So-Wacko Jacko Rule of Medicine:

If medical research is tainted, then the authenticity of medicine as a profession is questionable.

The foundation of medicine should be based on solid, truthful information. If that does not happen, then the authenticity of the entire profession is questionable. If medical research is bogus, then the profession becomes a farce.

My second way of ascertaining someone's intelligence is: Are they witty? One can be intelligent without being witty, but one cannot be witty without being intelligent.

Witty people are ingeniously creative and clever in a good way. They see through political correctness and view things as they are. They see humor in our stupidity. They know they don't know enough. They see through the BS and are not as easily bamboozled, duped, or hoodwinked by half-truths. They are critical and independent thinkers who see things differently than the conditioned masses. Witty people do not unquestioningly believe what they are told.

Science as God

Some scoff at those who believe in God, believing that such people are intellectually inferior and feeble-minded. Everyone seems to have a god, someone or something in which one places faith and trust and looks for meaning and guidance.

For some, that god is themselves. They possess *all* the necessary answers in their human brain, even though many of them have imperfect SAT or ACT scores. For some, science has become the god they don't think they need. They don't think they need God, yet they create one, unknowingly, out of science to explain life. Thus, science becomes their god, forming the center of a secular pseudo-religion, as Zuby alluded.

Some do not realize the science they follow is misrepresented and, in some cases, fake, which makes their god a false and most deceptive god. Yet, they perceive themselves as "enlightened" because they believe and "follow science."

Science is useful but has shortcomings. Frequently, it serves as a good starting point and guide. It cannot, however, explain two of man's most fundamental questions: "Why am

I here?" and "What is my purpose?" If science fails to answer those two questions, it will likely fall short on others too. If you believe in evolution, evolution may tell you *how* you got here but not *why*. And the why is far more important than the how.

Plus, as stated earlier, science is conducted by flawed people, which leads to flawed results. In most cases, the best science can do is approximate the truth. Something tells me the speed of light is not precisely 186,000 miles per second, but it is probably close enough to satisfy mere human comprehension.

Science in the Bible

Some consider the Bible a collection of mythology. Though certainly not a science book, there are two critical points to make about the Bible and science.

One, the science the Bible does address predates modern scientific acceptance, sometimes by centuries. Leviticus discusses the need for quarantining or isolating those with contagious disease. The circulatory system was not described by Harvey until the seventeenth century, while Leviticus 17:11 discussed the importance of blood long before this. It was not until the mid-1800s that hand washing prior to surgery became procedure, though Deuteronomy 23:12-13 discussed the need for sanitation and hygiene much earlier.

Thus, we can say science tends to move slowly, frequently slower than we have time to wait.

Secondly, and perhaps more significantly, the Bible does not include the science of its day that subsequently was proven wrong. Think about this carefully. If the Bible includes science of its day that is wrong, could it be trusted to represent the Word of God?

For instance, Ptolemy reported 1,022 stars in the sky in the second century AD, but Hebrews 11:12 and Jeremiah 33:12 discuss the stars as numerous as grains of sand on the beach long before Ptolemy. At that time, man could not know that there were more stars than could be counted with the naked eye; the first telescope was not invented until 1608.

How Much Should We Trust Science?

We all need to be careful with how much we fall in love with science, especially when it's conducted with impure intentions. We should view drug studies with the most skepticism, especially those that are industry-generated or industry-funded. Such studies are masterfully manipulated.

The phrase "the science has changed" is a bit of a misnomer. What has changed is our understanding. And if our knowledge is changing, then the outcome of science is always tenuous.

During the pandemic's peak, it was not unusual for me to go to my office and see an email from our medical director relaying the latest guidance on COVID-19. Then, at noon, there would be another email saying, "Forget the earlier email; the science has changed." No, more accurately, it was our understanding that changed. Science is only as good as our understanding; thus, it is limited by our understanding. And again, we are not as smart as we think.

The Olympic Fever

Consider our lack of understanding the weakness of "following the science." We have gone from locking down society to distancing, masking, and canceling sports, including postponing the Summer Olympics. Now, we allow athletes to participate in the Olympics with COVID-19 and a 102°F fever (Noah Lyles in 2024). What a dramatic turnaround in thought. Was our understanding wrong then, or is it wrong now? Was science wrong then or wrong now? One thing is for sure: the truth did not change; our perception did.

Not-So-Wacko Jacko Rule of Medicine:

Science changes, but truth does not.

We can only design studies to get to the truth based on our limited current knowledge. Because we are not as smart as we think, science is always wrong until it gets it right.

Science Can Take Us Backward

Science in medicine does not always propel us closer to the truth. Sometimes it takes us backward or further from the truth. When that happens, science does more harm than good. Bad science can stifle progress and take us down a pathway that leads to a dead end and even death.

Let me share a few examples related to my practice illustrating how science took medicine backward.

In 1942, Premarin (conjugated estrogens) became commercially available, and since then, it has been common to treat women with it for postmenopausal symptoms. Fifty years later, Premarin had become the number-one-selling drug in the United States, an impressive feat when you consider its use is limited to women only.[172]

But such hormonal replacement or treatment for men who suffer from the male counterpart called andropause was considered taboo and dangerous.

Why? Because of science.

In 1941, Huggins and Hodges treated three males suffering from prostate cancer with testosterone and used a new and what turned out to be an unreliable test to monitor the response. The disease in one patient worsened based on this test. One patient did fine, and the third was lost in the follow-up.

Based on a single patient arose the belief that testosterone feeds prostate cancer. Eventually, that belief was interpreted as testosterone causes prostate cancer. This interpretation makes little sense because prostate cancer rarely occurs in the segment of the male population with the highest testosterone levels—teenagers and males in their twenties.

In 1981, a more extensive study from Memorial Sloan Kettering involving fifty-two men came up with similar conclusions—that testosterone can worsen prostate cancer. However, both studies suffered from a knowledge gap that would not be filled till years later.

During the intervening forty years, studies that showed that men with prostate cancer did better clinically when given testosterone, but, for some reason, those studies did not change the perception that testosterone fed prostate cancer.

Largely based on the work of Abraham Morgentaler, MD, a Harvard urologist at the time, the connection between testosterone and prostate cancer was finally debunked. Dr. Morgentaler chronicled his journey debunking this pervasive idea in *Testosterone for Life* (which I believe all men should read) and in his article, "Testosterone and Prostate Cancer: An Historical Perspective on a Modern Myth," published in the European Association of Urology, July 27, 2006.

His journey is complicated but suffice it to say that we no longer believe that testosterone causes prostate cancer. However, it was not until 2006 or so that the mindset began to gain traction. Thus, for six decades, men were not readily afforded a similar treatment provided to women.

Science had let men down.

> As a quick aside:
>
> Premarin comes from **pre**gnant **mar**e ur**in**e. Now, consider that the FDA discouraged (which is not its role) people and physicians from using ivermectin, the horse dewormer, for treating COVID-19.
>
> Yet, that same agency approved the use of horse estrogens from horse urine for women. It seems somewhat contradictory. Whenever people or organizations flip-flop their positions, many times, it is because they have an ulterior motive.
>
> I will go into this Premarin/ivermectin example again in the chapter, "The Pharmaceutical Funded FDA." The chemical structure of some horse estrogens differs from those of women. So why do we give horse estrogens to women? Money.

Hydration vs. No Hydration

For decades, the athletic and medical communities did not think athletes should hydrate or replace fluids during practice or competition, that doing so might make them cramp up or waterlog them. Many football players and other athletes succumbed to varying degrees of heat illness during these "dark ages." It was not until the 1970s that fluid replacement was put into practice with any regularity.[173]

I did a medical rotation with Robert J. Murphy, MD, the head team physician for Ohio State's football team. He practiced during this transition from no water to water and told of giving players tablespoonfuls to see how they would react, gradually increasing the "dose."

Dr. Murphy was one of the early physicians to recognize the need for water replacement and promote its use.[174] What clued Dr. Murphy in on the need for fluids is that he noticed his patients who were farmers rarely developed heat illness despite hours working in the hot summer sun, yet many of the football players (younger and healthier than farmers) succumbed to the heat. He asked the farmers about that, and they told him they carried water coolers on their tractors in the fields and drank it liberally. Farmers, based on experience, knew what experts needed and wanted science to verify.

These days, we take the need for fluids for granted. Medicine and sports did not always recognize that need, but now, college football teams go through several hundred gallons of water in practice. (Today, sports drinks may replace water, but in the old days, it was water from a hose.) When you go from zero to several hundred gallons, your original thinking is way off. But that is medicine.

Common sense dictates that if you are losing fluid, you should replace it. One should not need science to reach that conclusion.

Science vs. Common Sense

We seem to want science to verify everything before we make decisions. We probably would be far better off if we "led with common sense," unless and until legitimate science provides legitimate results. However, that approach takes common sense, and many would want science to verify that approach with a randomized, double-blind, placebo-controlled study before deciding to lead with common sense. We would find ourselves trapped in a circular argument.

Not-So-Wacko Jacko Rule:

Science doesn't happen overnight, but common sense does.[IP]

This Not-So-Wacko Jacko Rule is common sense. Waiting for science to catch up to common sense seems unwise. Employing common sense until science catches up would be a more common-sense approach.

In the middle of a pandemic, common sense says we should repurpose drugs already determined to be safe by the FDA *decades ago,* like ivermectin and hydroxychloroquine, while awaiting the development of monoclonal antibodies, antivirals, and vaccines, which then must be tested for safety and effectiveness. When the death rate is low from an infectious disease, common sense says maybe we should only vaccinate high-risk patients.

Farmers and athletes have one thing in common: They employ common sense and keep things simple, and built within that simplicity is wisdom, which is more valuable and useful than science. Part of wisdom is the ability to make sound decisions in the absence of information or the presence of conflicting information.

To Exercise or Not Exercise If over 40

Here is one last example of conventional medicine where the wisdom attached to it is off course. After my medical training, my first position was at the Cooper Clinic and Aerobics Center in Dallas, Texas, founded by Ken Cooper, MD, PhD.

Dr. Cooper is world-renowned. In 1968, he wrote *Aerobics,* a book that discussed the health benefits of cardiovascular exercise. Actually, he coined the word *aerobics.* He is the person most responsible for the global fitness movement.

Aerobics was based on thirteen years of research while a flight surgeon for the US Army and US Air Force. He was the director of the Aerospace Medical Laboratory and developed the early exercise programs for NASA and its astronauts.

Dr. Cooper felt that exercise could be used to prevent and treat many chronic medical conditions and believed people of all ages could safely exercise if adequately screened and monitored.

In 1970, he left the Air Force to open a preventive health clinic in north Dallas. In the process, he pioneered the executive health examination and started to build the world's largest database on the health benefits of exercise, benefits that no group of medications can match.

But he faced a significant problem: The medical establishment did not believe in the concept of preventive medicine, and some doctors felt it was dangerous for individuals over forty to exercise, despite writings dating back to Hippocrates that physical activity is beneficial.

Dr. Cooper found himself in front of the Dallas Board of Censures, which considered revoking his medical license because he was conducting treadmill tests on people with heart disease, an uncommon practice at that time. Fortunately, Dr. Cooper had the data showing the benefits of these tests, and the board decided against revocation.

Nowadays, we take for granted that exercise is beneficial, but Dr. Cooper's struggles show how backward and out-of-touch medicine can be. We get mired in stale and traditional thoughts.

Medicine Is Often Wrong

These are just three examples of cases when medicine has been wrong. The need for exercise and fluids seems so basic and commonsensical that one should not need science to verify it. Prevailing thought and conventional wisdom in medicine is sometimes wrong; when it is wrong, it is frequently 180° off from being right.

Not-So-Wacko Jacko Rule of Medicine:

Science is always at least partially wrong until it gets it right, which may never be.

Complicated Science Complicates

We tend to make things more complicated than necessary. Take exercise. We talk about time, duration, and frequency of exercise as well as muscle confusion and developing muscle endurance, strength, and power. We talk about supersets. We talk about Zone 2 Training up to Zone 5 Training. All of that is good for the competitive athlete or the motivated weekend warrior.

If we liken the body to a machine, it is the only machine that breaks down faster from lack of use.

But for the average person, if I had to distill exercise to one simple concept, I would say "Do Not Sit." Not sitting does not imply standing only. It implies moving as much as possible.

Consider Newton's First Law of Motion: a body (object) in motion tends to stay in motion unless an external force acts upon it. If we liken the body to a machine, it is the only machine that breaks down faster from lack of use. Sitting is that external force that stops a body in motion.

And if you want something a little more advanced concerning exercise, "Lift until your muscles really burn, then do two or three more reps." That is more than forty years of training, practice, and expense distilled into a few sentences.

We sit far more than we do anything else these days. Try not sitting for an entire day except for eating and going to the bathroom. I bet you cannot do it. And if you can do it, you are most likely highly fit and healthy.

It's easy to lose the forest for the trees with science. Remember the people living in Blue Zones. They intuitively and indirectly apply and simplify science through living day-to-day life. If you want to stay active, be active. If you want to learn to hit a baseball, swing a bat. The point is we can often achieve the results of science indirectly and without strictly applying the science. I hope that makes (common) sense.

Keeping Things Simple

When I practiced in Dallas, I worked with the Dallas Independent School District (DISD) athletes. We four doctors cared for 22 high schools. I would cover two or three football games a week. (You can read about my experience with DISD on JackoMD180.com.)

I saw some of the country's best high school football and athletes. One school, David W. Carter High School, was the topic of three movies and documentaries, including *Friday Night Lights, Carter High,* and *What Carter Lost.* The school was a factory for producing college-caliber football players.

As a medical staff, we decided to verify any association between fitness and conditioning to injury patterns that we were seeing in the football players across the entire district.

We modified much of the NFL Combine Testing for high school athletes. In one day, we measured 1,500 athletes for bench press reps, squat reps, vertical jump, shuttle run (electronically timed), 40-yard time (electronically timed), 800-yard run, grip strength, various flexibility measurements, body fat, and a few other things.

As we designed our testing and study, we called strength and conditioning coaches at some of the major college football programs for any input they might share.

Having attended medical school at Ohio State, oops, *The* Ohio State University College of Medicine, I tried to call its strength and conditioning coach and struck out. So, I called the strength and conditioning coach at the University of Michigan, also known as "That Team Up North," to OSU fans. Though I don't remember the strength coach's name, I remember the conversation practically verbatim. I explained what we were doing with the study and that we were getting input from strength and conditioning coaches. He told me

> I don't put a lot of stock in some of those tests. Here, at the University of Michigan, we only care about three things. A true height. A true weight. And a true 40-yard time. That means electronically timed because we know how to interpret those. Other than that, if a kid looks like hell on film, that's all we need to know.

Basically, he was saying that a kid is either a football player or not, regardless of his vertical jump, bench press, squat, or even body fat. It doesn't matter how high one can jump if he is afraid to get hit.

He kept things simple. He did not lose sight of what truly matters. He did not get distracted.

He was looking at what we wanted to do from a performance standpoint. We were looking at it from an injury perspective, but I found his comments intriguing and insightful. You can learn something from everyone, even your rival.

Not-So-Wacko Jacko Rule of Medicine (and Sports):

We test what we can measure, and we think it is relevant because we can measure it. That is not always true.

That is what the strength coach at the University of Michigan intuitively understood.

Some of the "greatest of all time" athletes, including Tom Brady and Wayne Gretzky, tested poorly at their league's Combine.

There is more to treating and preventing heart disease than controlling blood pressure and cholesterol. Those are easy to measure and they are important, but their importance may be overstated. More on that in "You Are Not Likely to Die of Anything But Will Die from Something." Medicine has still not identified all relevant risk factors for most diseases; we just think we have.

Modern Medicine Kills a Lot of People

Doctors and hospitals have been the third leading cause of death until COVID came around.[175] Now, doctors and hospitals are only the fourth leading cause of death, but not because we've gotten better. It took a new disease to supplant us. Some of those deaths are related to our treatments, which are not as safe as science suggests, including "safe and effective" FDA-approved medications.

Below is a partial list, by brand names, of drugs taken off the market that the FDA originally approved.[176] Earlier, I explained how the FDA and medical journals make decisions based on the information the pharmaceutical companies provide. Editors don't control what information they receive. The FDA likely did receive and review all the information pharmaceutical companies had on this list of medications. However, it is likely that the pharmaceutical companies kept the FDA in the dark.

Baycol	Hismanal	Pondimin	Rezulin
Belviq	Lotronex	Posicor	Selacryn
Bextra	Meridia	Propulsid	Seldane
Cylert	Merital and Alival	PTZ and Metrazol	Trasylol
Darvon (Darovcet)	Micturin	Quaalude	Vioxx
DBI (phenformin)	Mylotarg	Raplon	Xigris
DES	Omniflox	Raptiva	Zantac (ranitidine)
Duract	Palladone	Raxar	Zelmid
Ergamisol	Permax	Redux	Zelnorm

The history of medicine is quite fascinating. Our predecessors did some unusual things, and they did some innovative things. They have done some brutal things, and some of what we do today, future generations will consider barbaric.

Some of our medical treatments, like lobotomies, have been inhumane. There was a time when we treated female maladies with a hysterectomy. Chemotherapy and radiation therapy, the mainstays along with surgery of today's cancer treatments, are severe when you think about it. We kill normal cells in the process of killing cancer cells; such treatments can have significant and toxic lingering effects.

Is Medicine a Pure Science?

Not-So-Wacko Jacko Rule of Medicine:

Medicine is not the pure science we are making it to be. There is a reason it is called the "practice of medicine." Science does not address human interaction, while medicine is based on it.

One of our fundamental mistakes in medicine is attempting to turn it into a pure science. It is not. It is part science and part art. And it is a lot of trial and error, or practice.

There is a reason we call it the "practice of medicine." Science can tell you how well a drug works (if it is honest science), but it cannot tell you if it will work in an individual patient.

Valuable knowledge comes from science but loses clinical usefulness when applied to the individual patient. Numbers like 83 percent or 14 percent have little meaning. When treating a particular patient, it is either all or none. A procedure or medication may have a 2 percent chance of death but, in any given patient, the patient is either going to die (100 percent) or not die (0 percent) from the intervention.

We have eight billion people on this planet, each with a different physiology. Math and physics are sciences where one correct answer exists. Medicine, frequently, has more than one answer. Medicine is eight billion shades of gray, which makes taking results from a population-based study and applying those results to the individual patient challenging.

Science loses some of its inertia when the rubber hits the pavement. In the end, what matters is what works for the patient. That sometimes means "experimenting" with the individual. We may find that an uncomfortable thought, but when we perform a study on three thousand patients, are we not performing three thousand individual experiments at a time and compiling them into one study to obtain a composite patient profile that few in the real world will match?

When a study shows that an intervention tested on three thousand patients was effective, it does not mean that all three thousand patients responded positively. When a study on three thousand patients shows an intervention did not work, it does not mean that all three thousand patients did not respond. Some likely did, possibly even a significant number, but not enough to satisfy "statistical significance."

We want studies on three thousand patients but forget that we can see what works in the patient in front of us by using them as their own test and control.

The Power of the N of 1

The patient can serve as an N of 1. That is, they can serve as their own test and control. The information you get from that approach is far more valuable because it pertains to the individual. In that case, you're practicing personalized medicine, which is the goal, is it not? Biohackers use this approach. They "experiment" on themselves.

Not-So-Wacko Jacko Rule of Medicine:

Data on an individual is more valuable than the results of a study of a few thousand.

Essentially, you get a baseline on a patient, try an intervention, and see if it works. If it doesn't, you try something else. It may not sound scientific, but how else do you know what will work on an individual? A study on three thousand patients does not tell you what will work for the individual before you.

Two apples a day can lower cholesterol by up to 23 percent, which is on par with some statins.[177] Let's imagine what could happen if you went to a doctor who feels you need to be on a statin to lower your cholesterol, and you mention that you want to try apples. That doctor may say, "Well, apples are not FDA-approved for lowering cholesterol. So, I still want you on a statin."

You then ask, "Is it true that statins can cause muscle aches and fatigue and be hard on the liver?"

And your doctor responds, "Yes, those can be frequent side effects, but at least we know what they are. We don't know what the long-term consequences of eating two apples a day might be, so I want you on a statin."

You say, "Well, apples have been around since the beginning of time."

Your doctor says, "Maybe so, but we still do not know any long-term consequences of eating two apples a day, so I still want you on a statin."

You ask, "Well, can I at least try the apples and have my cholesterol levels and liver tests monitored, and maybe even my coenzyme Q10 level, because I read statins lower it and cause muscle aches and fatigue?"

Your doctor says, "Well, now you are just being difficult. You should not do your own research. The guidelines call for a statin, not two apples a day. I want you on a statin, or you are free to find another doctor."

I meant to be humorous, but it is not far from the truth. Many patients can identify with such a scenario. It seems foolish, but that is how many physicians practice medicine these days. Doctors find more comfort in following guidelines and data from a study of three thousand patients than in data they obtain directly from an individual. They feel more comfortable prescribing medication right out of the gate rather than trying something simpler and more natural.

I would say, "Sure, try the apples. I am curious to see how well that works. Come back in a month." (Studies show that Brazil nuts can lower cholesterol quite well too.[178])

Vinegar has been shown to improve blood sugar and lipid control,[179] but you rarely see a doctor try it before reaching for the prescription pad. No Bragg's Apple Cider Vinegar sales reps visit doctors' offices, bringing in lunches.

I can monitor my patients more closely than a principal investigator involved in a drug study can. I consider this individualized approach to patient care superior to strictly relying on medical studies to guide care, particularly since we cannot trust science to provide valid results.

Here is another Not-So-Wacko Jacko Rule of Medicine:

We test what we can measure, and because we can measure it, we think it is relevant. That is not always true.

We measure blood pressure, in part, because it is easy to measure. But how important is it? And how important is treating it?

To prevent one cardiovascular event, 86 to 140 patients must take blood pressure medicine for five years, which raises the question about the validity of measuring blood pressure, especially at rest.[180]

To be transparent, I treat patients with elevated blood pressure. However, I wonder whether doing so matters in many of them, especially those with mild elevations and no other risk factors. It likely matters in a few but not the majority.

Why Are We Turning Medicine Into a Pure Science?

If medicine is a combination of science and art, why are we trying to make it a pure science? The short answer is that the results of science can be manipulated to control the narrative.

Medicine as an art gives too much control to the "artist," and the powers in medicine likely do not want to allow for too much "artistic leeway."

But there are other reasons. Some physicians like having a single right way of treating a condition. It removes thinking from the equation.

Once we have guidelines, we no longer need physicians.

We have developed a strong aversion to thinking, which is hard work, and we shy away from hard work these days. Steve Jobs supposedly spent three hours a day just thinking about the next game-changing product. At one point, Apple's slogan was "Think Different". Perhaps we should simplify it to "Think!"

Here is the thing about guidelines: Anyone who can read can follow them. Once we have guidelines, we no longer need physicians. Lesser-trained professionals can implement the guidelines. That frees up more money for those who employ medical professionals, which are large hospital systems nowadays.

From 1975 to 2010, the number of physicians in the US increased by 150 percent, keeping up with population growth. During those thirty-five years, the number of healthcare administrators grew 3,200 percent. Why do we need so many? Do you think all these administrators improve the quality of care or outcomes?

How can the system support and feed them? The pot contains only so much money.

Here's how: Change the system to allow for more "less expensive" mid-level providers and reduce the number of "expensive" doctors that hospitals employ. Implement guidelines so that mid-level providers don't have to think. Their decisions are all pre-determined by clinical practice guidelines. That is where medicine is headed.

I suspect the push to use and strictly enforce clinical guidelines is to eventually reduce or eliminate doctors, particularly in the primary care fields. That will become easier with emerging AI. One way or another, some doctors are going to be replaced, but most haven't realized it yet.

Strictly following guidelines can cause adverse effects. Frequently, clinical practice guidelines presuppose a routine problem is being dealt with, but that can only be determined after the fact. To some degree, strict following of practice guidelines is like "teaching to the mean" and ignoring the outliers.

Why Do You See a Doctor?

This seems like a silly question. But why see a doctor rather than another health professional? That is a more complex question to answer than it appears. The main reason you see a doctor, whether you realize it or not, is in case your routine problem is not as routine as you thought. You want to see someone with more training to avoid misdiagnosis.

Most pregnant women prefer to see an OB-GYN as opposed to a midwife. Why? At some level, the patients realize that they may not have a straightforward pregnancy or delivery. Many women would prefer someone to deliver their child who can manage any complications that may arise.

Clinical guidelines do not address the 10–20 percent of patients who do not have straightforward problems. A system that relies on mid-level providers will mismanage some of those outliers.

Clinical guidelines will address 80–90 percent of patient problems. Is that good enough? When I was in school, 80 percent was B-minus work. Most patients want a minimum of a 95 percent success rate and probably closer to 99 percent.

So, in my opinion, one key to being a good doctor is knowing when *not* to follow clinical guidelines, if a doctor's employer will allow them.

Medicine as an Art

The art of medicine and the art of life center around one act: the act of valuing people. On the JackoMD180.com site is the article "Valuing People: The Art of Medicine and Life." It is a story of my first encounter with Dr. Hughston during my sports medicine fellowship interview.

When I was just a tyke, my pediatrician's office was in the Southgate Medical Arts Building across the street from the Southgate Shopping Center near Cleveland, Ohio. The Southgate Shopping Center was one of the nation's first large shopping centers.

Our family moved to Solon, Ohio, when I was six, but I still went yearly to the Southgate Medical Arts Building to see the pediatrician to get whatever vaccine was recommended.

Science does not address human interaction. Much medicine is based on human interaction. Human interaction is an art.

As a teenager, I started to see a primary care doctor at the Solon Medical Arts Building. Then, I needed braces for my teeth, and I saw an orthodontist at the Solon Professional Arts Building.

I broke my tibia at fourteen and herniated a lumbar disk two months before turning sixteen. Both required surgeries, so I saw an orthopedist at a building simply called The Medical Arts Building.

Do you detect a theme? We no longer see the word "arts" on any medical office building. What happened to medicine being an art? The word has been "artfully" eliminated from medical lexicon. Have you wondered why? (Nor do we see charity hospitals anymore because charity, apparently, is demeaning.)

My answer would be that medicine, as a science, is more easily controlled and manipulated. As an art, medicine gives too much control to the "artist," and the powers in medicine likely do not want to allow for much "artistic leeway."

Any career that deals with people is an art. Teaching is an art. Practicing law is an art. Math is a science. Physics is a science. Medicine is a hybrid. It is both a science and an art. If I had to put percentages on it, medicine is 70 percent science and 30 percent art, maybe even 60/40.

We no longer see the word "arts" on any medical office building. What happened to medicine being an art? The word has been "artfully" eliminated from medical lexicon.

This push to make medicine a pure science is not healthy because the science is not pure. Additionally, you are dealing with people, and people are unpredictable. You can raise two kids the same way, and they will become entirely different adults. When dealing with people, we must treat them individually. So it is in medicine, but that is not happening.

Physicians rely on the patient for information, and that information may be incomplete, misrepresented, wrong, and sometimes, intentionally wrong.

As a physician seeing a patient, the first thing to determine is why the patient came to the office. Some patients have hidden agendas and are not always truthful. Other times, you must peel back a few layers of onion to discover the genuine concern.

Nowadays, we lump every patient into the same clinical practice guidelines regardless of individual circumstances and then seem perplexed when they don't achieve the expected outcome.

Doctor-Patient Relationships

Taking the art out of medicine has weakened the doctor-patient relationship, the cornerstone of nearly everything in medicine.

The art of medicine, in my opinion, centers around making the doctor-patient relationship a partnership rather than the paternalistic model commonly employed today. I never understood the benefit of that approach.

Practicing medicine well is very much an art. We overrate the value of science in a profession predicated on human interaction.

We want to force treatments on patients directed by guidelines. However, it is the patient's health, and the patient has a right to say how they are treated, regardless of the guidelines. That does not mean a physician should simply do what the patients want, but the patient's desire should be considered.

The stronger the doctor-patient relationship is, and the more the patient trusts the doctor, the better the outcome will likely be. The placebo effect in medicine *is* real, and patients are more likely to get better if they trust their doctor.

Documenting in an electronic health record (EHR) is time-consuming. To be efficient, physicians will commonly use a computer in the exam room, which takes away from the encounter between physician and patient.

Over the years, I have learned that if I talk to a new patient long enough and go beyond their medical problem, I typically discover that we share an interest or know someone in common. I try to talk to a patient long enough on that first visit to find that commonality. Then, I can build the doctor-patient relationship, in part, off that common feature.

Personalized Medicine Through Guidelines?

What I find interesting and contradictory is the need to provide personalized patient care while using guidelines. How can we do that? Treating all patients the same way does not make sense to me.

David Sackett, MD, was a Canadian physician and a father of evidence-based medicine.[181] He found himself, many times, clarifying what he meant by evidence-based medicine.

He says evidence-based medicine is not

- cookbook medicine, which is what it has become;
- meant to supplant or override physician experience; and
- does not mean that the patient does not have a say in how they are treated.

It would seem obvious that a patient should have a say in their treatment, regardless of what the evidence might suggest. And a patient's experience should be treated as evidence because it is personal to them.

Art of Communication

Another big part of the art of medicine is communication. Much of that is simply listening, a difficult skill for most of us to master. Along with listening, maintaining direct eye contact is essential.

Listening and maintaining eye contact are more challenging during this era of electronic health records. Earlier, I mentioned physicians using a computer in the exam room to reduce the amount of time they spend documenting the office visit. By trying to kill two birds with one stone, they do not make eye contact and only half-listen.

Back when we used paper charts, I could see a patient, give them my undivided attention, scribble a few notes, and, after the office visit, dictate a thorough note in a minute or two, have it professionally transcribed, and the information was in the patient's chart the following day.

Many office notes from electronic health records look unprofessional these days and are unnecessarily lengthy, so finding the information you want is difficult.

I once saw a physician (as the patient) on the first day that office went live with an EHR system. This highly-regarded doctor barely came up for air to look at me. He spent nearly 90 percent of his time looking at the computer screen.

Another part of the art of medicine is going beyond the patient's medical problems. I probably spend more than 50 percent of the visit talking to the patient about topics other than their medical problem. Patients appreciate that.

I learned much about the art of medicine and the importance of patient education when I did my sports medicine fellowship at the Hughston Clinic in Columbus, Georgia. Patients need to be educated, which is a time-intensive exercise less doable in today's insurance-based healthcare model. Patient education was paramount. At the clinic, we took as much time as needed with the patient and went home when the waiting room was empty, regardless of the time. The Hughston Clinic website regularly posts articles on wellness to educate their patients and the public (www.hughston.com/wellness).

A Patient's View of the Art of Medicine

I also learned much about the art of medicine as a patient from my encounters with the orthopedist who operated on my fractured tibia and lumbar disk herniation. Karl Alfred, MD, is the primary reason I decided to study medicine. You were not schlepped into a cold and drab exam room when you saw Dr. Alfred. You were escorted to his private, carpeted office outfitted with wooden bookshelves. Two chairs, one for the patient and one for a family member, faced his desk.

When I saw him for my back, he took out a piece of paper and handwrote some notes. I had just turned sixteen but had been dealing with back and radiating leg symptoms for two months.

He looked at me and asked the necessary questions, occasionally glancing at my dad. He seemed genuine and caring. He did not seem rushed, though he had a waiting room full of patients who raved about him. He exuded confidence with humility.

From there, I entered the exam room off his private office and changed into a gown. After the examination, I dressed and returned to his private office. He explained that I had a herniated lumbar disk, relatively rare for my age, but something he saw occasionally. He discussed diagnostic and treatment options.

I asked some questions. So did my dad.

Then I had one *big* question for him. Baseball was my sport; it was June, the peak of baseball season. I asked whether I could still play baseball while I weighed my options. I thought he would say, "What? Are you crazy? No, you should not play."

Instead, his reply was one I often used with some of the high school athletes I would later treat.

He said, "Yes, you can play, but a day will come when you won't want to (because of the pain). And when that day comes, call me, and I will admit you to the hospital. We will do a myelogram (injection of dye into the spinal canal because this was before MRI and CT scanners) to confirm the diagnosis and then place you in traction."

Traction was the standard of care based on the science of the times. I can testify it does not work. The science was not entirely right. A few months later, I had the first of three lumbar spine surgeries spanning 48 years, but I have avoided having any hardware placed in my spine to date.

At the time of that office visit, whenever I bent over, pain shot down my leg, which would tingle and go numb. Coughing and sneezing would shoot electrical pain down my leg, and simply tilting my head to look down did as well. Somehow, I thought I could still play baseball.

The night following my visit with Dr. Alfred, I had a baseball game. I played, but not well. For an athlete, not being able to perform at their highest level is extremely frustrating. On the car ride home, I looked at my dad and said,

"That day has come. Can we call Dr. Alfred tomorrow and have him admit me to the hospital?’

What I respect about Dr. Alfred is his allowing me to make my own decisions. He treated me like an adult. He did not steer me one way or the other. He did not make me seem foolish for asking a question, even though he knew the eventual outcome. He allowed me to prove to myself that "that day had come."

His approach with me became my approach with my patients. Rarely do I tell patients they *have* to do something. I present options, answer questions, and let them make the best decision. I try to understand their goals and work with my patients to achieve them.

Years later, when I was early in my career, I ran into Dr. Alfred at a hospital event (he was retired). I thanked him for treating me, and for his influence on me going into medicine.

Technology is replacing the physical examination. I cannot tell you how many times I hear a patient who saw another doctor say, "They didn't even touch me."

We don't always know who we might influence. I try to keep that in the back of my mind when I encounter anyone, especially patients. That's part of the art of medicine—recognizing your potential influence on patients beyond their medical problems.

As we force medicine down this pure science path, the art of medicine is disappearing. Medicine is becoming less personable, which adversely affects care and outcomes. In addition, technology is replacing the physical examination. I cannot tell you how many times I hear a patient who saw another doctor say, "They didn't even touch me."

There are times, especially during a follow-up visit, when an exam is unnecessary, but I make a point to listen to their heart and lungs or examine another body part related to the problem for which they came in. Touch is important.

The generation of physicians before me had excellent clinical exam skills. They needed those skills because they did not have today's technology. It was amazing to watch them perform an exam. Many could make accurate diagnoses by feeling a patient's pulse, and they could tell you how big the liver or heart was by percussing them with a tap of a finger.

The Hughston Clinic owned two airplanes and would fly teams of doctors to provide medical coverage for college football games. The clinic simultaneously served as team physicians for Auburn University, the University of Alabama, the University of Kentucky, the University of Virginia, Valdosta State University, and Troy State. During my sports medicine fellowship, six days a month, we would fly to rural outposts in Alabama and Georgia to hold free clinics in gymnasiums or cafeterias at the community colleges.

Throngs of patients awaited our arrival. We had no technology to assist with making a diagnosis. We performed exams with our hands, eyes, ears, and ability to take a thorough history. It was a fantastic learning experience and made us better clinicians. Plus, I learned a little about flying from Bill and Stan, the pilots, but only enough to be dangerous.

Suffice it to say that the physical exam has also become a lost art—one that does not cost any money to perform and could save a lot of money by avoiding unnecessary diagnostic testing.

The art of medicine is far more critical than those who now run medicine may believe. Thinking we can rely on and need only science and technology is a half-truth, and it is a major half-truth.

Medicine and Sports

What is going on with medicine is going on elsewhere, like sports. Nowadays, you barely need to know much about some sports to coach one of them; just follow the analytics. But the analytics do not factor in that your two best offensive linemen are hurt, and you are facing the best defensive line in the league when they say, "Go for it on the fourth with less than a yard."

Analytics do not consider a fifteen-mile-an-hour cross-wind, and your placekicker has already missed an extra point and a field goal, and whose head is not in the best frame of mind when they say, "Kick a field goal on fourth and five from the 32-yard line."

Coaching is an art, too, as is practically everything else.

We do ourselves a disservice when we remove the *art* of doing anything. Despite clinical practice guidelines and analytics, you should *think* as a physician and treat patients respectfully by giving them the necessary time, attention, and understanding of their goals.

You Are Not Likely to Die of Anything but Will Die from Something

I guess it comes down to a simple choice, really.
Get busy living or get busy dying.
—Andy Dufresne in *The Shawshank Redemption*

The title of this chapter seems contradictory, but it will make sense by the end.

One thing we are good at in medicine is making you feel as if you are sick or have a problem that needs attention. We are good at making situations seem dire. Here is some good news.

You are not likely to die of heart disease, cancer, or Alzheimer's. You are not likely to die from a motor vehicle accident or be a victim of murder. You are not likely to die from diabetes or its complications.

Yet, you will die from something.

Despite the impression that medicine gives, even deaths from heart disease and cancer are relatively low. That is not to say we are a healthy population. We are not. How detrimental something is depends on how you look at the numbers.

Medicine is like the law in one respect. Legislators pass many laws because a small group of the population, say 1–2 percent, is engaged in a behavior that the remainder of society feels is detrimental or inappropriate.

But all of us (supposedly) must comply with the law. Interestingly, the people least likely to comply with such laws are those for whom the laws were intended, as well as those who write them. This should not surprise us. Liars lie, cheaters cheat, thieves thieve, and killers kill. All of them do what they desire despite the law.

Those of us in medicine have developed the mindset that everyone dies of everything every day. So, what do we do? We treat everyone for every condition. We blast you with a regimen of medications to prevent you from dying of everything, yet you will only die of one thing, and even so, only once.

We treat you for every chronic condition we can think of, but only a small percentage of those treated will benefit from the treatment. The number of patients to be treated for one person to benefit is called the number needed to treat (NNT) and is surprisingly high for many medications, much higher than you expect. I reviewed some of those numbers to treat in earlier chapters. The lower the number needed to treat, the more effective a drug is.

Many of you who are taking prescription medications for chronic conditions will not benefit from those medications. You have been bamboozled, duped, and hoodwinked into thinking those meds are making a difference.

We now have a grossly overmedicated society. We are the most medicated country on the planet. Yet, we are one of the sickest countries among industrialized nations despite our "healthy diet of drugs."[182]

Not only have we taken a shotgun to the individual with medications, but we have also taken a shotgun to society with medications.

Know the Odds

Much of practicing medicine is simply playing the odds. What is the most likely diagnosis for this patient? What are the odds of the patient improving without treatment? What are the odds of improvement with treatment? Do the risks of treatment outweigh the benefits? What are the odds that the worst thing that can happen from this treatment happens? And so on.

You need to know several things when weighing any medical intervention. You need to understand your tolerance for risk and uncertainty. You need to know how likely a bad event will happen if you leave your issue untreated. How common is this disease? What is the disease's incidence baseline? Reducing something with a 1 percent incidence by 50 percent is insignificant. You have taken something rare and made it slightly rarer, but at what cost to your overall health?

Natural Frequency

You need to know the natural frequency of the disease. Let's say four men out of a hundred over the age of fifty with standard blood sugar control will suffer a heart attack. But in men over fifty with diabetes, six men out of a hundred will suffer a heart attack. That's a 50 percent increase in heart attacks, which sounds dire. Yet, if you are a male of over 50 with diabetes, your risk goes up 2 percent, that is, from 4 percent to 6 percent. An additional 2 percent increase does not sound as bad as a 50 percent increase, though both numbers describe the same outcome.

The two additional heart attacks are called the natural frequency. The 50 percent figure is the relative risk increase due to diabetes; the 2 percent is the absolute risk increase. Pharmaceutical companies, doctors, and the media like to highlight the relative risk increase (from not intervening) or relative risk reduction (from intervening with a treatment).

Here is where a significant assumption is made, and one that is not necessarily true. We assume that if we treat blood sugar in men over 50, we will lower the risk of heart attacks from six to four. That seems logical. But there may be something about men with diabetes that does not lead to a reduction in heart attacks despite lowering blood sugar to normal levels. Factors we don't understand may make diabetic men less responsive to heart disease reduction despite normalizing their blood sugar.

One would have to study several diabetic men over 50 to know for sure. Such a study will show that sugar-lowering medication lowered their blood sugar, but that is not the study's primary goal. Lowering your blood sugar is not the reason you are taking the medication; your goal is to reduce heart attacks.

Before weighing the possible benefit of a treatment, you need to know the natural frequency if left untreated. However, finding that information is challenging.

Playing Poker and Tilting the Odds in Your Favor

Learning to play poker well is a good skill for those who want to become physicians. Physicians must know the odds in life and medicine. If I were on the medical school's admissions committee, I would inquire about an applicant's poker ability.

As a patient, you must understand your risk tolerance, as that weighs in on nearly every decision you make in life, not just medicine. Do you purchase an extended warranty on every product you buy? If so, you probably have a low risk tolerance and vice versa.

Despite our poor health as a nation, the odds are still in your favor as an individual because you exert much control over your health. On the contrary, you have no control over the general population's health, the people the study results are based on.

Also, many physicians look at medications for chronic problems as a lifelong process. Once they put you on one, you likely are not coming off it, and in fact, there may not even be an attempt to determine whether you still need to take it.

Being on any medication chronically is not a desirable position. Over time, it changes your biochemistry.

In many cases, you will have time to improve your health habits and reverse whatever medical problem you have, so you do not need to resort to medications on a long-term basis. If you work hard, getting off some of these chronically prescribed medications or at least reducing the doses is possible.

Frequently, I will start a patient on medication for a chronic condition with the goal of using it for a short period. I will treat a patient's blood pressure or blood sugar to get the numbers standardized while they work on changing their habits. Then, I reduce the dose of medication to wean the patient off it.

You *do* have control.

Fear

One thing we did not do with COVID-19 is heed President Franklin D. Roosevelt's words, "The only thing we have to fear is fear itself." Instead, we went into all-out panic mode.

Fear drives many decisions in life, and in medicine, that fear is driven by both physicians and patients. We tend to feed off each other's fear. You don't want to have a heart attack. and your physician does not want to have one either. Because we have something that might reduce that risk, we prescribe it, even though it may not be that beneficial.

Fear drives many decisions, period. People are easily manipulated through fear. The mainstream media makes a living fomenting fear, and many individuals rely on mainstream medicine for their health information in addition to their general news. Fear draws viewership, which draws ratings, which draws money. Fear is used to gain control and money.

The antidote to fear is knowledge and action, not medication. You must know the odds of what you are dealing with. If the odds are not in your favor, you must take action to tip the odds back in your favor. When it comes to your health, that means adopting healthier habits.

Life is nothing more than tipping the odds in your favor to achieve or obtain whatever you want. If you want to be an Olympic athlete or a concert pianist, you must devote a minimum of ten thousand hours of practice. Anything less than that and you will fall short. But just because you practice ten thousand hours does not mean you will achieve your goal; you only greatly improved your chances.

Figure out what you want, learn what it takes to get it, and then get busy going after it. Having a plan lessens fear. You need a personal wellness plan.

Many times, we fear the wrong things or have unfounded fears. Let's look at some real-life events and the low probability of them happening despite our fears.

- The probability of a plane crash is 0.000001, and the chance of dying in a plane crash is 1 in 816,545,929.[183]
- Getting hit by a meteorite is more likely at 1 in 700,000.[184]
- The odds of being struck by lightning in a given year are 1 in 1,222,000, with a 90 percent chance of survival.[185]
- The odds of dying by a shark attack in a year is 1 in 300,000,000 with a lifetime risk of 1 in 4,332,817.[186]

The odds of getting killed by sharks are nil if you don't go in the water, which highlights that, in some cases, you have complete control of the odds.

Despite whatever lousy genetics you may have inherited, genes are turned on and off by our health habits and, in some cases, environmental factors. Thus, you are not destined to experience the same health issues as your ancestors. Take the precautionary actions to tilt the odds in your favor and decrease your need for drugs.

Death from Shingles

Do you know how many people die from shingles every year in the US? Less than one hundred.[187] Your doctor doesn't want you to be one of those one hundred. One hundred out of nearly 335,000,000 (the US population) are good odds you will not die from shingles.

Yet, all medical organizations, health agencies, and most doctors recommend vaccinating everybody eligible with Shingrix (a shingles vaccine). Indiscriminately vaccinating everyone for shingles seems inappropriate to me, especially for those in good health.

According to the CDC, one in three Americans will get shingles in their lifetime. About 10–18 percent of those who develop shingles can also develop nerve pain. Based on my experience with my patients and everyone I know, I would say those numbers are lower. But let's stick with the CDC numbers.

First, one out of three Americans is over one's lifetime. So, about 111,600,000 Americans will get shingles in their lifetime, and less than one hundred will die each year from shingles. So, if you live to be eighty, eight thousand would have died of shingles in your lifetime. Those are still pretty good odds that you will not be one of them.

One might argue that deaths from shingles are low because of vaccination, but that is a half-truth. In 2018, according to the CDC, 34.5 percent of the population over age sixty (a high-risk group) were vaccinated for shingles.[188] If we assume that those one hundred deaths occur among the unvaccinated over 60, and if we assume the shingles vaccine is 100 percent effective, that means there would have been 135 deaths in those over 60 from shingles in the unvaccinated.

What Is Your Risk Tolerance?

Fear of dying or having residual nerve pain sells the vaccine. As a patient, you need to decide how much uncertainty or risk you are willing to accept, but you cannot do that if you don't know the numbers. We all have our risk tolerance. Your choice depends on how much risk you are willing to take.

If one-third of the population gets shingles and 10–18 percent get the worst complication (outside of death, which approaches zero) of nerve pain, then there is a 3–5 percent chance of getting nerve pain if not vaccinated. Those are still very good odds if you are not vaccinated and better odds if you are healthier than the average person. You need to decide whether the risk of vaccination is acceptable.

To do that, you need to know the treatment's downside. The risk of death and getting nerve pain must be counterbalanced by any adverse reactions that the vaccination might cause.

Look at the VAERS data (Vaccine Adverse Event Reporting System) during the first eight months of Shingrix post-marketing use. (The CDC and the FDA jointly manage VAERS.)

Of approximately 3.2 million doses of Shingrix given, 4,381 reported adverse reactions, which is low. The overall number of adverse reactions was small.

Yet, 3 percent of the adverse reactions were considered serious, and another 4.5 percent developed shingles after vaccination. Additionally, seven patients died within six hours to six weeks of receiving Shingrix.

The overall safety profile for the Shingrix vaccine is favorable, but what are you trying to prevent with it? The seven who died shortly after being vaccinated likely would not have died if they had not vaccinated even if they developed shingles.

Rather than relying on a vaccine for patients at average and below-average risk, perhaps we should provide more patient education on recognizing the early symptoms of shingles. Then, we couple it with prompt treatment to minimize death and nerve pain.

There is a downside to every treatment we can minimize with risk stratification, which I discuss later in this chapter.

COVID: Don't Go to the Hospital

Much less common, we scare people into not seeking treatment.

COVID-19 was unique because it may be the only time in modern medical history that we discouraged people from going to the hospital, whether they had COVID-19 or not.

During the pandemic's peak, patients were advised to avoid the emergency rooms, if possible, out of fear of contracting COVID-19 at the hospital. In the meantime, we did nothing outside of symptomatic care for those with COVID-19 and told them to stay home. Dr. Fauci and the medical establishment discouraged other alternative treatments for the disease, nor did any of our federal health agencies develop any outpatient treatment/prevention protocol for COVID-19 outside of masking, social distancing, and symptomatic treatment. That's irresponsible and shocking.

The Frontline COVID-19 Critical Care Alliance (FLCCC) had protocols for prevention of COVID-19 as well as treatment. Much of FLCCC's prevention protocols involved the use of over-the-counter vitamins and supplements, along with some prescription drugs. Vladimir Zelenko, MD, who managed several hundred patients in Upstate New York, had a similar protocol as did Peter McCullough, MD.

Out of my two thousand patients, only one died from COVID-19 (or, at least, COVID-19 contributed to his death). This patient happened to be high-risk (obese, diabetic, and hypertensive). He was unvaccinated.

I had three other patients hospitalized for COVID-19. Two were vaccinated and hospitalized for COVID-19. They happened to be sisters. They had a third sister (vaccinated) who was also hospitalized for COVID-19, which would seem to indicate that their genetic makeup was a factor in contracting the disease.

My third patient (mid to late thirties) was hospitalized for COVID-19 and was not vaccinated.

Peter Kory, MD, a critical care physician (and FLCCC member), said: "Dr. Fauci's suppression of early treatments will go down in history as having caused the death of half a million Americans in the ICU." And Peter McCullough, MD, stated the same.[189]

How significant are half a million deaths? A half million deaths are 435 times greater than the 1,150 deaths of victims from mass shootings over forty years. As I said earlier, a bad healthcare policy can potentially be more damaging than many other things.

Those preventable deaths occurred through May 2020, five months of the pandemic. More have died since then, many more.

Scaring patients by telling them not to go to the hospital made it difficult to treat patients for other medical conditions. Patients opted to have their strokes and heart attacks at home, and some of them now have complications due to delays in treatment or no treatment at all.

Was that advice warranted?

In October 2020, our medical group reported that six of our seventy-five hospitalists contracted COVID-19 between March 2020 and September 2020, during the first seven months following the lockdowns. Hospitalists care for patients while they are in the hospital. Hospitalists are exposed to lots of germs and diseases. Frequently, they managed patients in the intensive care units, including those who had COVID-19.

Six of seventy-five hospitalists may seem like a high number, but let's look at their hours of exposure in the hospital. Take a forty-hour work week, multiply it by seventy-five hospitalists, and again by 26 weeks for 78,000 man-hours of hospital exposure. Six cases in 78,000 man-hours equals 0.000077 cases per hour of hospital exposure. If we assume that a patient spent an entire day in the ER, that number goes to 0.0018 chance of getting COVID-19 for 24 hours of hospital exposure. That's just to get COVID-19, which has a 99 percent overall survival rate for most.

The chance of dying or having a serious complication from an untreated stroke or heart attack far outweighs the risks of possibly getting COVID-19 by going to the hospital. Patients who avoided the ER out of fear of getting COVID-19 were done a disservice. We scared them unnecessarily. Once I had this information about our practice's own COVID-19 numbers, I had a much easier time reassuring patients that going to the ER was in their best interest.

In medicine, we tend to play on patients' emotions. This is wrong. We can do better.

Heart Disease and Cancer

Heart disease is the most common cause of death each year; cancer is a close second. That has not changed in years, despite the claim that we are "winning the war on heart disease and cancer." Despite winning these wars, we actively build more heart hospitals and cancer hospitals. So, are we really winning?

Each year, death totals from those two conditions continue to rise, yet remain relatively low. How can that be? Let's look at some numbers from the CDC and US Census for 2021–2022.

- The population of the United States, as of July 2022, was 333,271,411.
- The number of people who died in 2021 was 3,464,231, or 1.04 percent of the population.
- Deaths from heart disease were 695,547, representing 20 percent of the deaths, yet only 0.21 percent of the population, or one in five hundred.
- Deaths from cancer were 605,213, representing 17.5 percent of deaths but only 0.18 percent of the population, or about one in 550.

So, while deaths from heart disease and cancer combined represent 37.5 percent of the deaths, the total number of deaths from all causes each year hovers around 1 percent of the US population.

Based on deaths from heart disease, representing 0.21 percent of the population, you would need to know five hundred people to know one person who died of heart disease in the past year. Think about it. Many of you will not know one person who died of heart disease in the past twelve months.

Even though heart disease is the most common cause of death each year, its incidence is still relatively low, despite the poor health of many Americans.

This is not to suggest we should not address or prevent heart disease; it is to put the odds in perspective, so you can make a more informed decision about any care recommended to you. You may have the time to correct your health habits and reverse the trajectory of the course you are headed before jumping to medications.

If you can do that with the number one killer, you can take that approach with most other diseases.

Now, I know what some of you are thinking. "Hey Wacko Jacko, you are cherry-picking the data. Heart disease increases with age and deaths from heart disease go up with age. How about the data for the elderly?"

Fair point. Heart disease deaths *are* more prevalent in the over-sixty-five age group.

- The population of those aged sixty-five-plus is 62,655,025.
- Heart disease deaths in 2021 in this age group were 553,214, representing 80 percent of all deaths from heart disease (695,547).
- The number of deaths in those over sixty-five was 2,491,684 or 72 percent of all deaths in 2021, which numbered 3,464,231.
- Thus, death from heart disease represented just 0.9 percent of this age group and represented 16 percent of the total deaths in 2021 but 22 percent of all deaths for those over sixty-five.

So, yes, death from heart disease accelerates after age sixty-five but even then, 78 percent of those older than sixty-five who die each year will avoid heart disease as their cause of death.

You could argue that all these heart disease and cancer numbers would be worse if we did not try to intervene. That is true, but it is half-true. That half-truth must be balanced by the fact that each of us is still going to die. If one cause of death goes down, then another cause of death goes up because...we all die eventually. We have a 100 percent mortality rate in medicine.

Plus, we must balance the benefits of our treatment with the harm of our treatments. In some studies, iatrogenic causes of death—deaths caused by doctors and hospitals—are the third leading cause of death.[190] Barbara Starfield, MD, of Johns Hopkins School of Public Health, reported these numbers to be

- 12,000 from unnecessary surgeries;
- 7,000 from medication errors in hospitals;
- 20,000 from other hospital errors;
- 80,000 from hospital-acquired infections; and
- 106,000 from FDA-approved, *correctly prescribed* medications.

Thus, the healthcare system causes 225,000 deaths annually, making it the third leading cause of death. COVID-19 deaths recently supplanted this figure.

A study in the *British Medical Journal* published May 3, 2016, came to similar findings. They reported 250,000 deaths in the US were iatrogenic in nature, making it the third leading cause of death at that time (until COVID-19 came around).[191]

Everything you put in your body and on your body (foods, fluids, medications, vaccinations, and cosmetics) either help or cause harm to your health. Few things in these categories are "neutral" to your health.

The point of this exercise is not to suggest we should not intervene with treatments to prevent disease; the question becomes to what degree do we do it? And are there other approaches we can use to get better results?

Should we treat everyone to prevent heart disease? And by treat, I mean doing more than lifestyle changes. Or can we be more selective in who we treat and target those individuals most likely to benefit? This is called risk stratification.

Risk stratification is an attempt to limit interventions to those most likely to benefit but we are far from reaching that goal. Part of the reason is that we don't understand, recognize, or accept all risk factors for a disease.

Risk Factors Are Like Vocabulary

If you only have one thousand words in your vocabulary, you are limited in how you perceive the world as you can only describe it in the context of those words. You are also limited in how you communicate with the world—remember, you have only one thousand words. That makes living challenging and frustrating.

When we think of this, we are not surprised that studies show that people with behavior problems typically have a low vocabulary.[192]

I'm sure we all have moments when we want to say something, and we know what we want to say, but we don't know how to say it because we don't have the vocabulary. That's frustrating. I have encountered several such moments in writing this book. Imagine going through an entire day like that—some people do.

Something similar happens with risk factors and medical problems. If you only recognize a few risk factors for a disease, see that disease only in the context of those risk factors, and you address only those risk factors, then you will get limited results because you have a limited vocabulary.

Let's use heart disease as an example. The traditional risk factors for heart disease according to the American Heart

Association are family history, high LDL cholesterol, low HDL cholesterol, high blood pressure, diabetes, smoking, and obesity.[193] Certainly, there must be other risk factors.

We can't do anything about family history. That is non-modifiable. But do you see anything in common with the remaining modifiable risk factors? Mostly, we treat all with pharmaceutical solutions.

Do we really believe that only the risk factors with pharmaceutical solutions contribute to heart disease? If we physicians don't have a drug to treat the risk factor, we don't know what else to do, so we ignore other potential risk factors.

Exercise and healthier eating can reduce all those risk factors except for smoking (though exercise is a good habit to replace a bad habit) but typically we pay only lip service to exercise and nutrition. Many physicians feel that your risk of heart disease has been optimized if your blood pressure and LDL cholesterol are at the target goal. But are they really optimized? Not likely.

As for other risk factors for heart disease not considered by the American Heart Association, some have pharmaceutical solutions, and some do not:

- elevated homocysteine
- elevated C-reactive protein
- low vitamin D
- low vitamin K
- elevated triglycerides
- low EPA/DHA
- low testosterone (males)

- high estrogen (males)
- elevated insulin
- nitric oxide deficiency
- excess fibrinogen
- apo B
- cardiovascular fitness

If we were to see heart disease in the context of all these additional risk factors plus the traditional ones, then each risk factor takes on less weight or importance. If all these risk factors are at target except for LDL cholesterol, then maybe having an elevated LDL cholesterol becomes less concerning.

Why is that important?

Statin drugs, used for lowering cholesterol, work remarkably well at lowering cholesterol but provide only marginal benefits when you look at their absolute risk reduction of heart attacks. In studies, as many as one hundred people must take a statin to prevent one heart attack. That's a 1 percent absolute risk reduction even though statins can lower cholesterol by 25–40 percent.

That suggests that there is more to reducing heart disease than lowering cholesterol. Maybe some of these ignored risk factors are more important than previously thought. However, it makes sense that you will get better results if you target ten to twelve risk factors rather than five to six.

Drugs and Diabetes

Type 2 diabetes is largely a lifestyle disease, and, frequently, we treat it to reduce the many complications of diabetes, including reducing the risk of cardiovascular disease. Let's look at some of the numbers to treat.

Metformin is the most commonly used medication to treat diabetes as well as those with pre-diabetes. The ten-year number to treat with metformin to prevent death is 14, and the ten-year number to treat to prevent one heart attack is also 14.[194]

In patients at increased risk for developing type 2 diabetes, the number to treat is seven compared with counseling on standard diet and exercise when taken for one to five years. However, we do not see a significant reduction in diabetes in patients taking metformin compared to those counseled on intensive diet and exercise.[195]

According to TheNNT.com, the new SGLT-2 inhibitors and GLP-1 agonists used for diabetes fare no better in clinical outcomes (though very effective in lowering blood sugar) when directly compared to metformin other than greater weight loss occurs with newer classes. TheNNT.com coded these newer medications "green" compared to the patient's current diabetes regimen, but "yellow" when compared to metformin, which is far less expensive. The site also recognized there are important increases in harms with newer drugs, particularly "genital infections with SGLT-2 inhibitors and severe gastrointestinal adverse events with GLP-1 medications, if exclusively comparing the medications to metformin we would assign a color of yellow."[196]

Cardiorespiratory Fitness and Mortality

The need for fitness is frequently overlooked when we look at risk factors for any disease and mortality. Over ten years being in the lowest 20 percent of cardiorespiratory fitness (CRF) increases your risk of death by 400 percent.

Hypertension increases your risk by only 14 percent, cardiovascular disease increases your risk by 28 percent, cancer increases it by 33 percent, diabetes increases it by 34 percent and smoking increases it by 40 percent.[197]

The risk factors we do address only minimally increase mortality compared to being in poor fitness, which we rarely address.

Go back and look at the ten-year risk of death from hypertension. It's relatively low, which explains blood medications' high numbers to treat of 86 to 140 to prevent one cardiovascular event. The lower the risk of premature death, the higher the numbers needed to treat to prevent a death. TheNNT.com codes treating mild hypertension for primary prevention of cardiovascular disease are coded red.

We spend a lot of money addressing a risk factor that, relative to others, seems to have a minor impact on mortality rates. We do not get a lot of bang for the buck treating high blood pressure, yet all physicians do it, including myself, though I drag my feet when the elevation is mild and no other risk factors are involved.

Being in the next lowest quintile for CRF increases the risk of death over ten years by 288 percent, which is still high, but with just a little improvement in cardiorespiratory fitness, mortality risk dropped from 400 percent to 288 percent.

Fitness has a far greater impact on mortality than disease states. Dr. Ken Cooper recognized this fifty-plus years ago, which placed him at odds with the medical establishment, and even today we still do a poor job of addressing fitness. We eagerly treat diseases but not fitness levels.

In the 1970s, the Cooper Clinic was classifying patients into fitness quintiles as "very poor," "poor," "fair," "good," "excellent," and "superior" (the top 5 percent). These were further categorized based on age and gender.

Exercise is free and its few side effects are predictable and avoidable. As I said earlier, our biggest gains in life expectancy stem from the least expensive interventions, some of which also improve quality of life and function.

Not So-Wacko Jacko Rule;

We get the most significant gains in life expectancy from the least expensive interventions.

Dr. Cooper was ahead of his time. Or perhaps I should say mainstream medicine is way behind the times and has still not caught up with what Dr. Cooper and the Cooper Institute knew and implemented so long ago. Mainstream medicine is antiquated in its thoughts on the importance of fitness as well as other topics. We make things more complicated than they actually are.

Accept Questionable Science; Ignore Good Science

In medicine, we physicians tend to embrace questionable science (i.e., drug studies) and ignore solid science. The science on exercise is not influenced nearly as much by industry as the science on drugs. The data on exercise are legitimate and have been reproduced by others but promoting exercise is not financially profitable for the medical establishment. It is somewhat time-intensive from an education standpoint to discuss exercise during an office visit. It is much easier and more convenient to send a prescription in a few seconds instead of spending time discussing exercise.

Taking a blood pressure medication, cholesterol-lowering medication, or a drug that lowers blood sugar, will not improve your fitness level.

Guess what happens when you improve your fitness level? Your blood pressure improves and you see improvements in monitoring blood sugar and lower cholesterol. It's easier to control your weight. The opposite does not happen with medication. Taking a blood pressure medication, cholesterol-lowering medication, or a drug that lowers blood sugar, will not improve your fitness level.

Know Why You Really Take a Drug

If I were to ask someone why they are taking a statin, they would likely reply to lower their cholesterol. But that is not correct. You take a statin to lower your risk of heart attacks, strokes, and premature death.

Taking a statin to lower cholesterol is a half-truth. It is the carrot to get you on the medication and that it works in lowering your cholesterol motivates you to stay on it, but it may not reduce your risk of heart disease or stroke as much as you think. I am not suggesting you do not take one, but you need to be aware of that.

Eighty-six to 140 patients need to take a blood pressure medicine for five years to prevent one cardiovascular event. Is that relevant for you? That depends on your risk tolerance and your cardiovascular risk profile.

Results of a study published in November 2024 showed that a reduction of blood pressure medications or dose by greater than 30 percent in long-term care residents did not increase the risk of hospitalization, heart attack, or stroke. This is another example that questions our tendencies to prescribe medications to reduce risk factors.

Risk of Stopping a Medication

There is a risk if you stop taking medication for a chronic condition, so you should not do that without first speaking to your doctor. The risk of stopping is commensurate to the benefit obtained by taking it, however. If there was little upside to taking it to begin with, then the risk of stopping it is relatively low compared to stopping a medication that has a more significant benefit.

A Danish study on patients older than 75 looked at *major adverse cardiovascular events* (MACE) in whom statins were stopped after being on one for at least five years.[198] There was a 25–30 percent increased risk of a major adverse cardiovascular event in those who discontinued a statin. That sounds dire, doesn't it? Let's take a closer look.

We call this a *relative increased risk,* but the absolute risk was small. This parallels the relative risk reduction and absolute risk reduction we see when starting someone on a statin. To put the results of that study in perspective, there was *one excess* MACE per 112 patients who discontinued a statin per year. Think of 112 as the opposite of the number needed to treat and it turns out to be on par with the numbers needed to treat with statins.

The other point of this exercise is to highlight the many times patients do not receive the information to make a truly informed decision. Some people will jump at the chance to take a medication if it may remotely help, others want extremely convincing evidence. Most of the time, you get only the relative risk numbers, which are more likely to lead you and your doctor to start a medication.

You want to know the absolute risk reduction and the number needed to treat to prevent death or significant complications of a disease if left untreated.

Benefits of Some Long-Term Medications

Sometimes, being on a medication long-term becomes necessary and can be quite beneficial. Sufferers of rheumatoid arthritis and other autoimmune disorders realize a significant improvement in their quality of life with the many biologics now available to treat those disorders. Yes, the pharmaceutical companies occasionally provide us beneficial drugs but they typically benefit only a small part of the population. Autoimmune diseases affect 3 percent of the population compared to heart disease (20 percent).

Reverse Pareto Principle

In medicine, we're applying Pareto's Principle in reverse.[IP] We spend more time and money on things that provide the least benefit. Improving cardiovascular fitness is the single best thing you can do for your health along with healthy eating (which is harder to quantify and qualify). As I said earlier, a good personal trainer will do more for your health than a good doctor. And they are less expensive.

We Need a More Comprehensive Approach

We would get better results with heart disease, or any disease for that matter, if we took a broader approach. Unfortunately, the system is not built for that.

In our medical system, we have divvied up medical problems into silos, compartmentalizing everything. We have specialists and subspecialists, which is fine. However, each specialist tends to look at a particular problem through a very narrow prism.

Lifestyle improvement addresses all medical problems, yet the foundations of health, like exercise and diet, are not considered parts of conventional medicine. They are considered complementary and alternative medicine (CAM).

Conventional medicine focuses on its two main interventions—surgery and medication—neither of which patients desire. So, why do we focus on them? Because doctors are largely trained in those two modalities only.

Not-So-Wacko Jacko Rule:

If you control the brains of physicians,
you control medicine.
Big Pharma owns the brains of physicians.[IP]

Much of what I do in my practice I didn't learn in medical school or residency training for the simple reason that it was not taught. (It still isn't.) I went "out of my way" to learn it.

As physicians, we know why patients come to us, but rarely do we know why they won't come to us. A large segment of the population tries to avoid physicians, sometimes at all costs, and physicians don't even realize it.

According to the NIH, about 38 percent of the population will receive some of their healthcare needs from complementary and alternative providers.[199] This would include massage therapy, acupuncture, chiropractic care, naturopathy, homeopathy, yoga, tai chi, herbal medicine, electromagnetic therapy, biofeedback, meditation, and more.

Thirty-eight percent is a pretty healthy chunk of the population that, for one reason or another, is skeptical about what conventional medicine provides and delivers. I think they have good reasons to feel that way.

Complementary and Alternative Medicine (CAM)

Many of those alternative and complementary forms of medicine have been around a lot longer than allopathic (MD) medicine, which is only about two hundred years old. Acupuncture is not going away. If anything has survived for millennia, it is not going away.

Time will tell whether we say the same about allopathic medicine. I have a feeling allopathic medicine will give way to something else because it is on a self-destructive course. An entire population exists that does not want what conventional medicine offers. Physicians, for the most part, do not know CAM exists nor how to reach out to individuals wanting that treatment. Would you really want to be treated with medication or surgery if there were viable options? I assume most of you would say, "No."

An entire population exists that does not want what conventional medicine offers.

I mentioned complementary and alternative forms of medicine in "Does Medicine Matter?" Some of these treatments have found a home in today's medicine because they do work and science supports their use.

Let's take acupuncture, for example. It has been discovered that at the body's meridian points, where acupuncture needles are placed, reside a high concentration of stem cells. Stem cells are a key to healing. Acupuncture dates to 6,000 BCE. It would not have lasted this long if it did not work well enough in enough people, even if we don't know how it works.

Magnets are used in diagnostic imaging (MRI scans) and used to treat depression via transcranial magnetic stimulation. Pulsed electromagnetic therapy (PEMF) is FDA-approved and promotes tissue healing and treats pain. Electric current is used in physical therapy to treat musculoskeletal problems and implanted spinal stimulators are used in those who suffer from chronic pain. Dermatologists use phototherapy to treat skin disorders. Light therapy treats depression and other mood disorders.

Not understanding how something works doesn't mean it doesn't work. Do you care how the combustion engine works, or do you only care that the engine starts and runs when you turn the ignition? Remember, it is our understanding that changes with time.

Patients eventually stop treatments that don't work. Elite athletes do not use treatments that do not work. If elite athletes are doing something, especially on a large scale, it is because it works. We can use elite athletes to determine a standard of care or as a litmus test to determine gaps in your care.

Find out what elite athletes are doing for a particular medical condition and then try to get the same treatment. You may have to pay out of pocket for it, but it will be worth the cost.

Goal: To Die Functional

No matter what you do, in the end, you are going to die. Your goal is to die at the slowest rate possible while maintaining all functions as long as possible. You are not going to get there relying on prescription medications. As Bill Maher stated, "Ask your doctor if getting off your ass is right for you."

PART IV

The Pharmaceutical Funded FDA

First, it is providing a means whereby key individuals on its payroll are able to obtain both power and wealth through granting special favors to certain politically influential groups that are subject to its regulation This activity is similar to the "protection racket" of organized crime: for a price, one can induce FDA administrators to provide 'protection' from the FDA itself.

Secondly, as a result of this political favoritism, the FDA has become a primary factor in that formula whereby cartel-oriented companies in the food and drug industry are able to use the police powers of government to harass or destroy their free-market competitors.

And thirdly, the FDA occasionally does some genuine public good with whatever energies it has left over after serving the vested political and commercial interest of its first two activities.

—G. Edward Griffin

Those are strong words by Mr. Griffin. You will have an opportunity by the end of the book to determine if you agree, partially agree, or disagree with his view.

As you likely know, the FDA is one of our nation's federal agencies and part of the Department of Health and Human Services (HHS). The FDA regulates and oversees more industries than you may think. It is tasked with regulating food safety, caffeine products, tobacco products, dietary supplements, prescription and over-the-counter medications, vaccines, biopharmaceuticals, blood transfusions, medical devices, cosmetics, electromagnetic radiation emitting devices, animal food and feed, and veterinary products.

It has a lot on its plate. I will focus on that part of the FDA that oversees the drug approval process.

Big Pharma Funding of the FDA

Surprisingly, your tax dollars do not fully fund the FDA. Many people, including doctors, do not know this, but the FDA receives a substantial part of its funding from the industries it regulates, and specifically, from pharmaceutical companies, in the form of user fees. It also receives funding in the form of user fees from tobacco companies, medical device companies, companies in the food industry, and so on.

The FDA's 2024 budget is $7.2 billion with $3.3 billion (46 percent) of funding coming from the industries it regulates.[200] However, user fees fund the remainder of the FDA's budget set aside for regulatory activities involving human drugs.

Reviewing the table below, we see that in 2023, $1.49 billion of the $2.22 billion (64 percent) for human drug regulation came from user fees. (In the chart, BA stands for Budget Authority.)

Table 1. Food and Drug Administration (FDA) Appropriations

(in millions of dollars)

Program Area	FY2017 Enacted	FY2018 Enacted	FY2019 Enacted	FY2020 Enacted	FY2021 Enacted	FY2022 Enacted	FY2023 Request
Foods	**1,037**	**1,053**	**1,071**	**1,100**	**1,110**	**1,145**	**1,232**
BA	1,026	1,042	1,060	1,089	1,099	1,133	1,220
Fees	12	12	11	11	11	12	12
Human drugs	**1,330**	**1,619**	**1,881**	**1,973**	**1,997**	**2,116**	**2,220**
BA	492	496	663	683	689	714	790
Fees	838	1,123	1,218	1,290	1,308	1,402	1,430
Biologics	**340**	**360**	**402**	**419**	**437**	**457**	**475**
BA	215	215	240	252	254	260	275
Fees	124	144	162	167	183	197	200
Animal drugs and feeds	**195**	**198**	**225**	**239**	**245**	**255**	**301**
BA	163	173	179	191	192	202	242
Fees	32	26	46	48	53	53	58
Devices and radiological health	**448**	**507**	**576**	**600**	**628**	**648**	**698**
BA	330	330	387	395	408	420	466
Fees	118	177	190	205	220	228	232

Figure 3. FDA appropriations for 2023.

The following graph shows the FDA's funding history. Notice that user fees make up an ever-increasing amount of its funding. Thus, more and more, the FDA is being supported by the industries it regulates, which would seem to be a potential recipe for corruption.

FDA Funding History and FY2022 Appropriations

Since the enactment of PDUFA in 1992, FDA's spending from user fees has generally increased, both in absolute terms and as a share of FDA's total budget, accounting for over 45% of the agency's FY2020 total program level (see **Figure 1**).

Figure 1. FDA Spending, by Source, FY1992-FY2020

(in millions of dollars)

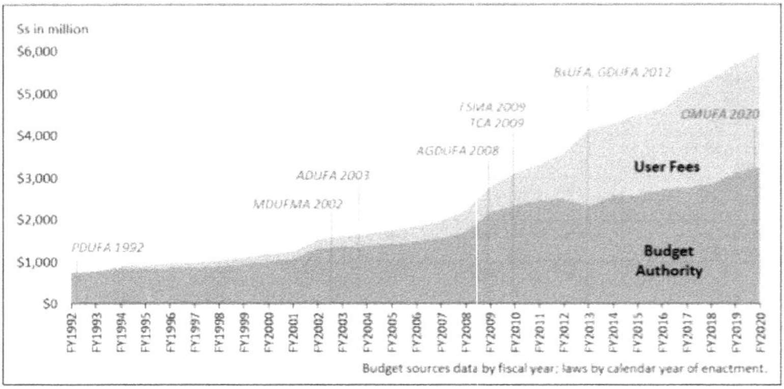

Source: Figure created by CRS using the FY1992 through FY2022 FDA CJs.

Notes: These amounts have not been adjusted for inflation. The purpose of this figure is to show how FDA's spending has changed over time to include a greater proportion from user fees compared to budget authority. The amounts used in this figure are from the "Actuals" columns in the FDA CJs, which, according to the FY2005 CJ, reflect FDA's actual spending rather than what was provided in the enacted appropriation. "Actual" amounts beyond FY2020 are not available from the FDA CJs. PDUFA= Prescription Drug User Fee Act; MDUFMA= Medical Device User Fee and Modernization Act; ADUFA= Animal Drug User Fee Act; AGDUFA= Animal Generic Drug User Fee Act; TCA= The Family Smoking Prevention and Tobacco Control Act; FSMA= Food Safety Modernization Act; BsUFA= Biosimilar User Fee Act; GDUFA= Generic Drug User Fee Amendments; OMUFA= Over-the-Counter Monograph User Fee Act.

There is a reason the graph's data begins in 1992.

Why User Fees?

In 1992, Congress passed the Prescription Drug User Fee Act allowing the FDA to collect fees from companies that produce certain human drug and biological products. The fees are levied when drug companies file a new drug application. The user fees "provide" the FDA with the means to hire more staff, significantly improve review times for drugs and biologics, and enhance access to new therapies for patients.

That all sounds nice, and it may be true. Nevertheless, doesn't that arrangement of the drug companies partially funding its regulatory agency lead to a situation where the "tail wags the dog"? This is known as *regulatory capture,* where the agency that regulates an industry falls under the control of said industry.

User fees are not unusual and most, if not all, of the fifty-two federal agencies collect user fees of one type or another.[201] The price of a stamp is considered a user fee. The fee you pay for a passport is a user fee. If you go to a National Park, you will pay a vehicle fee, that is, a user fee. The cost of an airline ticket includes a user fee that goes to the US Customs and Border Protection.

Certainly, there must be money somewhere precluding the need of the FDA to rely on pharmaceutical funding.

Let's look at the amount of money the US Government printed during COVID-19, the money it has given to Ukraine, and the money it has spent on illegal immigration. Could some of those monies fully fund the FDA by adding $3.3 billion and get the pharmaceutical companies and other industries out of the FDA funding process?

- Depending on the source, the US government "printed" $3 to $5 trillion during the COVID pandemic. Using the entire FDA budget of $7.2 billion for 2024, the entire amount of the newly printed $3 trillion and the government could fully fund the FDA for 417 years.[202]

- According to CNN, the US spent $113 billion on Ukraine as of September 2023, which could fund the entire FDA for 15.7 years.[203]

- According to the *New York Post*, the US has spent $451 billion as of November 2023 on illegal immigrants during the pandemic, which could fund the FDA's entire budget for 62.6 years. New York City alone spent $12 billion as of September 2023 per *Politico*.[204]

If it had the desire, Congress could find a way to entirely fund the FDA without using the pharmaceutical industry money.

The FDA and Big Pharma Relationship

We do know that, over the years, a cozy relationship has developed between FDA commissioners and Big Pharma.

Ten of the last eleven FDA commissioners took positions with drug companies upon leaving the FDA.[205]

NAME	Years as FDA Commissioner
• Steven M. Hahn, MD	2019-2021
• Scott Gottleib, MD	2017-2019
• Robert M. Califf, MD	2016-2017 and 2022 to present.
• Margaret A. Hamburg, MD	2009-2015
• Andrew C. von Eschenbach, MD	2006-2009
• Lester M. Crawford, DVM	2005
• Mark B. McClellan, MD, PhD	2002-2004
• Jane E. Henney, MD	1999-2001
• Frank E. Young, MD, PhD	1984-1989
• Arthur H. Hayes Jr., MD	1981-1983

Three of these former FDA commissioners serve on the Board of Directors or medical directors for the companies making COVID-19 vaccines. This includes Scott Gottlieb (Pfizer), Mark McClellan (Johnson & Johnson), and Stephen Hahn (Moderna).

Would these former commissioners get these cushy opportunities at drug companies if they were not pleasing the drug companies during their tenure as FDA commissioners?

The one former FDA commissioner in the last forty-plus years who did not subsequently take a position with a drug company was David A. Kessler, MD, who served as FDA commissioner from 1990 to 1997.

When you look at this relationship between the FDA and Big Pharma, it is much easier to understand Herbert Ley's words that I quoted earlier about the FDA protecting Big Pharma. Mr. Ley simply pointed out the half-truth about the FDA's role in "regulating" pharmaceutical companies.

The Drug Approval Process

It helps to understand the drug approval process. Consider the expense of bringing a drug to market; pharmaceutical companies will spend from $1 billion to $2.6 billion per drug, and they have more losers than winners.[206] We will learn later, though, that the federal government does much of the basic research on many drugs that the pharmaceutical companies develop. Thus, the pharmaceutical companies are *not* footing the entire bill for drug development. Taxpayers are.

Once a potential promising molecule is identified, it goes through a process. First, preclinical research is performed by studying a compound on animals. Then, an investigational new drug application (IND) is submitted and reviewed by the FDA before human clinical trials can begin.

Once the FDA gives the green light, the investigational drug enters several phases of clinical trials and then post-marketing approval. There are four phases of clinical trials.

Phase 1 assesses the safety of an investigational drug. Typically, the drug's safety profile is studied on 20 to one hundred healthy volunteers. This phase looks at the metabolism and excretions of a drug as well. Phase 1 takes about one year to complete.

- 70 percent of the drugs will move on to Phase 2 trials.

Phase 2 assesses the effectiveness of a drug, that is, how well it works. Usually, one hundred to three hundred volunteers with the specific condition are enrolled in phase 2 studies. Phase 2 takes about two years to complete and will also include a placebo group for comparison. Safety and side effects are determined too.

- 33 percent of the drugs will move on to Phase 3 trials.

Phase 3 trials begin if the drug is shown effective in the Phase 2 trial. Phase 3 trials include three hundred to three thousand patients who are monitored for drug effectiveness and further identify side effects. Different doses may be studied. Phase 3 trials take about three years to complete.

- 25–30 percent of the drugs go on to Phase 4.

Phase 4 is also known as the post-marketing phase and begins *after* a drug has been approved. Phase 4 is designed to gain additional information on drug safety, efficacy, or optimal use after approval. Rare side effects that may not be evident during phase 1, 2, and 3 trials can be more readily identified during the post-marketing analysis.

As you can see, pharmaceutical companies have more losers than winners.

I will discuss this further, but Pfizer combined phases 1 and 2 studying forty-five healthy volunteers for its mRNA COVID vaccine. Short-term two-month results of its phase 3 study were only available before its vaccine being permitted for use and available to the public under emergency use authorization.

What Does Drug Effectiveness Mean?

Drug effectiveness may be one of the biggest half-truths in medicine. It does not mean what you think. When you hear that a drug is effective, you probably interpret that to mean that the drug works in a vast majority of the patients who take it. Right? That certainly seems like a logical conclusion.

In the eyes of the FDA, drug effectiveness simply means a drug works better than a placebo, which of course, isn't expected to work at all. In clinical trials, one group of patients receives the drug, and a second group of similar numbers receives a placebo. That is a somewhat meaningless exercise comparing a drug to something you know should not have an effect and it is risky to half the patients who have a condition and are being treated with a "dummy pill."

In the eyes of the FDA, drug effectiveness simply means a drug works better than a placebo, which of course, isn't expected to work at all.

But that is how most drug trials are designed. Sometimes drugs are compared to existing approved drugs. This is usually done when a drug company is certain its drug is superior to its competition or can make it look superior through various tricks.

A drug must outperform a placebo to have a chance of being FDA-approved, which makes sense on one hand. But it also means that a drug does not have to work in most patients to be FDA-approved. Do you follow me?

The difference between how well a drug performs compared to a placebo must reach *statistical significance*, meaning that the outcome of a study was not likely to have occurred by chance alone. It means the results of a study are legitimate. You can count on it. But it does not mean the results are relevant.

It is quite possible, and happens often, that a drug outperforms a placebo, the difference being statistically significant, yet the drug is not effective in most patients. That possibility makes sense when you consider that besting a placebo is a low bar to achieve.

Thus, statistical significance does not imply clinical relevance.

Clinical relevance means just that—the results are relevant or meaningful in a clinical setting and can change a clinical outcome. In the end, something can be statistically significant without being clinically relevant.

Allow me to use a fictitious example showing one extreme. Suppose you have a concoction to grow hair and you compare it to a placebo. The placebo happened to grow hair in 1 percent of the patients and your concoction grew hair in 15 percent of the patients, and that difference met statistical significance. Assuming it was safe, then your concoction could be FDA-approved even though it will not work in 85 percent of the patients. Your concoction bested the placebo and that is what matters, so there must be something in the concoction that stimulates hair growth in some patients.

Let me now use a real-life example. Three statistics are important when evaluating the results of drug studies:

relative risk reduction, absolute risk reduction, and the number needed to treat.

Lipitor, for many years, was Pfizer's number-one-selling drug. In the phase 3 trial known as the ASCOT LLA study,[207] patients with high blood pressure and three other risk factors for heart disease, but without known heart disease or prior heart attacks, were studied to see if the addition of 10 mg of Lipitor would lower the rate of heart attacks over forty months. This is called a primary prevention trial. If this same study were done on patients who already had heart attacks, coronary bypass surgery, or coronary artery stenting, it would be called a secondary prevention trial.

In that study, for every one hundred patients who received the placebo, three had heart attacks over the 40-month period or 0.9 heart attacks per one hundred people *per year.* For every one hundred patients who received Lipitor over the forty months, 1.9 had heart attacks. That is 0.57 heart attacks per one hundred people *per year*. (40 months = 3.33 years; 1.9 divided by 3.33= 0.57.)

The first thing that should stand out is that for being the leading killer in this country causing more than 690,000 deaths a year, heart disease/heart attacks are still relatively uncommon. Of all the people you know, how many had a heart attack this past year? Many of you probably cannot think of a single person.

In its ads, Pfizer promoted a *36 percent relative risk reduction* in heart attacks in those taking Lipitor. This is a true statement, but it is a half-truth. Is a 36 percent relative risk reduction relevant? Maybe. Maybe not. If everybody died of heart attacks, then a 36 percent relative risk reduction is certainly impressive.

Here's how we get to that 36 percent relative risk reduction. Subtract 1.9 heart attacks in the treatment group from

3.0 in the placebo group and we get 1.1. Then divide 1.1 by 3.0 and we get 36.67 percent.

That's an impressive number if everyone suffers heart attacks. But only a relatively small number suffer heart attacks, as we alluded to above. What we want to know is not the relative risk reduction but the absolute risk reduction.

Calculating that is easy. Simply subtract 1.9 heart attacks/100 in the treatment group from 3.0 heart attacks/100 in the placebo group for an *absolute risk reduction* of 1.1 percent. That 1.1 percent does not sound nearly as impressive as 36 percent, which is why pharmaceutical companies rarely mention the absolute risk reduction.

For the sake of illustration, let's round up the 1.9 heart attacks per one hundred patients in the Lipitor group to an even 2.0. This means that for every one hundred patients that took Lipitor for forty months only one patient received the intended benefit (3.0 minus 2.0). Thus, in the ASCOT-LLA study, the *number needed to treat* is one hundred.

One hundred patients had to take Lipitor for one person to be spared a heart attack, meaning 99 did not get the intended benefit of Lipitor, at least, for those forty months of the study.

Yet, Lipitor performed better than a placebo and that difference was statistically significant. But was it clinically relevant? It might be for someone with a very strong family history of heart disease who also has several cardiac risk factors. For many, though, that statistical significance would not be relevant to their medical care.

Science breaks down when applied to the individual.

The number to treat is a function of time on a medication as well as the dose. The longer you take a medication, the more likely you are to obtain the intended benefit, but that is offset by the fact that you are also more likely to get a side effect. Higher doses may lower or improve the numbers to treat but also come with the potential for more side effects.

For primary prevention (those without established heart disease), the ten-year NNT for a moderately strong statin ranges from 20 to 26 and 12 to 16 for a high-intensity statin.[208] Using the lowest number to treat provided, twelve patients would need to take a high-potency statin for ten years to prevent a cardiac event. Is that relevant? Again, that is up for you to decide when considering your risk tolerance level and your overall cardiovascular risk.

Again, this study applies only to those who were at risk for heart disease but did not have it at the time of the study. These numbers do not apply to those who have had heart attacks or coronary artery bypass surgery. Statins are more beneficial for those who have had heart attacks or have heart disease.

Now, if you hear about a 36 percent risk reduction in heart attacks you would probably want to be on that drug, right? But if you hear a number needed to treat of one hundred, or even twelve, you might think twice about starting a medication.

We see similar results with rosuvastatin, made by AstraZeneca, which is a more potent statin than Lipitor or atorvastatin. In its study, there was a 54 percent relative risk reduction in preventing heart attacks at 1.9 years, but the absolute risk reduction was 1 percent.[209]

One study found the five-year NNT from statins to prevent one cardiac event in low-risk patients was 146, and in high-risk patients, the five-year NNT was 53.[210]

In "Does Medicine Matter?" I mentioned we believe that because we do well in the treatment of acute conditions, such as infections with medication (primarily antibiotics), that we can treat chronic problems successfully with medications. The NNT to eradicate H. pylori (a bacterium) which causes stomach ulcers is 1.1. That means for every 11 patients treated with an antibiotic, H. pylori will be eradicated in 10 of those cases with six to ten weeks of treatment but the NNT is five to get a stomach ulcer to heal. But an NNT of five is much more impressive than we see for blood pressure and cholesterol-lowering medications.[211]

Drugs are effective at lowering blood pressure, cholesterol, and blood sugar levels. They are not nearly as effective in preventing complications of those conditions, which is the main reason you take such medications.

Not-So-Wacko Jacko Rule of Medicine:

You are more likely to become financially healthier by buying stock in pharmaceutical companies than you are to become physically healthier by buying their drugs.[IP]

As physicians, we feel like we must do something and, because the only skill most physicians in non-surgical fields have is writing prescriptions, we write prescriptions.

Drug Safety

Determining drug safety is more complicated than determining effectiveness. Pharmaceutical companies must consider how many side effects are associated with a drug, how serious they are, and how often they occur. The average drug label shows seventy side effects as opposed to one or two intended benefits.[212]

Because heart disease is the number one killer in the US, any drug that increases heart attacks, despite being effective in treating the condition it is intended for, will usually not be approved following the phase 3 trial. Or, if a drug is seen causing an increase in heart attacks not detected in phase 3 (like the drug Vioxx or Avandia), it will be taken off the market during the post-market analysis.

Vioxx was an extremely effective nonsteroidal anti-inflammatory. When the decision was made to take it off the market, I had patients stating they would sign a waiver exempting the pharmaceutical company if it caused them to have a heart attack because it was helping their joint pain better than anything else ever did.

The Tail Wags the Dog

Do you ever take a step back and look at some of the ways things are done and shake your head? I do, all the time. Why do we allow drug companies to tell the FDA their drugs are safe and effective? Why not have an independent organization do that?

Let's look at our tax system. The IRS (a.k.a. the government) asks us to tell it what we owe. What other business does that? There is so much fraud and abuse in the government because, rarely, is any government agency run like a business.

Asking the taxpayer how much tax he or she owes seems like a recipe for fraud. But that's how the government works, and it does the same with drug approval. It relies on the information the drug companies give the FDA to determine whether a drug is safe and effective enough to be "FDA-approved." Basically, the FDA is asking the drug companies, "Should we approve your drug?" Or telling them, "Give us only the information you want us to have so that we approve your drug."

Are Compounded Products FDA-Approved?

If a medication is *not* FDA-approved, you may assume that the FDA evaluated it and determined that it is not safe or effective. It can mean that, but it does not necessarily mean that. The FDA is exempt from evaluating some treatments from a safety and efficacy perspective.

New drugs must undergo the FDA approval process involving pharmaceutical companies conducting clinical trials to demonstrate that a new drug is safe and effective. Compounded drugs are considered new drugs but do not undergo clinical trials.

Many physicians look negatively upon compounding pharmacies and drug companies and frequently speak negatively of them because they are competitors. All they hear is that compounded drugs are not FDA-approved without understanding the reason. They assume compounded drugs are unsafe.

Compounding pharmacies produce *custom-made* drugs for a *specific individual* called compounded drugs. Each compounded drug is considered a new drug. The compounding pharmacy knows the name of the patient and where they live when they compound a medication. Big Pharma has no idea who the end user of their products will be.

The answer to the question, "Are compounded products FDA-approved?" is "No," but that is a half-truth. The reason compounded drugs are not FDA-approved is because the FDA does not approve compounded drugs.

That may not make sense, so let me put it another way. Congress specifically and *intentionally* exempted compound medications from the FDA approval process via Section 503A of the Federal Food, Drug, and Cosmetic Act.

This isn't as bad as it sounds. Compounded medications are out of the FDA's jurisdiction when it comes to approval, but compounding pharmacies must use ingredients that come from FDA-registered facilities and manufacturers. The compounding labs and equipment are subject to regulation and are inspected by state pharmacy boards and the FDA.

There are practical reasons for exempting compounded drugs from the FDA approval process.[213] Compounded medications are custom-made for a specific patient, so it is not possible to conduct a clinical trial for safety and efficacy on a study group, even though the ingredients are coming from FDA-registered facilities. How would we conduct a clinical trial on a compounded drug made for one individual? How could we verify the dose without destroying the compounded product for use? The FDA can easily verify the dose of commercial products (by testing a sample of pills), but how do we verify the dose and safety of a compounded medication without destroying it and thus making it unavailable to the patient for whom it was intended?

Advantages of Compounding Pharmacies

Compounding pharmacies have several advantages over commercially mass-produced drugs. Big Pharma manufactures drugs by the thousands in limited dosage options. The pharmaceutical companies also do not know the names of their product's end users, unlike compounding pharmacies.

Compounding pharmacies can compound medications in a wide range of doses not commercially available. For example, let's say a commercially available patented drug comes in two doses, 100 mg and 200 mg. The 100 mg dose is not quite effective for you, but the 200 mg dose causes side effects. A compounding pharmacy could make a 150 mg dose for you that may give you the benefit without the side effects.

Compounding pharmacies can also compound drugs in unique delivery systems like lollipops, dissolvable tablets, suppositories, injectables, and topical products. Compounding pharmacies have more flexibility in dosing and a drug delivery system than pharmaceutical companies.

FDA Protection of Big Pharma

When the FDA states compounded medications are not FDA-approved, it implies that the drugs are not safe or effective without clarifying that it is not given jurisdiction to approve compounded medications. It takes a leap in logic to reach that conclusion based on what I have explained. However, many physicians make that leap because they are poorly educated on this topic. Big Pharma does not want physicians using compounded products, and physicians are getting the half-truth on compounded medications.

Other Compounded Products

The majority of chemotherapy agents are compounded. The dosage is, frequently, based on a patient's weight, kidney function, and liver function. Those chemotherapy agents are custom-made for a specific cancer patient. They are compounded and, likewise, not FDA-approved though the ingredients must come from FDA-registered facilities and manufacturers.

If the government made compounding illegal, it would destroy the cancer treatment business. And you will find out soon how large a business it is.

The same is true for many IV bags administered in the hospital, ER, or urgent care center. If anything is added to a standard IV bag, like potassium or an antibiotic, that bag of fluid is now a compounded product. There is no way for the FDA to assess whether that IV bag truly contains 40 milliequivalents of potassium or 500 mg of amoxicillin without testing it, thus making the IV bag unavailable to the individual patient for whom it was intended.

Even mixing two or three medications in a syringe, as is frequently done for soft tissue and joint injections, ends up being a compounded product. There is no way for the FDA to verify that the syringe contains what it is stated to contain without making the syringe of medication unavailable for use.

Many physicians avoid using compounding pharmacies because of the lack of FDA approval but have no problems with chemotherapy agents and IV bags. These are hypocritical actions due to a lack of knowledge. Again, my Not-So-Wacko rule is in play—**if you control the brains of physicians, you control the practice of medicine.**

Physicians have been bamboozled, duped, and hoodwinked by the FDA, pharmaceutical companies, and the medical education hierarchy. They have a blind spot in their education.

A Company Must Request FDA Approval

When you hear that something is not FDA-approved, it does not necessarily mean that a medication or device is not safe or effective, although it could mean that. The FDA does not take it upon itself to approve or not approve medications. An entity must apply for FDA approval before the FDA enters the approval process.

It is not always cost-effective for a company to seek FDA approval for its product. For example, testosterone is not FDA-approved for use in women, but frequently, it is prescribed by physicians who specialize in hormone replacement. The reason testosterone is not FDA-approved is because, to the best of my knowledge, no pharmaceutical company has applied for FDA approval for testosterone use in women. The market for testosterone in women is not big enough to justify the expense of doing phase 1, 2, and 3 clinical trials.

By keeping a product a nutritional supplement, a company cannot make any health claims on the label. Some manufacturers of nutritional supplements have proven health benefits based on double-blind placebo-controlled studies but elect to keep the product as a supplement. A drug can only be marketed for the FDA-approved conditions. A supplement can be marketed to everyone.

Plus, the expense of clinical trials precludes supplement manufacturers from seeking FDA approval. The reality is big business likes regulation because regulation is expensive to comply with and that expense limits competition. Few entities, outside of pharmaceutical companies, have the financial resources to conduct the clinical trials that the pharmaceutically funded FDA requires for FDA approval. It is another way the FDA protects the pharmaceutical industry.

Big business shuns competition, so it tries to eliminate it in any way it can, or the company will buy the competitor if it must. Pharmaceutical companies own some nutritional supplement companies too.

TA-65 is a supplement from TA Sciences. The product lengthens telomeres, which play a role in the aging process and therefore, indirectly, in nearly all chronic diseases. The company has published several placebo-controlled studies showing the product works on several conditions. It has elected to keep the product as a supplement.[214]

It is easy to be misled by the phrases "FDA-approved" or "Not approved by the FDA." Hopefully, you now have a better understanding.

Why Do You Take a Medication or Vaccine?

Before you agree to start a medication or receive a vaccine, you should ask yourself a series of questions. What are you trying to accomplish? What are the upsides to taking it? The downsides? And how common are they? What is the best thing that happens if I take a drug or vaccine? What is the worst thing that happens if I take it, and what if I do nothing? Are there other alternatives that might be just as effective or safer?

If it's a vaccine, what are you trying to prevent? How common is a particular infection? How many die from it if not vaccinated? Short of death, what is the worst complication of an infection?

We prescribe medications and vaccines so often that we rarely stop to consider that they are not innocuous.

Physicians can easily demonstrate that a medication is lowering your blood pressure, or lowering your cholesterol, or lowering your blood sugar. That makes the drugs look very effective and reinforces your use of them. "See how much your blood pressure has improved!"

But proving that you have been spared a heart attack or a stroke by taking those medications is not easy and when such endpoints are looked at many people will not receive the REAL intended benefit of being spared a heart attack or stroke.

Modifying a risk factor for a disease does not necessarily modify the risk of getting the disease in all individuals. Some will benefit from medications used in chronic disease management, but many will not, as demonstrated by the number of cholesterol and blood pressure medications. The challenge is knowing who will benefit and who will not. We are not smart enough to know that currently, so we err on the side of treating everyone.

Drugs Are Approved in Isolation but Prescribed in Clusters

Drugs are approved in isolation but, frequently, are prescribed in clusters. Unfortunately, clusters have never been studied in double-blind placebo-controlled studies to determine safety and efficacy. You may be on three medications and each of those medicines may be safe and effective in isolation, as determined by the FDA, but it does not necessarily follow that the trio remains safe and effective when taken concomitantly.

Pick any three drugs you can think of. Go to PubMed.com and search for a study involving those three drugs. Look for a study that shows that taking those three drugs concomitantly is safe and effective. You will not find any. So, I wonder how evidence-based medicine is being practiced when those three drugs are prescribed simultaneously. The concept of evidence-based medicine is based on a half-truth and is not always attainable and physicians do not realize that they are deviating from the concept when prescribing a cluster of drugs.

Over time, some drug-drug interactions are recognized, and some medications need a dosage adjustment when prescribed with another medication, or certain adverse reactions may be more common. That is not the same as studying that trio of meds in a double-blind, placebo-controlled study. Nobody knows how a trio of medications will affect your metabolism, your neurotransmitter production, your gut microbiome, your immune function, or your hormonal milieu will be affected.

Admittedly, it is not practical to conduct such studies on various combinations of drugs being prescribed simultaneously. With this in mind, perhaps, we should be more judicious in our use of drugs and not prescribe and dispense them like they are Halloween candy.

Vaccines

What I discussed with medications also applies to vaccinations. Vaccines are studied and approved individually but administered sometimes in clusters and sometimes in stacks. While each approved vaccine is safe and effective, we have no studies regarding the accumulative effects of multiple vaccinations over a lifetime on the human body. Despite what you read or hear, the effects of most vaccines can last a lifetime.

Vaccine safety is a nebulous term and is defined relative to the patient's health. According to the Federal Code of Regulations § 600.3, *safety* is defined as

> the relative freedom from harmful effect[s] to persons affected, directly or indirectly, by a product when prudently administered, taking into consideration the character of the product in relation to the condition of the recipient at the time.[215]

This means a vaccine is considered safe to the degree you are healthy. The problem with this definition is vaccines are frequently studied on healthy individuals and approved on that basis but then given to the general population including those with cancer, diabetes, heart disease, autoimmune disease, neurodegenerative disease, and so on. Are vaccines safe for those individuals? I'd go further and question whether they were even studied in those individuals.

Also, such a definition makes it very difficult to ascribe a bad outcome or adverse effect from a vaccine to the vaccine outside the not uncommon fever and sore arm. Most adverse effects will be dismissed as being related to any pre-existing condition one may have.

As discussed earlier, there has been no appreciable reduction in deaths from infectious diseases since the passage of the Vaccine Assistance Act of 1962. That raises the question, then, what are we trying to accomplish with many of the vaccines now given?

A main problem with vaccines is that it is hard to study their long-term effects in a controlled environment because nearly everyone is vaccinated. We don't have a large unvaccinated control group to compare with, except, maybe, the Amish population. And such studies are impractical, extremely costly, and take a decade or two to conduct.

In its six-month study on its mRNA vaccine, Pfizer largely eliminated its control group after just two months of data when it unblinded the study prematurely (with the FDA's approval) making analyzing safety and efficacy challenging. I will go over this more in "Pfizer's Deceptive COVID-19 Vaccine Trial."

While the CDC and World Health Organization (WHO) may say there are no health risks with receiving up to 72 or more vaccines in a lifetime, there is no evidence of the highest level to support that opinion.

Vaccine manufacturers now have a cradle-to-grave business, and one that is most lucrative, because there are now vaccines for every stage of life. Not only that, but if a vaccine fails or gives subpar results, what do we do? We give you boosters. Vaccines that are subpar in performance and durability are more lucrative than those that are effective at a single dose because of the need for boosters.

It seems we are trying to vaccinate against any possible infection and disease these days. I'm not sure that is so wise.

We seem to want medication and vaccinations to take the place of healthy living practices and take the place of Mother Nature. I believe we should focus on facilitating normal function and enhancing our immune systems in other ways.

Physician Education on Drug and Vaccine Approval

I do not recall any lectures in medical school or residency training related to how the FDA approval process works, the funding of the FDA, the role and benefits of compounding pharmacies, how vaccines and drugs are manufactured, and why drugs are designed the way they are which has more to do with getting patents. I will address that patent aspect in the next chapter.

FDA Speeding Out of Its Lane

The FDA has several tasks. One of them is not to tell physicians how to practice medicine or advise patients on medical treatment. That is left to state medical boards and specialty boards.

Many of you may have seen this FDA message discouraging the use of ivermectin, the horse dewormer, because you are not a horse. What the message does not tell you is that ivermectin was discovered in 1975, and the FDA approved ivermectin for use in humans in 1987.

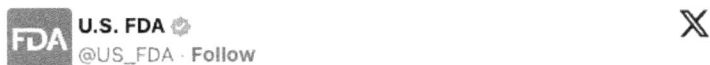

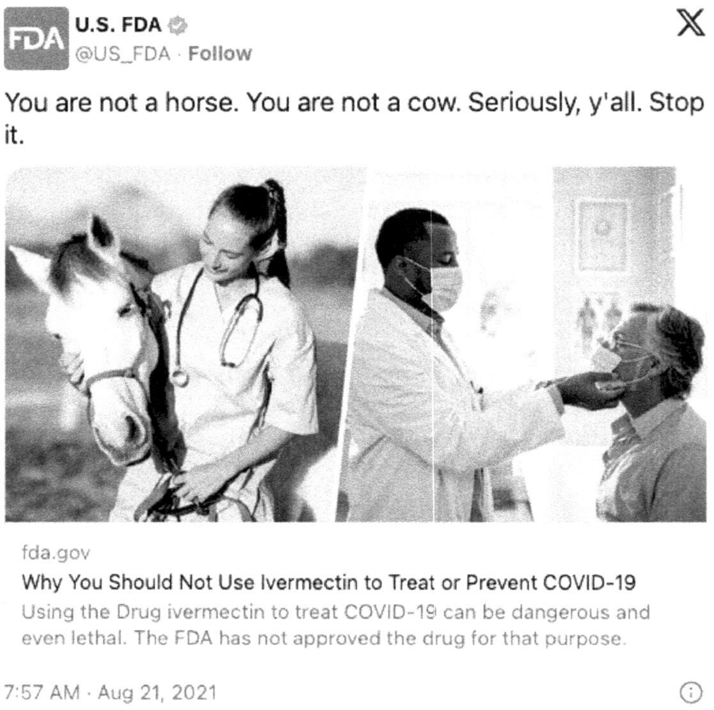

Ivermectin's developers, William Campbell and Satoshi Omura won the 2015 Nobel Prize in Physiology and Medicine for their discovery and applications. Do you think they would have won the Nobel Prize if ivermectin were as dangerous as the US medical establishment made it out to be with COVID-19? It was the first time in 60 years that the Nobel Prize was awarded to an infectious disease medication.

Japan's Kitasato Institute referred to ivermectin as one of the few wonder drugs, along with penicillin and aspirin, which have had the greatest impact on health.[216] In July 2021, the *Wall Street Journal* questioned why the FDA would attack a safe and effective drug.[217] For 33 years, from 1987 to 2020, ivermectin was determined safe for human use, then COVID-19 came and then it became dangerous even though it was still being prescribed for parasitic infections during the pandemic. (More on this when we get to *COVID-19: Confusion, Chaos, and Coercion.*)

Doctors fell for the ad, as did patients.

What was not widely known is that the FDA did not need to approve ivermectin's use for COVID-19 for a physician to prescribe it for that use. The FDA-approved indications of a drug limit how a pharmaceutical company can *market* a drug, not how a physician can *prescribe* it.

Once a drug is FDA-approved, a physician, in his or her better judgment, can prescribe it for any disease recognized by the Health and Human Services, with some exceptions. This became an issue years ago when human growth hormone (HGH) was popular and was being prescribed for anti-aging purposes.

Since aging is not considered a recognized disease by HHS, human growth hormone (or any other medication) cannot be prescribed for aging, but it can be prescribed for any recognized condition related to aging, such as loss of muscle mass or bone density, depression, and so on.

Some state medical boards have limited the conditions for which human growth hormone can be prescribed, and, in those states, a physician can prescribe it only for those limited conditions. State medical boards could do the same with ivermectin and hydroxychloroquine if they want to, but none have, as far as I know.

Writing prescriptions for a condition not FDA-approved is called off-label use and is commonplace. About 30–40 percent of prescriptions are written off-label.

The question that must be asked is, why did the FDA go this route of discouraging ivermectin for COVID-19? The FDA fully knows doctors can prescribe it for COVID-19. So, why did they discourage its use?

In my opinion, the FDA employed a deliberate scare tactic to run interference for the mRNA COVID-19 vaccine makers (remember, they partially fund the FDA). It took advantage of the unknowing public and many unknowing physicians who did not or would not know that the FDA was operating outside its scope with this ivermectin scare tactic.

On August 27, 2024, Project Veritas caught, on camera, the Department of Justice attorney who defended the FDA, stating that the FDA's campaign against using ivermectin for COVID-19 was misguided and an overreach of its authority.[218]

Remember the quote earlier in the book by Herbert Ley, the former FDA Commissioner:

> The FDA protects the big drug companies[, *delete*] and is subsequently rewarded, and using the government's police powers, they attack those who threaten the big drug companies. People think that the FDA is protecting them. It isn't. What the FDA is doing and what the public thinks it is doing are as different as night and day.

But the FDA does not discourage women from taking a horse piss pill (Premarin) for menopause. Why the different FDA attitude toward women swallowing pills made from horse piss? Whenever people or organizations flip-flop or are inconsistent in their thoughts and actions, a hidden agenda is motivating them.

As more comes out about COVID-19, the FDA and CDC will look very bad, as will a few individuals. Those agencies will lose credibility, and it appears to be already happening.

Here is another example of the FDA protecting the pharmaceutical industry.

Merck's MMR Vaccine

In 2010, a False Claims Act was filed against Merck, a pharmaceutical company. The suit was brought by whistleblowers and alleged that Merck, in collusion with the FDA, falsified the potency of the mumps component of the measles-mumps-rubella (MMR) vaccine and, in the process, misled the CDC, which was buying its vaccine. A Federal Appeals Court dismissed the case in August 2024 and concluded that Merck may have made false claims to the CDC, but those claims didn't play a role in the agency's (CDC) decision to purchase the vaccine. The Court found the alleged violations "minor and insubstantial."

The judges said that, even if the evidence showed the government knew about Merck's representations and data falsification because the FDA was aware of Merck's deception and the CDC continued to purchase the vaccine with that knowledge, Merck did not commit fraud and, thus, there was no violation of the False Claims Act.[219]

It is not fraud if the government knows it is being defrauded.

Patented Drugs: Where the Money Is

I rob banks because that is where the money is.
—Willie Sutton

Becoming and staying healthy is not all that complicated (we make it more complicated than it is), but it does take discipline. Many people would rather find it in a pill rather than with lifestyle changes, thinking they are getting the same benefit, but they are not.

When you exercise and eat healthily, your entire body benefits. Such universal benefits do not happen when you take a drug. Before you jump to a pill, you need to understand why drug companies make their drugs the way they do.

Simply, drug companies make drugs the way they do to get patents to make money. That is where the money is. Generally, a drug company cannot receive a patent for something the body naturally makes, so it employs what I call work-around strategies to get patents.

I have received a patent for an invention, and I know something about patent law. I am far from an expert on patent law but probably know more about it than most lay people. Patent law is very complicated, so I am going to speak in general terms at the risk of oversimplifying it too much.

A drug that can be patented, even if minimally effective, is more beneficial to a pharmaceutical company than a drug that is highly effective but not patentable or one in which the patent has expired.

Companies design drugs so they can be patented, not necessarily to match or replicate normal human physiology. They are designed the way they are to make money. Newer, patented drugs are not necessarily more effective than older, off-patent drugs, but they are more profitable.

If depression is simply a matter of having a serotonin deficiency (it is not), why not make a serotonin pill? Cannot be patented, thus no money in it.[220]

Not-So-Wacko Jacko Rule to Live By:

Just because a drug may work doesn't mean it's the only thing that works or the best thing that works.

How to Get a Drug Patent

Because companies cannot receive a patent for a naturally occurring product or substance, they must employ a couple of work-around strategies. Three of the more common include:

1. Preventing the breakdown of a naturally occurring molecule or blocking a natural physiological process from occurring.

2. Modifying a natural molecule enough to receive a patent while retaining much of the benefit of the natural or original molecule, while minimizing side effects. Rarely is that modification successful.
3. Using a closely related molecule from animals.

These work-around strategies frequently lead to the development of drugs that fight against normal physiology, which may be okay in the short term, but what are the long-term effects of an altered physiology?

Big Pharma's Drugs

Let's look at a list of some of the more common drug classes:

- Selective serotonin reuptake inhibitors
- Angiotensin-converting enzyme inhibitors
- Angiotensin II receptor blockers
- Beta-blockers
- Proton pump inhibitors
- HMG-CoA reductase inhibitors
- 5-alpha-reductase inhibitors
- SGLT-inhibitors
- GLP-1 agonists
- COX-2 inhibitors

Do you see a trend with the names of the classes? With one exception (GLP-1 agonists), they all block or inhibit a biochemical process that the body was designed to have. Most drugs do not facilitate normal physiology. Blocking something for the short term is one thing, but blocking something long-term may not be so benign.

It has been my observation that once a patient goes on one long-term medication, it is only a matter of time before they need a second and then a third. Why is that? I don't have a definitive answer, but my hunch is that the altered physiology from the first long-term drug plays a contributing role leading to other medical problems, though certainly some of the need for additional future drugs is related to ongoing unhealthy habits a person has.

We have an epidemic of diabetes and obesity in the US. Could an overreliance on medications for chronic problems be a contributing factor? Part of the liver's job is to metabolize drugs and toxins, and part of its job is to process glucose (sugar). A question that comes to my mind is: If the liver is spending more time breaking down drugs and toxins, does it have less capacity to handle sugars and, thus, contribute to diabetes and obesity?

Though pharmaceutical drugs may have benefits, they are all toxins to some degree as well, and the body must detoxify itself to remain healthy. Detoxification requires resources that can be depleted during the process, making the body more vulnerable to other insults.

Whenever we use a blocker or inhibitor, downstream metabolites are not being made, and those would-be metabolites have functions.

Earlier, I questioned whether depression is caused by a serotonin deficiency. If so, why not prescribe a serotonin pill? Why make a medication that blocks the breakdown of serotonin and has the unintended consequence of blocking serotonin's downstream metabolites, some of which have health benefits?

Drug making is about making money, not necessarily improving human physiology at its root.

Work-Around Strategies

Let's dive deeper into some of these work-arounds.

The first work-around strategy is preventing the breakdown of a naturally occurring molecule or blocking a physiological process.

Examples of these work-arounds include:

- selective serotonin reuptake inhibitors (SSRIs)
- angiotensin-converting enzyme inhibitors (ACE inhibitors)
- angiotensin II receptor blockers (ARBs)
- beta-blockers
- proton pump inhibitors (PPIs)
- HMG-CoA reductase inhibitors (statins)
- 5-alpha-reductase inhibitors
- SGLT-inhibitors
- COX-2 inhibitors

No one has a deficiency that would require taking any of these classes of medications. SRI deficiency, PPI deficiency, statin deficiency, and so on do not exist.

Blocking a Drug's Breakdown

Consider some of the side effects when the metabolism of a naturally occurring molecule is blocked or inhibited. Some antidepressants are associated with an increased risk of suicide. You would think the opposite would be the case. Our bodies need a metabolite of serotonin, 5-hydroxyindoleacetic acid or 5-HIAA. If serotonin is not being broken down, then our bodies aren't making 5-HIAA at healthy levels. Low levels of 5-HIAA occur from serotonin reuptake inhibitors (SSRIs), and low levels are associated with aggressive behavior, suicide, and homicide.221 (Note: There may be more to gun violence than just guns, given our propensity to prescribe SSRIs. We now have elementary-aged kids on SSRIs.)

Proton pump inhibitors (PPIs) decrease acid production in the stomach, which is useful for those with peptic ulcer disease and other acid-related disorders. But when our stomachs don't produce acid, food is not broken down properly, and nutrients are not absorbed. PPIs interfere with the absorption of calcium, magnesium, and B12 and are associated with an increase in hip fractures.[222] They are also associated with certain kidney problems and, possibly, dementia.

Plus, changing the pH of the stomach and gastrointestinal (GI) tract changes the types of microorganisms that live in our GI tracts. We have one hundred trillion organisms living in our gut and on our skin—more than the 30 trillion cells that comprise the body.

Most of those microorganisms have health benefits. In fact, 80–90 percent of serotonin is made in the gut due to the gut microflora. We now consider the gut as the second brain. However, the change in the pH also leads to the overgrowth of unhealthy or disease-associated bacteria, contributing to conditions like small intestinal bacterial overgrowth (SIBO).

Second Work-Around Strategy

Examples of a second strategy, modifying a natural molecule enough to get a patent, include non-bioidentical hormones, including conjugated estrogens and progestins. While patients have hormone deficiencies, no one suffers from a deficiency in non-bioidentical hormones because the body does not make them. The body makes bioidentical hormones. That's what bioidentical hormones mean—hormones identical to what the body makes.

Both pharmaceutical work-arounds cause side effects and can lead to other health problems.

You can look up the numerous side effects of all these classes of medications. The average drug label lists seventy side effects per drug, with one hundred side effects for the more commonly prescribed drugs and up to 525 listed side effects for some drugs. This does not mean all side effects are serious.[223] Chances are, with most drugs, that a patient is likely to get at least one side effect.

Modifying a Naturally Occurring Molecule

Below is the chemical structure of progesterone, a natural hormone produced by men and women, frequently referred to as the pregnancy hormone.

Progesterone

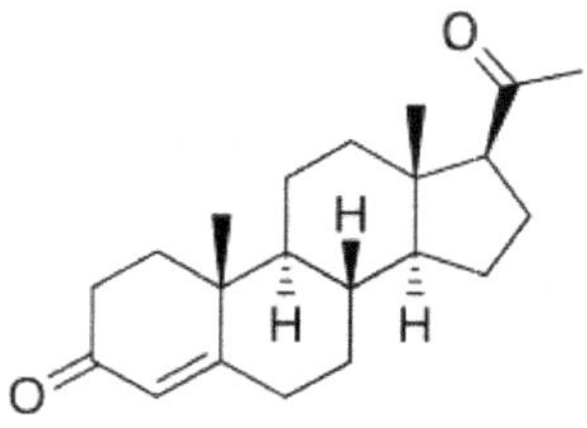

Below is a picture of medroxyprogesterone, which is a progestin commonly referred to as progesterone. It looks very much like progesterone but behaves quite a bit differently. It was used in the Women's Health Initiative (WHI) combined with Premarin in a pill known as Prempro. In the WHI, the use of Prempro was associated with a

- 26 percent increase in breast cancer related to Prempro
- 29 percent increase in heart attacks related to Prempro
- 41 percent increase in strokes related to Prempro

Medroxyprogesterone

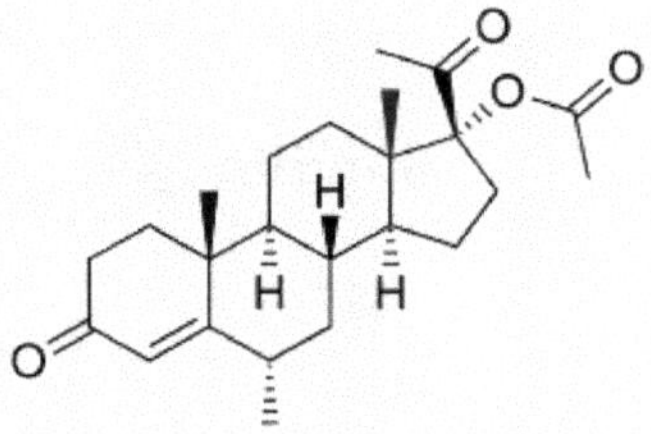

There is not much structural change between medroxyprogesterone and progesterone. The WHI used Premarin—conjugated estrogens from the urine of pregnant mares—which takes us to the third work-around to achieve a patented drug.

Using an Animal Compound224

Here is a drawing of 17 beta-estradiol or E2, an estrogen compound the human body naturally makes:

17 beta-estradiol

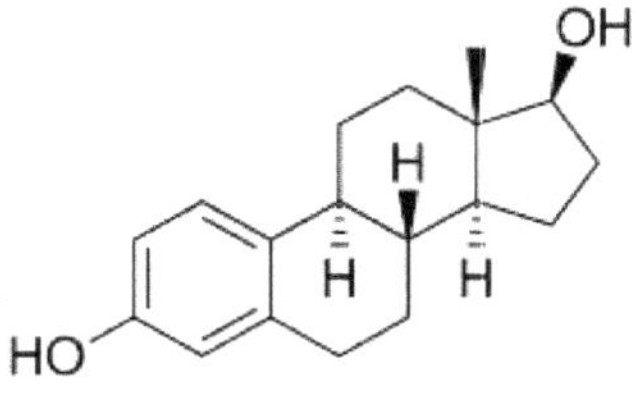

Below is a drawing of equilin sulfate, a horse estrogen that makes up 20–30 percent of Premarin. It is quite a bit different than estradiol but somewhat similar in structure. It is just one of at least eleven equine estrogens in Premarin. These estrogens are bioidentical to horses but non-bioidentical to women.

Equilin

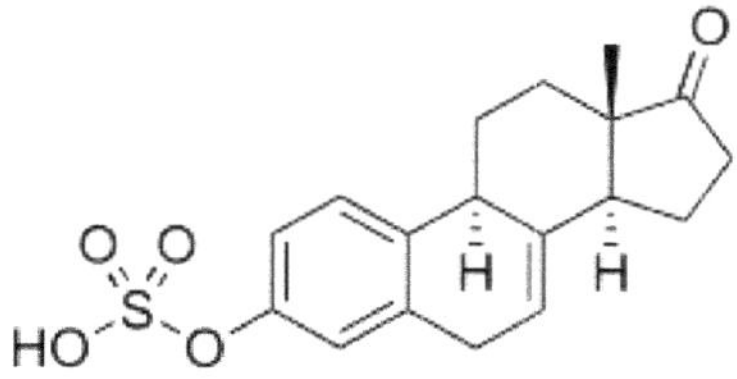

Equilin sulfate is carcinogenic in humans, increasing the risk of endometrial and breast cancer, heart disease, strokes, and blood clots.[225] The slight difference in structure between the molecules leads to a significant difference in effects on the female body.

Now, let's return to our discussion on compounding pharmacies. First, many conventionally trained-only physicians (all physicians are conventionally trained, but some go beyond that) do not believe in hormone replacement.

Somehow, they have come to accept that something your body is born with is unhealthy.

I think some of that view is shaped by some of the bad outcomes that develop from using non-bioidentical hormones, including Premarin and Prempro, as reported in the WHI study. Some physicians extrapolated the adverse effects of non-bioidentical hormones to all hormones.

Yet, many conventionally trained-only physicians will default to using FDA-approved non-bioidentical hormones because they misunderstand compounded products and why they are not FDA-approved.

Non-bioidentical hormones are FDA-approved, so many physicians prefer to prescribe them over a compounded hormone, completely identical to what the body once made in abundance. Thus, FDA approval of non-bioidentical hormones trumps bioidentical hormones in the minds of conventionally trained-only physicians.

After the findings of the Women's Health Initiative were reported, much hormone replacement therapy ceased. Women who felt better on hormone replacement therapy and wanted to continue it had difficulty finding a doctor to prescribe it. Eventually, a small group of physicians started using compounding pharmacies to compound bioidentical hormones. As more physicians started using compounded bioidentical hormones, the large pharmaceutical companies lost a significant amount of market share. Eventually, they began to make their own versions of bioidentical hormones.

Now, pharmaceutical companies make commercially available bioidentical hormones, but in a small number of fixed doses. This process does not allow for fine-tuning a dosage that compounded products can achieve.

Summary of Patented Drugs

Patented drugs are where the pharmaceutical companies make their bigger profits. Drugs are designed to be patentable, not to mimic or replicate normal human physiology. (Few drugs replicate normal human physiology.) FDA approval does not mean that a drug is safer or more effective than a compounded medication.

Anatomy of a Patent

Patents are issued or granted to individuals or inventors, not companies. Many times, researchers are developing inventions as part of their employment with a company. Typically, the company owns the legal rights to the patent, though the individual inventors may receive compensation beyond their salary for the invention. Every company has its own policy on handling this.

Some companies allow employees to work on their ideas, allocating a certain amount of company time and resources for employees to pursue their ideas in exchange for rights to the invention down the road. One such company is 3M, and it allows employees to spend 15 percent of their time on innovation.[226] Hewlett-Packard and Google operate with similar models.

On a patent, you will see *Assignee*—the entity to which the inventors have assigned the legal rights to the patent. In my case, I started a company called Jaggo, Inc. (a take on my surname), and I assigned the rights to it. A copy of my patent follows.

US005544430A

United States Patent [19]
Jacko

[11] **Patent Number:** **5,544,430**
[45] **Date of Patent:** **Aug. 13, 1996**

[54] **ATHLETIC SHOE COVER AND ANKLE SUPPORT COMBINATION**

[75] Inventor: **Joseph G. Jacko**, Dallas, Tex.

[73] Assignee: **Jaggo, Inc.**, Dallas, Tex.

[21] Appl. No.: **216,178**

[22] Filed: **Mar. 22, 1994**

[51] **Int. Cl.**[6] **A43B 5/00**; A43B 5/18; A43B 7/20

[52] **U.S. Cl.** .... **36/7.1 R**; 36/9 R; 36/89; 36/100; 36/101; 36/114

[58] **Field of Search** .... 36/7.1 R, 7.2, 36/9 F, 88, 89, 100, 101, 114, 1.5, 2.0

[56] **References Cited**

5,144,759	9/1992	Mascotte	36/7.1 R
5,165,182	11/1992	Michael	36/7.1 R
5,172,493	12/1992	Diaz	36/2 R
5,176,624	1/1993	Kuehnreich	36/101
5,251,386	10/1993	Diaz	36/2 R
5,311,676	5/1994	Hughes et al.	36/7.1 R

Primary Examiner—Paul T. Sewell
Assistant Examiner—Marie Denise Patterson
Attorney, Agent, or Firm—Harris, Tucker & Hardin, P.C.

[57] **ABSTRACT**

The present invention relates to a shoe cover that can be attached to a selected athletic shoe to provide an improved appearance of the upper portion of the shoe. The lower edge of the shoe cover attaches to the bottom of the shoe upper or to the side of the sole portion, so the bottom surface of the sole is not restricted. The top of the cover is retained tightly against the top of the shoe upper to give the cover a snug fit

Patents Listing Dr. Fauci

I go into this because one controversy that has arisen relates to patents on drugs for which Anthony Fauci, MD, is listed as an inventor. He is listed as an inventor on fourteen patents that I could find, and possibly more. The dates on the patents range from 1995 to 2016. (The appendix includes a listing of patents for which Dr. Fauci is listed as an inventor.)

Two or three names are listed on each of those patents, and he is listed as the last inventor. Many patents show the same two or three names. The controversy relates to any money he may have received for those drug inventions while serving in his role as NIAID, and if so, whether that conflict of interest guided the decisions he made.

The distribution of royalties received by federal agencies is addressed in 15 US Code § 3710c. This code allows federal employees listed as inventors to receive up to $150,000 annually.[227] The question is not whether it is legal for Dr. Fauci and other federal employees to receive royalty payments. The question is whether the possibility of royalty payments affected his decisions to promote certain drugs as NIAID Director and influenced his decision to suppress the use of repurposing existing drugs that might compete with those for which he is an inventor.

During Dr. Fauci's tenure as director of NIAID, the agency became an incubator for drug development. Early research on many molecules would be done through NIAID and not the pharmaceutical companies. Clinical trials would be conducted through principal investigators (PIs) at approximately 1,300 academic centers. Then, the NIAID would transfer some, or all, of its share of the intellectual property to the pharmaceutical companies through the HHS's Office of Technology Transfer.[228]

Once a drug is successfully marketed, royalty payments flow back to the NIAID and, subsequently, to the individual inventors per 15 US Code § 3710c. Academic centers and PIs also receive their share of royalty rights.

From 2010 to 2016, every drug the FDA approved—210 in total—originated, in part, from NIH-funded research. The NIAID is one of 27 institutes and centers that comprise the NIH.

The dollar amount to support the research on those drugs was $100 billion, and over 90 percent of the funding represented basic research more related to the biologic targets than the drugs themselves.[229]

That amounts to $476 million per drug (of the 210 approved drugs) that the pharmaceutical companies did not have to spend on basic research and drug development.

As I write this, we have learned from the COVID Select Subcommittee Hearings in May–June 2024 and information from Open the Books that the NIH received $710 million. NIAID received $690 million of that $710 million in royalty payments from pharmaceutical companies in 2022 and 2023.[230]

From 2009 to 2021, the NIH received only $325 million, with NIAID receiving just $23.9 million. Was the big jump related to the COVID-19 vaccines?

Taxpayer money makes these drug patents possible. Thus, the government subsidizes the pharmaceutical industry. Some people will think it reasonable for the federal government to engage in such a relationship with the pharmaceutical industry. Those relationships, to an extent, may be unavoidable.

Just like we have partnerships with industry and academic research, we have partnerships between government and industry. Given the complexity and expense of research, the partnering of government and industry may be unavoidable, much like the relationship between industry and academic centers.

Another possibility would be for the pharmaceutical industry to collaborate on its own, do the basic research, and then determine which pharmaceutical company will bring an individual drug to market. The current arrangement with the NIH and the pharmaceutical industry is ripe for conflicts of interest and abuse to occur.

An important issue, in my mind, is whether one person (Dr. Fauci) should have so much control of that partnering and be the person making decisions on what drugs are to be used, especially during pandemics.

For a more in-depth discussion of Dr. Fauci's close ties to the pharmaceutical industry, I refer readers to Robert F. Kennedy Jr's book, *The Real Anthony Fauci: Bill Gates, Big Pharma, and the Global War on Democracy and Public Health*. The book contains a section on how the NIAID has become a pharma "subsidiary" under Dr. Fauci's leadership.

While one is supposed to have contributed to the concept behind the invention, one does not have to actively participate in the invention's development to be listed as an inventor. We see similar listings in academic research where, many times, the department head appears as an author on any study originating from that department, even if the only contribution was to the concept of a study.

The main reason to be listed as an inventor is to not only receive proper recognition but also to receive financial rewards. If your name is not on the patent, you will not receive anything. Dr. Fauci admits to receiving royalty payments for at least one drug patent.

In an interview with the Associated Press, Dr. Fauci reported that he tried to refuse royalties but was told he was legally obligated to accept the money. In addition, he should not disclose it on his federal financial disclosure as the payments are considered part of his federal compensation rather than outside income.

He further stated that he planned to donate the royalty payments, saying, "I am going to give every penny of it to charity—no matter what the yearly amount is."[231]

If Dr. Fauci's claims are true, he should be able to point to an employment contract or government policy stating he is required to receive royalty checks. Also, he should be able to provide evidence of how much money he donated to organizations, but that does not appear to have occurred.

Even so, it does not eliminate conflicts of interest as he would still be motivated to push certain drugs to enable his colleagues to be listed on those patents and receive royalties.

The fact that the NIAID is doing some of the early research and development (R&D) on new drugs is probably one reason Big Pharma can spend more on executive salaries and shareholders than R&D. In this sense, the taxpayer subsidizes Big Pharma. Just as Alaskans receive money from the state's oil riches, perhaps US taxpayers should receive a share of the pharmaceutical industry's profits.

For my little patent, I paid for everything. I paid the patent attorney. I paid to incorporate a company. I paid for the materials. I paid for prototypes. I paid the University of Dallas MBA Capstone program to develop a marketing plan. I did not have the luxury of using other people's money free of charge.

I am all for entrepreneurship and innovation, and I think people should be rightfully compensated for their inventions. In general, I have no issue with whether Dr. Fauci was legally entitled to royalty payments, assuming he contributed to the concepts of the drug inventions. However, he either needs to be a drug developer or the director of NIAID, not both simultaneously.

The taxpayer subsidizes Big Pharma.

And the royalty program for federal employees needs to be revisited, as federal employees are using other people's money, not their own, to develop products. They get to play with house money and reap potential rewards on the taxpayers' dime.

The system we have for drug development is ripe for conflicts of interest and abuse, with opportunities to promote certain patented therapies over off-patent therapies that still have clinical utility. And we have put much of that control in the hands of a single person.

Big Pharma needs an endless supply of patented drugs, and our government helps it. Yes, Bill Maher is right when he says the government is your dealer and it subsidizes illness in America. You and I subsidize it with our taxes.

Then, Big Pharma uses its vaults of money to control every other major aspect of medicine.

PART V

My Wake-Up Call

Beware of false knowledge; it is more dangerous than ignorance.
—George Bernard Shaw

We have reviewed how the medical system functions behind the scenes and revealed its dark side. When did I realize the medical profession was tainted and corrupt?

I have long questioned some of what we do in medicine, as early as my first month in medical school, but three events woke me up to the dark and corrupt side of medicine. One of them we all experienced—COVID-19.

Until 2007, for the most part, I followed the recommendations of the professional societies to which I belonged. While I did not agree with everything we were taught, I did not seriously call out the deceptions I encountered.

That began to change in February 2007 while I was practicing with the Steadman-Hawkins Clinic of the Carolinas. I was asked to give a talk on anabolic steroids to an audience of sports medicine physicians, physical therapists, and athletic trainers. I had a canned talk on the topic that was much the same as any talk you would have heard from a sports medicine physician: Anabolic steroids are dangerous, and athletes should avoid using them.

To save time, I contemplated giving the same talk. However, because the talk wasn't until June, I decided to update it, devoting some time to examining the topic from a user's standpoint. That decision took me down an unexpected road when I came across an interesting document.

Central to my talk was the testimony of Rick Collins, then the leading legal expert on anabolic steroids, given at a federal hearing in front of the United States Sentencing Commission on April 12, 2005.[232] He made ten points distinguishing testosterone from other anabolic steroids, and he stated that testosterone, when used properly, is safer than other prescribed hormones, like insulin, and safer than many commonly used over-the-counter medications.[233]

I ended up spending more than one hundred hours of research I had not anticipated. I spent many of those research hours trying to prove that Mr. Collins was wrong, but I concluded the opposite. I found myself agreeing with him—and he was a lawyer! I detailed my story in two articles on my website, JackoMD180.com: "My Unexpected Journey into Age Management Medicine" and "Why Is Testosterone a Controlled Substance?"

The issue surrounding testosterone, an anabolic steroid, is important because it became viewed as dangerous as other more potent anabolic steroids when the government classified it as a controlled substance under the Anabolic Steroid Control Act of 1990.

Being lumped into the category of a Controlled Substance, on top of the view (now known to be wrong) that it triggered prostate cancer, gave testosterone a bad reputation. This served as another deterrent to men using testosterone replacement for health purposes.

Mr. Collins suggested that the real reason anabolic steroids became a controlled substance had little to do with adverse health effects, but more with cleaning up cheating in sports.

I obtained and read the five hundred pages of transcripts from the Congressional Hearings on Anabolic Steroids that the University of Georgia Law School sent me. In the end, I reached the same conclusion as Mr. Collins. The sports medical community had lied, distorted, and misled physicians by overhyping the dangers of anabolic steroids. Certainly, these steroids have more risks than human-made testosterone, but athletes were not dropping like flies as the medical community was suggesting. (At that time, there had never been a long-term study to indicate that anabolic steroids were as dangerous as was stated.)

In his testimony to Congress, Charles Yesalis, PhD, the leading epidemiologist in the area of anabolic steroids, intimated that the medical industry feared a long-term study would show that anabolic steroids were not as dangerous as the medical community wanted society to believe, possibly fueling further abuse or use.

Essentially, it was easier to scare people from using anabolic steroids by stating they were dangerous than demonstrating they were unsafe. This is a classic example of the use and power of fear, similar to what we witnessed with COVID-19.

Fomenting fear is a control mechanism, and people use it when the truth gets in the way of their objectives.

I concluded that the impetus to curb cheating in sports was strong enough that *Congress relied on weak medical evidence to ascribe a legal remedy to what is, ultimately, an ethical issue.*

It is a dangerous slope we slide down whenever we use medicine as a means to justify an objective falling outside of medicine. I see parallels in the way things were handled with anabolic steroids and now in the management of COVID-19.

The outcome of those Congressional Hearings was the passage of the Anabolic Steroid Act of 1990, classifying anabolic steroids as a Controlled Substance. (HR 4568) The chairman of the Senate Committee on those hearings was then-Senator Joe Biden.

Unfortunately, the Anabolic Steroid Act created the perception that testosterone is dangerous, even for legitimate medical purposes, and it led physicians and patients away from using testosterone.

The Act did not curb cheating in sports, as evidenced by the proliferation of anabolic steroids, especially in baseball, since the Act's passage. It did land many bodybuilders and weightlifters in jail, though, which was not the Act's goal.

The half-truths of information physicians were taught about anabolic steroids and the ulterior motives of our government leaders and leaders of organizations (in this case, sports) left a sour taste in my mouth.

For the first time, I saw the dangers of medical professionals, medical organizations, government, the legal system, media, and private organizations colluding to address a relatively perceived minor problem in society.

Does that sound eerily familiar today on a larger level?

That experience made me start to question how much of what we physicians are taught is true, and I have been questioning many aspects of medicine since—the most recent being COVID-19 management.

The passage of the Anabolic Steroid Act of 1990, like many laws, had unintentional consequences. A hormone that every man, woman, and child makes was included in the Act, which is testosterone. Think about the folly of that. You and I are walking around producing a hormone our government has classified as a controlled substance. It boggles the mind.

That misperception of the dangers of testosterone is not insignificant. Those perceived dangers deterred many middle-aged and older males from seeking male hormone treatment for legitimate medical purposes, which was commonplace in women since the early 1940s.

To dissuade the use of anabolic steroids, professional groups like the American College of Sports Medicine (ACSM) in the 1960s and 1970s conducted studies to *intentionally* show that anabolic steroids do not work by using doses too small to make a difference and much smaller than what athletes use.

The ACSM's first position statement, in 1977, concluded, "there is no conclusive evidence that extremely large doses of anabolic-androgenic steroids either aid or hinder performance..."[234]

But athletes knew they worked. Everybody taking them knew they worked. All you had to do was look at someone to know anabolic steroids worked, so why even attempt a study that athletes would see through?

As a result, the sports and medical professions lost credibility with athletes and have never fully regained it. And we will see the same thing with COVID-19 once more people wake up, and some are slowly waking up. Eventually, it will become a tsunami, and when that happens, the medical profession will have a hard time recovering.

ACSM's research showed that the medical profession has little credibility among users of anabolic-androgenic steroids (AAS), with less than 10 percent perceiving physicians and pharmacists as knowledgeable on the topic.[235]

But times have changed; the illusion has burst, and reality has emerged.

This is from Michele LaBotz, MD, writing about the ACSM's consensus statement on "Anabolic-Androgenic Steroid Use in Sports, Health, and Society" on August 31, 2021.

> ...one piece of information that stood out to me was that users of anabolic-androgenic steroids (AAS) spent an average of 268 hours researching AAS before initiating use! That is a LOT of homework, and there is no way that the vast majority of us in sports medicine can match this degree of knowledge and research in an ongoing fashion. It can be intimidating when a patient or client knows more than we do on matters related to sports and performance. So, how do we keep up with all of this information?

That is extremely honest writing there. I give her credit. She includes a tidbit that patients should endeavor to achieve: Strive to know more than your doctor on aspects of health that matter most to you.

The deceptions to dissuade the use of anabolic steroids in sports and the surrounding ethical and legal issues represent half-truths.

Lessons Learned

This awakening taught me a few lessons.

- As much as possible, physicians need to review the original source of medical information. During COVID-19, many physicians were/are simply relying on CDC guidance, but the CDC is not the source of most medical information. Plus, the CDC has about 3,400 corporate sponsors, all "buying influence." Like everything else, the CDC is in bed with Big Pharma. The CDC owns over two hundred patents, with more than fifty of them vaccine-related.[236]

- Physicians need to do their own research, especially on topics related to their practice. You, as a patient, should do your own research, which is much easier in the Internet Age.
- Physicians need to develop an appreciation of the history of events that lead to certain medical conclusion,s sometimes passed down as gospel truth but are not.

During my oncology rotation during residency, the attending physician was from the Cleveland, Ohio, area, like me. He was a big baseball fan, and baseball was my sport. On rounds, he and I would fire baseball trivia back and forth, trying to stump the other.

We asked each other questions like, "What was the starting lineup for the 1927 Yankees?" Or "How many combined wins did Dizzy and Daffy Dean have for the 1934 Gas House Gang (St. Louis Cardinals)?"

One day, he said, "It's interesting that you and I know all this baseball history, but how well do we know the history of medicine?"

That always stuck with me, and since then, I have made the point of reviewing the history of medicine, especially topics that interest me or are relevant to my practice. The history of medicine is fascinating.

The second event opened my eyes to the dealings of pharmaceutical companies.

In 2012, I returned to Ohio and joined a large physician-owned primary care group. I took over the practice of a retiring internist. My goal was to transform the practice into a sports medicine and men's health practice, but I found myself doing more general internal medicine than I wanted.

I finished my residency in internal medicine in 1989 and had not practiced much internal medicine since then. When I was at the Cooper Clinic in Dallas, I did manage some patients with high blood pressure and high cholesterol, but that was the limit of applying my internal medicine training.

Meetings with Pharmaceutical Representatives

For 20-plus years, I practiced sports medicine exclusively. During most of my career, managing patients with athletic injuries, I did not need to write many prescriptions or interact with the pharmaceutical industry. The only prescriptions I wrote were for the non-steroidal anti-inflammatory of the year, muscle relaxants, short-term prescriptions for pain medication, and an occasional antibiotic.

By 2012, there was a proliferation of new drugs, many of which I knew nothing about or had even heard before. To get up to speed, I agreed to meet over lunch with pharmaceutical reps to learn more. The rep would bring lunch for our staff, and I would listen to their spiel and learn about their medications.

Quickly, I caught on to the deception used in marketing drugs.

I think most pharmaceutical reps genuinely believe they are providing a valuable service with the information they provide doctors, and most believe in the drugs they represent. I don't think they realize, however, that their pharmaceutical company has carefully conditioned them and trained them to share information most beneficial to the company by painting their drugs in the best possible light. In effect, the pharmaceutical reps are dealing in half-truths, likely not even knowing that the information they provide is carefully orchestrated to bamboozle, dupe, and hoodwink physicians.

Like physicians, pharmaceutical reps are pawns in the system.

Several key metrics are important in evaluating drug efficacy. They include relative risk reduction (RR), absolute risk reduction (AR), and the number to treat (NNT), among others.

Drug reps like to talk about relative risk reduction, the least important of those three metrics, but the one that looks most impressive for drug companies. We see the relative risk reduction prominently displayed in the drug's marketing material and hear about it in television commercials. It is the least valuable metric yet the most misleading.

Physicians are more apt to write prescriptions when the results of drug studies are presented in terms of relative risk reduction rather than absolute risk reduction. (MARCATTO). So, I guess it is our own fault as physicians that we are misled. We have told the pharmaceutical industry, "Here's how to dupe us: Couch your results in terms of relative risk."

Let me share real examples of the deception of pharmaceutical companies in how they report their efficacy data. The number needed to treat is the number of patients who must take a drug for one patient to receive the intended benefit of the drug.

Many of you are likely on an FDA-approved drug that boasts a 36 percent relative risk reduction in heart attacks (sounds impressive), but one hundred of you will have to take the drug for forty months for just one to realize that reduction (not so impressive). That one hundred needed to prevent a heart attack is the absolute risk reduction, resulting in an absolute risk reduction of only 1 percent. That drug is Lipitor or atorvastatin.

Let's now look at one of atorvastatin's competitors, rosuvastatin (Crestor), which is the most potent statin. It boasts a 44 percent reduction for all cardiovascular events at 1.9 years of use, a 54 percent reduction in heart attacks, a 48 percent reduction in stroke, a 46 percent reduction in revascularization (stents and bypass), and a 20 percent reduction in all-cause mortality. From a relative risk perspective, those are all impressive numbers.

Many of you are likely on an FDA-approved drug that boasts of a 36 percent relative risk reduction in heart attacks, but one hundred of you will have to take the drug for forty months for just one to realize that reduction.

But the numbers needed to treat to prevent heart attack, stroke, or death at 2, 3, 4, and 5 years are 95, 49, 31, and 25, respectively. What do those numbers mean in English? Ninety-five patients must take rosuvastatin for two years to prevent one of those events, 49 patients must take the drug for three years to prevent one event, 31 patients must take the rosuvastatin for four years for one person to benefit, and 25 patients must take it for five years to prevent one event.

In the context of those numbers, rosuvastatin does not look nearly impressive. As a patient, you most likely would be agreeable to take rosuvastatin based on the relative risk numbers, but would you feel the same based on the numbers to treat to receive the intended benefit of the drug?

One drug rep I met with was launching a new drug for heart failure. He proudly stated that the drug had a great number needed to treat, the only time I recall a drug rep willing to give that data. He said the NNT was 22. I almost choked on my food because 22 does not sound good to me. However, it is a good number to treat relative to the numbers needed to treat blood pressure meds and the rosuvastatin numbers to treat.

When it comes to drug efficacy, you are only getting the half-truth and, often, the half that is deceptive. Of all the entities engaged in the healthcare system, the pharmaceutical industry engages in the most half-truth tactics.

COVID-19

The third event, one we all encountered, endured, and became indentured to, and which became the final wake-up call for me, was the management of COVID-19. In a coordinated fashion, the entire weight of the medical establishment, with the help of the media, descended upon us, stoking fear for an infectious disease that has a 99 percent-plus survival rate.

Why? I will devote an entire chapter to COVID-19 and one chapter to Pfizer's vaccine trial. COVID-19 was the event that finally motivated me to write the book you are now reading.

What does a physician do once awakened?

What do physicians do when they realize that medicine has a dark side? It is difficult to walk away given the years of training, sacrifices made, and the debt that may have accumulated getting that training.

Waking up to the half-truth presents you with two issues: dealing with the half-truth and what you do career-wise.

When you see through the half-truths, you can be vocal or quiet. Or something in between. Thinking you can change the system likely isn't going to happen, at least very quickly.

Some physicians were outspoken about the suppression of therapies like ivermectin and hydroxychloroquine for COVID-19 and suffered the wrath of the medical establishment. Some were vocal about the vaccines and the vaccine mandates. And others kept quiet.

I suspect that how secure a doctor is in his or her position and whether they are employed might determine their approach. Some lost their jobs for sharing their opinions publicly. What I find troubling is how many physicians sided with the establishment's tactics to silence other doctors who expressed their opinions.

Medicine has always discussed differing opinions. But differing views suddenly were not tolerated. Any physician who acted or had an opinion that differed from the medical establishment was attacked and viewed as a quack, conspiracy theorist, illegitimate, and more.

Why did the medical establishment fear those doctors? Why did it muzzle them and refuse to debate them? If the truth is on your side, why fear, why muzzle, and why not debate?

In a nutshell, the establishment's agenda for control was more important than your health. You need to get this in your head: *To the medical establishment, you do not matter.*

Furthermore, if you cannot have an honest debate on medical matters, then you no longer live in a free society.

Once awakened, what does a provider do in the long term?

I've thought long and hard about this question because I lived it. In the end, providers have three options.

1. **Retire completely.** Some providers are doing that at earlier ages.

2. **Adapt.** Try to be in the world (medical system) but not of the world, and several awakened doctors have done that. They limit how much they participate in the system, primarily by not accepting insurance, but one cannot completely dissociate from the system.

   Many doctors in this adaptable group, in which I include myself, have obtained additional training in Age Management Medicine, Anti-Aging Medicine, Longevity Medicine, Functional Medicine, Integrative Medicine, and Alternative and Complementary Medicine.

   The above areas emphasize prevention and lifestyle, restoring hormones to healthy levels, performing more comprehensive physical examinations, obtaining more extensive lab work, and less reliance on pharmaceutical drugs. Such physicians focus on the fundamentals of health.

3. **Spend less time in patient care.** Many *Physician Side Gigs* followers do this and offset any lost income by either doing something else in medicine or something outside of medicine.

From Patient Care to Administration

One observation I have made, which is disappointing, is that some physicians leave practice to go into healthcare administration. In their new administrative role, you would think they would be physician-friendly and sympathetic to doctors, but they are not. To keep their jobs, they succumb to the medical establishment's pressure to keep doctors in line.

With 77 percent of US physicians now employed, the hospitals, health systems, or corporate entities can easily muzzle those who might want to be more vocal.

Employers have more sway over physicians than patients may think. These entities "own" physicians. We think physicians have autonomy and practice medicine the best way they see fit, but that is far from the truth. It was that way once, and patients would gravitate to physicians who shared their philosophy.

Nowadays, in the insurance-based model, it matters little who you see as your doctor. You will get the same advice. The only difference is whether you like your physician. The advice you receive has become cookbook medicine: Follow the recipe. Do not deviate from it.

To my surprise, many doctors like being told what to do. It takes the thinking out of the equation. They simply follow what perceived authorities, like the CDC, recommend without questioning those recommendations.

Recommendations for masking and six-foot distancing were not based on meaningful evidence. Yet, because the CDC recommended those practices, physicians and patients followed them because of the CDC's perceived expertise and authority.

Half-truths are more persuasive when coming from those in leadership positions considered to be experts and authority figures. The medical establishment takes advantage of that perceived authority and expertise to control physicians.

I love learning and being taught. While I consider myself to be teachable and coachable, I like to leave the application of that knowledge and skill to my own device. I think many of us feel that way. So much of everything is micromanaged these days, including medicine.

Physicians now deal with four years in college, four years in medical school, and three to five years in residency training, and then, about half the doctors will spend one to three years in a subspecialty fellowship, all while being brainwashed by the pharmaceutical-controlled medical education system. After completing this, those from federal health agencies, hospital administrations, and insurance companies—who do not care for patients—tell them how to practice medicine.

> *It doesn't make sense to hire smart people and tell them what to do; we hire smart people so they can tell us what to do.*
>
> —Steve Jobs

Perhaps medicine would be best served if the medical establishment listened to physicians more, especially those on the front lines who actually care for patients.

This micromanagement in society is now ubiquitous, and it is unhealthy.

Is it any wonder we have a society of people unable or scared to make their own decisions? I think workplace micromanagement is a key contributor to that indecision. We are creating a society of human robots. It is intentional, and the self-proclaimed elites are foisting it on us.

Rarely do I see patients who love their job, primarily because they are micromanaged and are not free to do it the best way they see fit. They are stressed, their careers are unfulfilling, and many keep job-hopping, hoping that the next job will be different. But it rarely is.

How Much Did My Drug Lunches Cost?

In "Big Pharma and Its Pursuit of Power," I mentioned doctors taking money or receiving gifts from pharmaceutical companies. The cost of those lunches provided to me and my staff by the pharmaceutical reps is tracked and documented on the OpenPaymentsData.CMS.gov website. You can research any doctor and see whether they have received any money or gifts from the pharmaceutical or medical device industries.

In the spirit of transparency, below are the costs of five years of lunches provided to me. The Open Payment system is updated every July 1.

Year	**Cost of Lunches**
2023	$92
2022	$1,781
2021	$2,296
2020	$2,091
2019	$2,418

If you play around on the website, you can zero in on individual transaction costs and see which pharmaceutical companies were involved. Interestingly, the reps of drug companies with diabetes drugs typically brought in the least healthy lunches.

The lunches were a nice perk for our employees and me, but it did cost me one patient appointment on the days I met with drug reps. This lost appointment was more costly than the value of the lunch, but the purpose of the lunch was to learn about the pharmaceutical reps' drugs.

And it is less likely that, without those lunches, this book would have been written.

Is Cancer a Parasitic Disease?

Half of writing history is hiding the truth.
—Captain Malcolm Reynolds, *Serenity*

> **Note:** The purpose of this chapter is to illustrate the business of cancer, not to encourage the use of what the medical establishment may consider unorthodox cancer treatments.

This chapter's title may seem like a ridiculous question. We all know that cancer is characterized by the unchecked growth of abnormal or aberrant cells. Right?

What if that concept of cancer is just a half-truth or at least not the full truth? Maybe the whole truth has been hidden. Maybe the cause of some cancer may be simpler than we realize.

This chapter's title is the same as that of an article published in *JAMA* on March 28, 1891.[237] However, it is not the first article to raise this question or explore the possibility that cancer, at least some cancers, may represent or result secondarily from a parasitic infection.

In 1890, in the *British Medical Journal*, microbiologist and pathologist William Russell, MD, reported finding parasitic spores within cancer cells. In his paper, *An Address of a Characteristic Organism of Cancer*, he formulated a hypothesis of how cancer is a parasitic disease. Today's larger medical community has dismissed this hypothesis.

The 1891 article called into question and challenged the previous year's findings but the possibility of micro-organisms possibly causing cancer goes back even to 1887.

My purpose in bringing up this topic is threefold.

1. As early as 130 years ago, medical findings and opinions were found to be at odds with one another, highlighting the uncertainty of science.
2. Our medical ancestors' thinking and actions were more advanced than we give them credit.
3. They seemed more open to questioning conventional mainstream thought than we are today.

Here are some things our medical ancestors did.

1. The first knee arthroscopy was done in 1912, though it did not become commonplace until the 1970s. Most orthopedic surgeons today may not know that.
2. The first instrument to evaluate a bladder interior was reported in 1806. Testicular transplants were being done by the mid-1800s. Our medical ancestors were quite advanced in their thinking in some ways but were limited by the technology of their days.

3. In the late 1800s, the thought that microorganisms may cause cancer was remarkable, given the limitations of technology, and it seems counterintuitive to our thinking today, but is it?

We know that some cancers are viral-related. HPV (human papillomavirus) is linked to cancers of the vulva, vagina, penis, anus, and throat. Hepatitis C is linked to liver cancer. And some cancers are linked to bacterial infections, like gastric cancers and H. pylori. Ovarian cancer has been linked to chlamydia and mycoplasma infections.[238]

Thus, the thought that parasites may cause some cancers (directly, or indirectly by changing a cell's metabolism or DNA) is not that far-fetched. Though I am not stating cancer is a parasitic disease, I am reporting what is in the medical literature and showing the rationale behind that stream of thought.

What is interesting is that more cancer studies today involve the use of anti-parasitic drugs. Drugs like ivermectin and hydroxychloroquine are used to treat parasitic infections. Might they have benefits in treating cancer? Possibly. Presently, they are being studied with that hypothesis in mind. To be clear, the cancer studies looking at ivermectin and hydroxychloroquine and other anti-parasitic drugs are not using them as stand-alone therapies but as adjunctive therapies to traditional cancer therapies.

Their use in cancer *is not misinformation*. Go to PubMed.com and search "ivermectin and cancer" and "hydroxychloroquine and cancer." For "ivermectin and cancer," I found 369 results at the time of this writing. For "hydroxychloroquine and cancer," I found 997 results, with more studies being published monthly.

Also, visit the Clinicaltrials.gov site and search "cancer and ivermectin" and "cancer hydroxychloroquine." The results are clinical trials already underway or recruiting cancer patients to study these two medications and cancer. Both medications are off patent, so there is not much profit in using them, and thus in studying them. But studies on them might lead to the development of the next generation of antiparasitic drugs that could be patented and become quite lucrative for pharmaceutical companies.

Why am I bringing up this topic of cancer as a parasitic disease? Because ivermectin and hydroxychloroquine might be useful in treating cancer. This might be a secondary reason why both medications were discouraged from use with COVID-19.

That may seem like an odd statement, a jump in logic, or a brain freeze. Let me explain.

By now, you know medicine is a big business, the biggest in the country. To thrive, it needs a sick and unhealthy population that can be treated, preferably with expensive therapies. Ivermectin and hydroxychloroquine are inexpensive. No one makes much money when physicians prescribe them.

Remember the Not-So-Wacko Jacko Rule:

Big Pharma makes it money on drugs that are still on patent. It manipulates the medical system to ensure these drugs become the first line of treatment.

Remember, ivermectin was successful in 97 percent of the COVID-19 cases in Delhi, India. But its use was discouraged here. As of March 3, 2020, China had protocols using chloroquine, a cousin of hydroxychloroquine, for COVID-19. It was found effective against coronaviruses as early as 2004.[239] Countries that used hydroxychloroquine for

COVID-19 had one-tenth the death rates as the US. But its use was discouraged here.[240] We have to ask why.

What would have happened if, instead of vaccinating masses of people for COVID-19, we had masses taking ivermectin and hydroxychloroquine to protect against COVID-19, and we then saw an unexpected benefit? For example, what if we saw a drop in cancer cases, especially early-stage ones, and those patients with cancer improving beyond what is expected on standard treatment?

You and I would think that would be great. But would that be good for the cancer business and for Big Pharma? Not at all.

No one reading this would want to believe that implication, including myself. However, based on what we know about how medicine works behind the scenes and the influence of Big Pharma on medicine, it does not seem an unlikely possibility.

You want health, they want sickness.

A study from *The British Medical Journal*, published in October 2023, found that US oncologists who accept money from pharmaceutical companies provided non-recommended and *low-value* cancer drugs to their patients. None of the non-recommended drugs cited in the study were anti-parasitic drugs, however.[241] Such oncologists are, essentially, rewarded for not keeping the patients' best interests in mind. For me, this is another example of corruption in medicine. Many people will engage in unethical activities for money; the powers know this and use it to enlist the help of ordinary people.

What you need to understand, if you don't already, is your goals for your health vary greatly from the goals of the entities that run medicine. Most providers do what they believe is in your best interest based on their controlled training. You want to prevent illness; the entities that control medicine want to treat you as expensively as possible for as long as possible.

Cancer is a money-making industry. Also, it seems you must read *The British Medical Journal* to discover how US physicians are paid off. (You may recall this journal also published payments made by pharmaceutical companies to US medical journal editors.)

Laetrile

The medical establishment has a history of squashing potentially inexpensive cures for cancer. In the 1970s, Laetrile (also known as amygdalin) was popular and inexpensive. Due to reports that Laetrile was ineffective and dangerous, it was banned for use in the United States, despite its use in other countries where it had been shown effective and safe and continues to be used.

Laetrile's story is eye-opening. It is worth watching the documentary *Second Opinion: Laetrile at Sloan-Kettering*. The documentary was produced in 2014 and focuses on Ralph Moss, PhD, assistant director of public affairs and hired as a science writer at Memorial Sloan-Kettering Cancer Center. He was closely following the work of Dr. Kanematsu Sugiura, who had been a highly regarded researcher at Sloan-Kettering for sixty years.

In the early 1970s, Dr. Sugiura discovered that Laetrile was effective in the treatment of metastatic lung cancer in laboratory animals. The results were impressive enough that the higher-ups (four physicians) at Memorial Sloan-Kettering approved and were coordinating a study to be done on humans with researchers in Mexico. But the study was never done.

In 1975, the US government stepped in and stopped the study before it could be started. Suddenly, three of the four physicians in favor of a human study did an about-face, coming out publicly against the use of amygdalin. They even stated that no animal study had ever shown it to be effective, which was not true.

Those four physicians were:

- Robert Good, MD
- Lloyd Old, MD
- Chester Stock, MD
- Lewis Thomas, MD

Dr. Moss found this about-face odd, primarily since Dr. Sugiura had provided Dr. Moss with copies of his research that showed amygdalin effective in approximately 80 percent of the cases. Because he had Dr. Sugiura's results that contradicted what the top physicians at Sloan-Kettering were stating, Dr. Moss suspected he was witnessing a cover-up.

Second Opinion portrays only Dr. Moss's side of the story, but he comes across as honest and driven to find the truth. There is a reason the four physicians were not interviewed for the 2014 documentary. All four had died by then—*all from various cancers.*

Dr. Moss was planning on writing a story on Dr. Sugiura's work on amygdalin and his impressive results when Sloan-Kettering told him to stop following Dr. Sugiura's work and asked that he lie about those results. They suggested that he instead write an article stating that studies on amygdalin were negative and that the substance was worthless.

Dr. Sugiura never claimed amygdalin to be a cure for cancer, but his several studies showed it kept cancer in check and from spreading.

Although he refused to write a negative piece on amygdalin, Dr. Moss held off on writing the story he wanted to write. He did not release any more press releases on amygdalin but continued to quietly research the reason for Sloan-Kettering leadership's abrupt turnaround. In the process, he uncovered the following:

- Sloan-Kettering's Board of Directors were investors in petrochemical and other polluting industries. The hospital was being run by people who made their wealth by investing in the worst cancer-causing things known.
- CEOs of top pharmaceutical companies that produced cancer drugs also dominated the Board. They had a vested interest in promoting chemotherapy and undermining natural therapies.
- The chairman and the president of Bristol-Myers Squibb, the world's leading producer of chemotherapy, held high positions on the Memorial Sloan-Kettering Cancer Center (MSKCC) Board.
- Of the nine members of the hospital's Institutional Policy Committee, seven had ties to the pharmaceutical industry.
- The hospital itself invested in the stock of these same drug companies.

- Directors of the biggest tobacco companies in the US, Philip Morris and RJR Nabisco, held places of honor on the Board. Six board directors also served on the boards of *The New York Times*, CBS, Warner Communications, *Reader's Digest*, and other media giants.[242]

That last discovery is important, as the media played a tremendous role in the narrative that Laetrile was ineffective and dangerous. We see similarities with COVID-19 and the media's role in denigrating the off-label use of anti-parasitic medications to treat that disease.

Also, what Dr. Moss uncovered nicely illustrates how the entities that control medicine protect each other, as discussed already in "Big Pharma and Its Pursuit of Power."

Finally, in November 1977, Dr. Moss held a press conference and blew the whistle on Memorial Sloan Kettering Cancer Center's suppression of positive results with amygdalin. He was fired the Monday following his press conference.

His firing is an example of what happens when a physician or key employee does not toe the establishment's line. We saw similar actions taken against those who were vocal about COVID-19 management. We are now seeing specialty boards revoking the certification of physicians who have not followed the medical establishment's preferred narrative.[243]

All of this serves to remind us of things we never seem to grasp. History, they say, repeats itself. People in power will do what they can to stay in power. Physicians do not control their profession.

The medical establishment controls physicians and medical information, but it is losing its grip on the latter. With the advent of the internet and open access to much medical information, the medical establishment is losing its monopoly on medical information. Consequently, it relies more and more on mainstream media and "fact-checkers" to steer the public to certain sources of medical information to help control the desired narrative. And now, it appears to have moved on to "punishing" physicians who express thoughts contrary to the preferred narrative.

You need to be aware of that and engage in your own research.

FDA and Laetrile

William W. Vodra, the FDA's former associate chief counsel, said, "No one is going to pay $70,000 for a new cancer drug if they can buy Laetrile for 75 cents." That statement would not be shocking if it came from someone representing Big Pharma, but that statement comes from the FDA's legal counsel. I guess we can say it does represent the pharmaceutical industry since it is largely funded by it.244

The FDA decides which drugs are banned. As stated before, even by a former FDA Commissioner, the FDA protects the pharmaceutical industry.

Mr. Vodra's statement is from the 1970s, when chemotherapy was far less expensive than it is today. Today, chemotherapy can run $200,000 and immunotherapy $300,000. Laetrile is probably still 75 cents.

It seems likely that, once the board of directors of Memorial Sloan Kettering Cancer Center realized there was little money to be made with Laetrile, they pressured physicians to abandon any studies on its use.

Recent studies done in other countries show that amygdalin is effective and safe in the treatment of cancer, but you still cannot get it in the US.[245]

Costs of Cancer Treatments

Cancer is a big business. So big that more people make a living from cancer than die from it, and it is the second leading cause of death. According to the National Cancer Institute, the costs of cancer care are expected to grow from $190.2 billion in 2015 to $246.6 billion by 2030.[246] The average patient's out-of-pocket expenses are:

- $43,516 for initial care;
- $5,516 for continuing care; and
- $109,727 in the last year of life.

National out-of-pocket expenses for the four most common cancers approximate:[247]

- $3.14 billion for breast cancer;
- $2.26 billion for prostate cancer;
- $1.15 billion for colorectal cancer; and
- $1.35 billion for lung cancer.

Keep in mind that these are only out-of-pocket expenses. They show that, indeed, cancer is a big business.

Once you build something, you have to keep it in business. The same is true in medicine. We have a proliferation of cancer and heart hospitals that must now stay in business. Just as we must feed the military-industrial complex, we must now feed cancer and heart hospitals. Preventing cancer or "curing" it in its early stages with non-profitable drugs is self-defeating from a business standpoint.

More money can be made by pushing vaccines and antivirals for COVID-19 than with ivermectin and hydroxychloroquine. Also, there are more lucrative cancer treatments than ivermectin and hydroxychloroquine and, potentially, more lucrative ones down the pipe.

Ivermectin and Cancer

Best known as the horse dewormer, ivermectin is approved to treat several human diseases and, not uncommonly, used to treat scabies and lice.

Ivermectin has several mechanisms of action useful in treating cancer, mainly acting on cancer-signaling pathways involved in cancer proliferation (the Wnt, AKT, and mTOR pathways).[248] Plus, it inhibits cancer stem cells. Ivermectin also

- inhibits the proliferation and metastasis of cancer cells;
- inhibits angiogenesis (disrupts blood vessel growth to cancer cells);
- promotes programmed cancer cell death through apoptosis, autophagy, and pyroptosis;
- reverses and prevents multidrug resistance; and
- optimizes effects of the concomitant use of other chemotherapy drugs.

Ivermectin has been studied as a treatment for twenty cancers. William Makis, MD, has explored these studies on Substack.com: bladder, lung, glioma, multiple myeloma, ovarian, prostate, colon, pancreatic, melanoma, cervical, hepatocellular carcinoma, osteosarcoma, gastric, leukemia, esophageal, cholangiocarinoma, breast cancer stem cells, chronic myeloid leukemia, renal cell carcinoma, and glioblastoma.

As you review the references to this section on ivermectin and amygdalin, pay close attention to the names of the researchers behind the studies. For a more complete picture of what is and can be done in medicine, you must get away from only reading research from the United States centers. You also need to get past the point of thinking that US medicine is the best and most advanced in the world. Remember, the US is 49th in life expectancy among developed nations despite spending the most money and our healthy diet of drugs.

Hydroxychloroquine and Cancer

Hydroxychloroquine and its cousin, chloroquine, also have several anti-cancer effects:

- They affect several pathways important for control of cancer growth, including the Toll-9/NF-κB receptor pathway, activate stress response pathways, enhance p53 activity, and CXCR4-CXCL12 expression in cancer cells.
- They normalize blood flow to cancer cells, which tends to be high.
- They activate the immune system by changing tumor-associated macrophages from M2 to M1.
- They stimulate cancer-associated fibroblasts.

Hydroxychloroquine is used to treat SLE (lupus) and rheumatoid arthritis and to prevent malaria. In many African countries, it is available over the counter. Is a once-a-week dose enough to prevent cancer or keep early-stage cancer in check? Maybe. Maybe not.

Fenbendazole and Cancer

This is another anti-parasitic medication that looks promising in the treatment of cancer. Fenbendazole has 12 proven anti-cancer mechanisms, according to William Makis, MD, an oncologist.[249] Fenbendazole belongs to the benzimidazole class of drugs. That class has been used since the 1960s to treat helminth (worm) infections in livestock and humans. Toxicities from benzimidazoles are very rare.

Fenbendazole is not FDA-approved for human use, but it is used in veterinary medicine. It is very inexpensive.

The twelve anti-cancer mechanisms of fenbendazole

- disrupt microtubule polymerization (a major mechanism);
- induce cell cycle (G2/M) arrest;
- block glucose transport and impairs glucose utilization by cancer cells (major);
- increase p53 tumor suppressor levels (major);
- inhibit cancer cell viability (mTOR);
- inhibit cancer cell migration and invasion (EMT pathway);
- induce apoptosis;

- induce autophagy;
- induce pyroptosis and necrosis;
- induce differentiation and senescence;
- inhibit tumor angiogenesis;
- reduce colony formation and inhibit stem-ness in cancer cells; and
- may sensitize cancer cells to radiation therapy.

No clinical trials using fenbendazole have been done. However, mebendazole, one of its cousins, is FDA-approved (brand name of Emverm) for human use and is much more expensive than fenbendazole.

Mebendazole is being studied in the treatment of colon cancer (phase 3 trials) and brain tumors FN (phase 1 trials) and in pancreatic cancers.[250]

To illustrate the cost difference between a non-patented drug and a patented one, one capsule of non-patented fenbendazole is $0.55.[251] One tablet of patented mebendazole costs $600 to $700.[252] That is a significant price difference. If you were a pharmaceutical company, which drug would you study to treat cancer?

Economics plays a huge role in the way medicine is practiced.

It is unlikely someone will pay millions of dollars to fund clinical trials unless the medications being studied can provide an acceptable return on investment. Fenbendazole is not a medication that will bring a healthy return on investment, even if it were approved for human use, but mebendazole can—and it is the one being studied in cancer.

That's another thing about drugs and medical research. Rarely will drug companies study things that are not potentially profitable. Your cupboards likely store inexpensive items that have health benefits that will never be studied.

Think back to my earlier comment on ivermectin and hydroxychloroquine being discouraged from use in the treatment of COVID-19 because they might provide secondary benefits with cancer treatment. Does it now seem less off-base?

What If Cancer Is Not a Parasitic Disease?

Again, I am not stating cancer is a parasitic disease or that it results secondarily from a prior parasitic infection. I am reporting what appears in the literature and shows a rationale behind the concept that some cancers may be caused by parasites.

But even if it can be proven, beyond all doubt, that no cancer is a parasitic disease or a result of a parasitic infection, it does not mean antiparasitic drugs cannot and do not work in cancer. One reason I listed the mechanisms of action for some of these antiparasitic drugs was to show the many ways they potentially stop cell growth, and that includes growth in cancer cells.

Researchers are studying them for a reason. There is something to their use.

We must abandon this antiquated view that antivirals are only effective against viruses, antibiotics are only effective against bacteria, antifungals are only effective against fungi, and anti-parasitic drugs are only effective against parasites. All of them kill cells or microorganisms, or at least, they stop their growth. Likely, there is some cross-over utility for them in infectious diseases, and other disease processes like cancer and autoimmune disease.

Azithromycin, an antibiotic, was found helpful in COVID-19, which is caused by a virus. Hydroxychloroquine treats autoimmune diseases like SLE and rheumatoid arthritis.

> **My prediction:** If some of these inexpensive anti-parasitic drugs are shown to be effective in some types of cancer, Big Pharma will make the next generation of patented anti-parasitic drugs that they can profit from. That is probably already underway.

Until Big Pharma makes the next generation of patented anti-parasitic medication, it cannot afford to have too many people benefit from the less expensive, off-patent ones currently available. They may be motivated to suppress such information and discourage any off-label use.

The purpose of this discussion is not to encourage using Laetrile or anti-parasitic drugs for cancer without first discussing it with a qualified physician. Instead, I want to highlight the business nature of cancer and medicine and the degree to which Big Pharma, with the FDA running interference, controls the medical field. Big Pharma will do whatever it can so that only profitable treatments will be used first.

Were the potential cancer benefits of anti-parasitic medications in the back of the minds of those who called the shots on COVID-19 when the use of anti-parasitic drugs was suppressed and discouraged? Based on history, it does seem plausible.

Cancer and infectious diseases are not the only areas where repurposed drugs may be beneficial. There are over nineteen thousand FDA-approved drugs, many of which have more than one mechanism of action, making it likely that physicians may prescribe these drugs for conditions for which they are not currently approved.

Drugs can be repurposed in about half the time it takes to research, develop, and test a novel drug therapy and at far less cost.[253] There are seven thousand rare diseases, 95 percent of which have no FDA-approved therapeutic agent. Potentially, repurposing can help those who suffer from these diseases rather than waiting for a novel drug to be developed.[254]

Note: Some patients request prescriptions of hydroxychloroquine or ivermectin to have on hand in the event they contract COVID-19. Most doctors are resistant to writing such prescriptions, and patients may be tempted to obtain these anti-parasitic medications through foreign online sites when unable to obtain them through proper channels in the US.

I strongly recommend against doing so. The drug's purity is paramount, plus there is a high probability your shipment will be confiscated upon arrival in the United States.

Where You Get Your Information Matters

In politics the truth is strictly optional and that also seems to be true in parts of the media.
—Thomas Sowell

As we inch closer to the topic of COVID-19, we need to look at the media and how the information we receive and believe shapes our thoughts. Some bamboozling, duping, and hoodwinking related to medicine comes from the media.

About the above quote, let me disclose that I do not hold career politicians and many of today's national news journalists in high regard. Both groups excel at telling half-truths, and I have little respect for such individuals.

I share the following thoughts because they come into play when we get to "COVID-19."

Career Politicians

Many career politicians feign doing good and being on the side of the people but are among the most corrupt in society. They enrich themselves at our expense. Many have sociopathic features. (I refer you to Dr. Stout's comments in "Observations of a Rapper.")

I think anyone who thinks politicians, as a whole, call the shots is quite naive. Politicians are merely the face of the real power players. They should don logos of the special interest groups they genuinely represent. Politicians largely exist to give us the illusion of choice. With some exceptions, we have a one-party system with two unpalatable flavors.

Just like much of the medical establishment has sold out to corporate interests at the expense of patients' well-being, career politicians have chosen to be well-paid corporate slaves rather than public servants.

The Media

As medical journals are marketing extensions of the pharmaceutical companies, the mainstream media are marketing extensions of the real powers in Washington, DC, and globally—those who control the politicians. Some refer to the politico-media complex. We seem to have many complexes that run and control society.

The media specializes in sensationalizing everything, whether in politics, medicine, sports, and so on. Most things are not as dramatic as the media portrays, and the media specializes in creating fear, which is what it does best. Also, when it comes to health information, the media are dependent on pharmaceutical ad money.

Someone once said they are more impressed with the person who sets out to improve their little corner of the world and ends up influencing the world, like Mother Teresa, than the person whose focus from the get-go is to change the world. Many politicians and some journalists fall into that group that needs to transform the world and make a splash while quenching their thirst for control and influence.

Politicization of the COVID-19 Pandemic

It is hard to discuss COVID-19 without wading into some of the unfortunate politicization of the pandemic. I think most readers realize that there is a political divide on views of COVID-19 and the vaccines. If you know someone's political party affiliation, you could probably accurately guess their views on COVID-19 and whether they were vaccinated, and if vaccinated, how many boosters they received. If, today, you see someone wearing a mask in a car, you can probably peg how they vote.

There may be a chicken or egg question on this topic. Do we believe the news we receive, or do we gravitate to the news sources we wish to believe? Some patients hop from doctor to doctor until they find one who tells them what they want to hear. Are we doing the same with our news sources?

But here is what we do know.

Journalists and Party Affiliation

Let's start with the party affiliation of journalists.

Every ten years, Syracuse University surveys journalists in the US, asking about their political party affiliation. The 2022 Syracuse study is called the "American Journalist Under Attack: Media, Trust, and Democracy: Key Findings."[255]

The first survey was done in 1971, and, at that time, 35.5 percent of the journalists were Democrats and 25.7 percent were Republicans, with the bulk of the remainder being Independents.

In 2022, only 3.4 percent of the journalists were Republicans, with 36.4 percent being Democrat,s and the bulk of the remainder Independents.

Thus, there has been a huge drop in the number of Republican journalists and a slight increase in Democrat journalists over the past fifty years. That likely affects how the mainstream media reports the news. The title of one article I referenced for this chapter is Astonishing Number of Journalists Align with Democratic Party, so a political slant to the news should not be unexpected. This is a polite way to say it is biased.

More journalists are college-educated than in 1971, which may explain more of the gap between the left (Democrats) and right (Republicans). Let's look at the reason for this gap.

Results of the Syracuse University findings prompted well-known reporter and political pundit David Brooks to say, "Now we're not only a college-dominated profession, we're an elite-college-dominated profession."[256]

In this era of diversity, equity, and inclusion (which may be reaching an end), college campuses may be the least diverse and inclusive segments of society. Thirty-nine percent of the top sixty-six liberal arts colleges had no registered Republican professor. In anthropology departments, the Democrat-to-Republican ratio was 133:1, and in social science, the ratio was 133:0.

Another survey of colleges showed that 72 percent of the faculty are liberal, with 15 percent being conservative. Also, they have more liberals than conservatives in every department surveyed, with business departments having the closest ratio of 49 percent liberals to 39 percent conservatives.[257]

Consequently, it is likely that the unbalanced exposure to liberal/democrat ideology affects the views of journalists.

"Elite" is frequently a self-description. Elite people like to do your thinking for you, one reason they refer to themselves as "elite," as in being superior to you and me.

Voter Party Affiliation

These 2022 numbers from the Syracuse study are out of alignment with the American electorate, however. In 2023, Gallup's weekly polls consistently showed that 29 percent of voters are Republican, 29 percent are Democrats, and 40 percent are Independents. (Party Affiliation, Gallup News.258

Party Affiliation and Views on COVID-19

Consider vaccination rates by party affiliation. According to Gallup, as of September 2021, 92 percent of Democrats had received at least one dose of a COVID-19 vaccine compared to 56 percent of Republicans.

Now, let me backtrack.

Near the time of the COVID-19 vaccine roll-out, in December 2020, a poll conducted on five thousand US adults through the Franklin Templeton-Gallup Economics of Recovery Study found that, regardless of party affiliation, most Americans overstated the risk of being hospitalized from COVID-19.

At that time, the risk of hospitalization was 1–5 percent, depending on the data source. Republicans scored better than Democrats on that, with 26 percent of Republicans giving the correct response as compared to 10 percent of Democrats. But both groups overstated the risk of hospitalization which seems to suggest that there was much misinformation being spread through the media regardless of source.[259]

In August 2021, about nine months after the vaccine rollouts, Gallup conducted a poll on 3,158 U.S. adults and asked two questions:

1. As far as you know, what percentage of unvaccinated people have been hospitalized due to coronavirus?
2. As far as you know, what percentage of fully vaccinated people have been hospitalized due to coronavirus?

The correct response is less than 1 percent of unvaccinated and less than 1 percent of vaccinated were hospitalized for COVID-19.[260]

That is not a misprint. Less than 1 percent of the vaccinated and less than 1 percent of the unvaccinated were hospitalized for the disease. Gallup calculated that information using data from the Department of Health and Human Services and the US Centers for Disease Control and Prevention (CDC).

I will go over more of these types of data in "COVID-19: Chaos, Confusion, and Coercion" and "Pfizer's Deceptive COVID-19 Vaccine Trial."

By subtracting the response to question 2 from question 1, Gallup calculated a respondent's view on vaccine efficacy, which I discuss in more detail in that chapter as well.

Misinterpreting Vaccine Efficacy

Democrats, regardless of vaccination status, were more accurate than Republicans, regardless of vaccination status, on the efficacy of COVID-19 vaccines. But how we define vaccine efficacy is misleading. (I will go into it in "Pfizer's Deceptive COVID-19 Vaccine Trial.")

More accurately, I should say the meaning of "vaccine efficacy" is misinterpreted by the media and many physicians.

When you hear that a vaccine is 95–99 percent effective in preventing infection and 96 percent effective in preventing hospitalization, you likely assume that 95–99 percent of those vaccinated will not contract COVID-19 and 96 percent of those vaccinated will not be hospitalized by it.[261] That is not what it means. It cannot possibly mean that. Here's why.

Less than 1 percent of the unvaccinated were hospitalized with COVID-19, meaning 99 percent-plus avoided hospitalization without the vaccine. Let me rephrase it this way. Not being vaccinated was 99 percent effective in "preventing" hospitalization from COVID-19.

That 96 percent efficacy means that the 1 percent of the unvaccinated who were hospitalized with COVID-19 would have been reduced by 96 percent had they been vaccinated. In other words, instead of 1 percent being hospitalized who were not vaccinated, it would be 0.04 percent had they been vaccinated. This will make more sense when we get to the chapter on Pfizer's vaccine trial.

It goes back to what was discussed in "You Are Not Likely to Die of Anything but Will Die of Something." You need to know the baseline incidence of a disease or condition and the natural frequency of something if left untreated.

The reported 95–99 percent are relative risk reductions, and they are intended to mislead. It has been shown that physicians are more likely to write prescriptions based on relative risk reduction rather than the more important absolute risk reduction. Based on relative risk reduction, physicians are also more likely to recommend vaccines. The main purpose of relative risk reduction is to make things look more dramatic than they are—like the media do.

Ask your physician for the absolute risk reduction and the numbers needed to treat. That is the information you want to make the best decision for yourself. Likely, your physician will not be able to tell you because they will not know, and they will not know because such information is not readily available.

If reducing your 1 percent chance of being hospitalized with COVID-19 by not being vaccinated to 0.04 percent by being vaccinated is significant enough to offset the unknown risks of a vaccine using a never-before vaccine platform in your mind, then getting the vaccine is worthwhile.

However, keep in mind that more side effects come with the vaccine as opposed to not being vaccinated. You need to know your risk tolerance. Outside of getting COVID-19 (which has a high survival rate), there are no side effects to not being vaccinated—and *the risk of getting a side effect is greater than the risk of avoiding hospitalization because you were not vaccinated.* You need to know the odds.

Thus, there are some minimal benefits to the COVID-19 vaccines but not nearly as many as most people were led to believe due to misinterpretation or intentional misleading of vaccine efficacy. We will find out soon, in the next chapters, that the benefit of the vaccines is short-lived and the vaccines are associated with more adverse effects than advertised.

When there is less than a 1 percent risk of hospitalization in the unvaccinated, vaccine efficacy numbers of 95–99 percent border on being meaningless. If 50 percent of the unvaccinated were hospitalized for COVID-19, then a 95–99 percent efficacy rate would have meaning, but not at 1 percent. That is true for all vaccines you might receive as an adult.

The net effect is that Democrats scored better than Republicans on a somewhat meaningless metric, at least as applied to the case of COVID-19 vaccines.

Unvaccinated Hospitalization Rates

But here is where things get interesting. For the *unvaccinated* hospitalization risk, only 2 percent of Democrats responded correctly compared to 16 percent of the Republicans. Again, the correct answer is less than 1 percent.

The data that stands out most is that 41 percent of Democrats felt that at least 50 percent of the unvaccinated were hospitalized due to COVID-19. That over 50 percent response was far and away the most common response given by Democrats.[262]

Where you get your information matters.

Why would the average Democrat believe that 50 percent of those with COVID-19 who were unvaccinated required hospitalization when it was less than 1 percent? It's doubtful they came to that figure on their own.

A huge difference lies between 50 percent and 1 percent. How can there be such a stark difference between perception and reality? My best explanation is that it relates to the journalists' party affiliation and, thus, the reporting of the news, coupled with the news consumer's bias and gravitating to certain news outlets.

We all have biases, and journalists probably have more than most. Those who own and run media companies, of which there are only a handful, probably have even bigger agendas. If you control the news, you control brains. And one way to accomplish that control is to stoke fear and misrepresent data. Fear paralyzes and allows individuals to condition and shape the thoughts of others. With the installation of fear, you can get people to believe almost anything and do almost anything.

Fear

Fear drove many COVID-19 decisions and much human behavior, but little for the good.

Sociologist Barry Glassner wrote *The Culture of Fear,* in which he talks about fearmongering. He explains that, over eight years, there was a 20 percent drop in murders, yet a 600 percent increase in reports of murders on network news during that same period.[263]

That much news coverage devoted to murders probably affects the outlook of many. This is not unlike medical publications. If all you read are positive outcome studies on antidepressants, you begin to believe they should be in the drinking water, when, in truth, they work only about half the time.

Fear is used whenever facts are not on the side of the narrative. In medicine, we saw it in the case of anabolic steroid use. "If we don't have facts, let's scare the athletes from using them."

Here is one example of the media stoking fear and trying to manipulate our thoughts from the *Washington Post Podcasts*:

> There's a pervasive idea that your body and your immune system can be healthy enough to ward off COVID-19, which of course is a novel coronavirus. No one's body can. No one's body is healthy enough to recognize and just totally ward this off without a vaccine.[264]

Do you see anything wrong or out of place with that statement? Look at it again, closely.

By October 2021, we were 22 months into the pandemic. When the *Post made* that statement, millions and millions worldwide had already had COVID-19 and survived without a vaccine, disproving the statement. Yet, people fell for not a half-truth but an outright lie spread by the media. Why did the media intentionally lie?

The government wants to control us with laws, and the media with propaganda—and they work together to achieve that goal, thus, the politico-media complex. That Washington Post quote highlights how little respect the media have for us, the public. They do not respect us, and yet, many of us keep going back to them for more deception and more distortions.

In response to a Gallup poll, which shows declining trust in the media and his decision not to have *The Washington Post* endorse a presidential candidate, Jeff Bezos, founder of Amazon and owner of *The Washington Post,* said

> We must be accurate, and we must be believed to be accurate. It's a bitter pill to swallow, but we are failing on the second requirement. Most people believe the media Is (sic) biased. Anyone who doesn't see this is paying scant attention to reality, and those who fight reality lose... What presidential endorsements actually do is create a perception of bias. A perception of non-independence. Ending them is a principled decision, and it's the right one.[265]

Some have far too much trust in the government, the media, and the medical profession.

We all need to accept that the powers that run the world have an ongoing desire to manipulate our thinking in all areas of life. There is a battle for control of our minds.

He who controls the media, controls the mind.
—Jim Morrison

Just as pharmaceutical companies control the brains of physicians, media companies attempt to influence your thoughts, and that is more likely to occur the more you watch or listen to the news.

We are, largely, nothing more than our thoughts. Protect what you allow into your brain.

Given the vast discrepancy Democrat voters perceived between COVID-19 hospitalization rates and the reality of the unvaccinated, coupled with the significant discrepancy in political party affiliation among journalists, we might conclude that Democrat voters get their health and other news from mainstream media outlets which seemed "all in" on COVID-19, painting a dire scenario.

You would think or, at least hope, that when it comes to your health, mainstream news would give accurate information because lives are at stake. That it did not occur makes you, or at least me, wonder how inaccurate the rest of the reporting may be from mainstream news on other topics.

The last place you expect deception is in medicine. That includes health information. If the media are deceptive with health news, what else are they willing to lie about?

Remember this Not-So-Wacko Jacko Rule of Medicine:

The people who control medicine are willing to risk your health in their quest for money, power, and control.

I rarely watch mainstream news or listen to talk radio. The few times I watched mainstream news during the peak of COVID-19, it reinforced and fueled the panic surrounding COVID-19, outlining a doomsday scenario not borne out by what I was seeing in my practice and my research.

The few times I listened to talk radio, I would hear nearly the opposite. Based on what I was seeing, the truth was in the middle, but much closer to the conservative side.

In the end, we panicked, or were led to panic, over a virus that had a 99 percent overall survival rate. And we scared people into vaccines and social isolation and stripped them of their ability to work. Through fear, we pitted family members and co-workers against one another.

Instead of feeling disbelief with that statement, we should feel anger, especially those who had a loved one die because we did not use all treatments available, lost jobs during the pandemic, developed severe reactions to the vaccines, developed depression and anxiety, or whose children, greatly affected by the changes in the education system, have fallen behind one to two years developmentally and socially. Some of you should be furious. You were bamboozled, duped, and hoodwinked.

Due to living in the Internet Age, we have gone from not having enough information to having too much information. Discerning the truth has become more challenging, and the media have decided to "help" you in this search.

Changing Opinions in 2024

We are beginning to see a bit of changing opinions when it comes to COVID-19 and the perceived benefits of the vaccines. This phenomenon probably cannot be explained by media influence, however, because the change goes against the narrative.

In January 2024, Rasmussen reported that 53 percent of American adults believe it is likely that side effects of COVID-19 vaccines have caused a significant number of unexplained deaths. Among adults, 24 percent say they know someone whose death they think may have been caused by the vaccine's effects.

In that survey, 54 percent of Americans believe there are legitimate reasons to be concerned about the vaccines' safety (69 percent of Republicans and 37 percent of Democrats). But another 33 percent think people concerned about vaccine safety are spreading conspiracy theories, and another 13 percent are unsure.

In June 2024, Rasmussen reported that 24 percent of American adults who got at least one dose of a COVID-19 vaccine *regret* getting vaccinated, with 69 percent having no regrets.

That same survey looked at Americans' trust in the medical and pharmaceutical industries. It found that

- 17 percent of Americans have a lot of trust for the medical and pharmaceutical industries;
- 37 percent have some trust;
- 25 percent don't have much trust; and
- 18 percent have no trust at all.

The survey also found that trust in the medical and pharmaceutical industries correlated with how many reported vaccine doses. Of those who received the initial round of vaccinations plus boosters, 80 percent have at least some trust in the medical and pharmaceutical industries, dropping to

41 percent among those who received just one dose and 30 percent among those not vaccinated at all.

Why do I say these opinions in 2024 are probably not influenced by the media? Because the media immediately label as a "conspiracy theorist" or "wacko" anyone who publicly states that the vaccines are harming people. The media has quashed negative news about vaccines. Consequently, the changing opinions about vaccine concerns in 2024 are being driven by something else.

Monopoly of Medical Information No Longer Exists

Before the internet, the medical community monopolized medical information. That is no longer true. You have access to nearly all the same medical information that I and other physicians have. *You no longer need to rely on the media for health news.* Many of you may not have realized this. A goal of this book is to make you less dependent on others for health information.

To control the desired narrative, the medical establishment relies more on the media and uses faceless and nameless "fact checkers," spin doctors, to steer the general population to the information the establishment wants people to see and hear. Also, doctors discourage you from doing your own research. These are all control mechanisms.

You no longer need to rely on the media for health news.

Doctors are trained in a limited space and know little other than medications and surgery. They don't want to be challenged on things they do not understand. By doing your research, you become a threat to them, and you will get an eye roll from your doctor.

Experience

What else is changing opinions on COVID-19 vaccines and leading to a decline in trust in the medical and pharmaceutical industries? I have no data to explain it, but I suspect it is based on personal experience and the experience of their close friends, family, and co-workers. Plus, their own research.

To me, much of this change in opinion on the vaccines is akin to politicians discussing the state of the economy. A politician can throw out all sorts of numbers trying to show the economy is strong and vibrant, but as people look at their bank accounts, bills, and rising prices, they know things are not as rosy as being peddled. Their personal experience evaluates the economy.

And I suspect the same is true with the vaccines. The establishment and media can talk all they want about how great the COVID-19 vaccines are, but...

People now have experience to draw upon and are less dependent on studies and news accounts. They have witnessed firsthand how the pandemic and vaccines have personally affected them. I alluded to this in "Science Is Always Wrong, until It Gets it Right." What matters is what works for the individual or what affects them, not any study's outcome.

Dr. Hughston was big on "trusting and believing your own experiences," which is not easy to internalize when your experience runs counter to mainstream thought, goes against the grain of your peers, and you find yourself solidly in the minority.

Experience and data are both important, but data can be manipulated. Do we really need to offer alternative explanations for what can be experienced? For example, do we believe politicians when they say, "I know you are about to go bankrupt, but the economy is doing well. Trust me"? To explain away experience, they peddle misinformation: "What you are experiencing is not real." You respond, "Well, I am flat broke. That's real."

Some of our politicians and media are not much different than Baghdad Bob, the Iraqi Information Minister, who made outlandish statements during his reporting of the US-led invasion of Iraq in 2003. You may remember hearing him say, "It has been rumored that we have fired Scud missiles into Kuwait. I am here now to tell you we do not have any Scud missiles, and I don't know why they were fired into Kuwait."[266] (You'll find more of his notable quotes online.) Many of us familiar with that time laughed at Baghdad Bob, but we fall for similar deceptions from our leaders and media. Although those deceptions are not quite as outlandish, some of them are every bit as untruthful.

Untrue is untrue regardless of how subtle or how outlandish the statement. The half-truth is a subtle lie. Our media, medical establishment, and government have mastered the art of the half-truth.

Not-So-Wacko Jacko Rule of Medicine:

Avoid mainstream media for your health news.

You have access to the same medical news doctors do. Take advantage of it.

Many who were vaccinated still contracted COVID-19, and some have gotten it three or four times. I have seen some of these patients. The vaccines are not working as advertised. Some individuals have developed new health conditions they did not have before being vaccinated, which, in and of itself, does *not* prove cause and effect, but when such occurrences are happening, many times over, with people they know, they begin to have doubts. I've seen reports of people whose cancer was in remission but has returned and is now untreatable, and I hear reports of unusual and more aggressive cancers.

New-onset autoimmune diseases have occurred in those vaccinated too.[267] Sudden deaths have increased fivefold in professional European soccer players since the vaccines, in comparison to the pre-vaccine era.[268]

OneAmerica, an insurance company providing group benefits, saw a 40 percent increase in deaths in the working-age population (ages 18–64), the group subjected to the vaccine mandates. To put that in perspective, the insurance industry sees only a 10 percent increase in deaths during a one in two hundred years catastrophe.[269]

But because the media says otherwise, viewers believe it.

Where You Go for News Matters

Where you go for your news does matter. Personally, I felt the world was better off when all we had was thirty minutes of local news in the evening, followed by thirty minutes of national/world news. Those thirty minutes were spent reporting the news, not shaping or creating the news and telling you how to think.

There was less time for "brainwashing." News 24/7/365, where topics are discussed ad nauseam, with people vegetating much of the day in front of the television and journalists trying to justify their existence, is shaping people's thoughts and behavior more than we realize.

Free yourself from someone else's interpretation. Recognize that you do not need the media to get health information. Go to PubMed.com or Cochrane Reviews (CochraneLibrary.com) and research whatever topic is important to you. You have the same access to medical information as I do—you may just not realize it.

I recommend you read studies on health topics important to you rather than relying on someone's interpretation. I have seen cases where reporters interpret a study's results incorrectly. As much as possible, and this is true for physicians who previously relied only on CDC guidance, go to the source. The media, frequently, are not the source of the news they report.

I also recommend gathering all points of view, pondering them carefully, filling in missing information with the best logic and common sense you can muster, and then periodically reviewing and challenging your views and opinions. You are searching for the truth. When you're done, you may not like what you've uncovered, but that doesn't change the truth.

The truth, likely, lies somewhere in the middle (but not in the dead center) of all you review. Be objective and cast aside your emotions. Emotionally charged people are more easily manipulated by those who know how to stoke emotions.

I respect doctors who are thoughtful in their approach to what they do and why they do it. They have excellent reasons beyond "That's the way we've always done it," or "That is what they told us to do." Rarely do they buy everything conventional medicine is selling. They don't take a one-size-fits-all approach; they personalize care to the individual. Simply put, they think.

Despite having several great mentors, I did not always agree with them, nor were they 100 percent right all the time. You must do your thinking, and thinking is hard work.

Importance of Critical Thinking

I read or heard that Steve Jobs would spend three hours a day just thinking of the next big idea. If you look at Apple's history, the company typically came out with a game-changing product about every five years during Mr. Jobs' tenure. That is a lot of thinking in between ideas.

What has Apple come up with since his death? Not much, which demonstrates the importance of thinking.

You have a brain. Use it! You should not simply be a sponge and passively absorb what you are told and take it at face value. You need to reject some of what you are being told. Engage in critical thinking. Do your research.

Our ability to think is what separates humans from every other living being. We seem to have developed a society where we gladly pass the baton onto others to think for us, including physicians who primarily relied strictly on CDC guidance during the pandemic, with nary a challenge to its recommendations.

You do not need the media to tell you what you should think. And there is little from watching mainstream news that is going to improve your life. The media are not any more of an expert on any topic or life than you are.

You are controlled by those who control your thoughts. Hence, be the one who controls your thoughts. You can never be your whole self if you do not think for yourself.

I encourage everyone to think!

The individual has always had to struggle to keep from being overwhelmed by the tribe. If you try it, you will be lonely often, and sometimes frightened. But no price is too high to pay for the privilege of owning yourself.

—Rudyard Kipling

PART VI

COVID-19: Chaos, Confusion, and Coercion

The urge to save humanity is almost always only a false-face for the urge to rule it.
—H. L. Mencken

Nothing speaks to being bamboozled, duped, and hoodwinked as much as the handling of the COVID-19 pandemic. Future generations of doctors will scratch their heads when they learn how we managed this pandemic.

Medicine's half-truths were probably never more prevalent and never more implemented than with COVID-19 but with the addition of fear and more fear.

Probably a higher percentage of patients expressed doubt about the handling of COVID-19 than expressed by those within the medical profession. Often, patients see the half-truths of medicine better than physicians.

I believe that physicians bought into the narrative that the medical establishment promoted at a higher rate because they were just better programmed by the system and had a higher level of trust. Physicians are so sure of what they have been taught that they rarely question anything.

We know the public is losing trust in the medical profession. A relatively high percentage of patients try to avoid seeing doctors as much as possible and gravitate to alternative and complementary providers due to a lack of faith in the medical establishment. About 38 percent of the US population receives at least some of its healthcare services from alternative and complementary providers.[270]

Patients seem to have a higher distrust of conventional medicine than physicians realize. That is borne out by the Rasmussen surveys reviewed in the previous chapter. Now, patients are more likely to question the effectiveness of the lockdowns, the masking, the social distancing, and the vaccines than physicians.

Conventional medicine has an image problem that it does not realize exists.

Freedom

One issue that came up with COVID-19 is that people want to exercise their freedom of choice. We have an incomplete view of freedom. We think of freedom as only being able to do what we want to do (as long as it is not harmful to others). It goes beyond that. *Freedom is also the ability to not do what you don't want to do.*

Many people did not want to mask, and many did not want to be vaccinated. Some were coerced into being vaccinated. The freedom of choice to not do what they did not want to do was taken from them. They were coerced into the vaccines, masking, and social distancing for the "good of society."

Given the corruption of scientific information and the realization that the media engages in misinformation, perhaps we should be careful about surrendering freedom for the good of society and in the name of public health. We slide down a slippery slope when we give up freedoms in the name of public health, yet many of us were willing to slide down during the height of the pandemic. The government can make anything into a public health issue with the aid of unscrupulous physicians, propagandizing media, and bogus science.[IP]

Freedom is also the ability to not do what you don't want to do.

Do you want to give up freedoms based on bogus science and not just medical science?

It may be wise to consider three things, Robert F. Kennedy Jr. said in his speech at Defeat the Mandates on January 23, 2022.[271]

- Every power that the government takes from us will never be relinquished voluntarily.
- Every power they take from us, they will ultimately abuse to the maximum extent possible.
- Nobody in the history of the planet has ever complied their way out of totalitarian control.

Living in our country, we tend to think that things Mr. Kennedy says could not happen in this country. But how many of you expected to learn of the deceptions and half-truths of medicine you are now learning?

Benjamin Franklin once said, "Those who would give up essential liberty to purchase a little temporary safety, deserve neither liberty nor safety."

During the peak of the pandemic, many were willing to give up many freedoms in exchange for safety. That safety was largely an illusion because it was based on half-truths. Thousands have died in the history of this country for us to have the freedoms we have, and overnight, we were quick to give some of them up.

Every time you give up a freedom, willingly or unwillingly, you become less of a human. If you give up enough freedoms, you become a slave or a puppet. You are no longer your own person. You become subhuman to those who pull the strings. With some of our freedoms disappearing these days unwillingly, it may not be wise to voluntarily give up more.

Coercion

In Robert Fulghum's book *All I Really Need to Know, I Learned in Kindergarten,* I happened to learn a valuable lesson a year after kindergarten. It's a story about coercion.

It was the winter of 1966-67, and my teacher was Mrs. Trimple. She was old. She looked older than my grandmother, who looked old herself, being 62 at the time, which is younger than I am now. My grandmother immigrated from Eastern/Central Europe in 1921, spoke broken English, wore no make-up, and a house dress with big cloddy black shoes was her daily attire. Except for the broken English and perhaps some make-up, Mrs. Trimple reminded me of her.

One day in the dead of winter, we took our afternoon "potty break." A spitball fight broke out in the boys' restroom that I had nothing to do with. When we returned to the classroom, Mrs. Trimple began her search to find the instigator.

Two other boys claimed I started it. Mrs. Trimple approached me and said I needed to apologize to the class for causing a disruption. Because I had not instigated or even participated in it, I refused.

She said, "If you don't apologize, you will spend the remainder of the day standing in the hallway." I held firm, saying, "It wasn't me. I had nothing to do with it." She gently took me by the arm, escorted me out of the classroom into the hallway, and said, "You can come back in once you apologize."

I thought to myself, "I'll show you."

It was probably one o'clock in the afternoon. So, I just stood in the hallway, occasionally sitting down against the wall, or walking up and down the hall, gazing into some of the other classrooms.

The upper half of the classroom doors had windows, and I could peer into the various classrooms but was too short to see much. I could see, however, the heads of some students and the clocks. I don't remember whether I knew how to tell time, but I knew when the little hand was on three and the big hand hit twelve, the school day was over. So, I stood there waiting for the little hand to be on three and the big hand hit twelve. It seemed like an eternity.

At some point, Mrs. Trimple opened the door to check on me and said, "When you apologize, you can come back in." I replied, "Mrs. Trimple, I DID NOT DO IT." She informed me that I would continue to stand in the hallway until I apologized.

I was determined to hold firm. I continued to stand, sit, walk, and gaze. I faced a predicament, though. It was winter.

And winter in northeast Ohio is cold, and unfortunately, my coat was in the classroom.

In those days, if you got into trouble at school, you got into more trouble when you got home. If I went home without my coat, I would have some explaining to do, plus I would be cold sitting on the bus ride home.

I hatched my plan. Right before the big hand would land on twelve and the little hand three, I would open the door and give a half-hearted apology, hoping that it would suffice.

About a minute before the big hand hit twelve, I busted through the door and said, "Mrs. Trimple, I am sorry." She said, "No, not to me. Apologize to the class!"

I looked at the class and said, "I'm sorry." Then I retrieved my coat and quickly scampered to get on the bus. I never told my parents anything about the incident. Why would I do that? If I had done that, I would have just gone home without the coat.

Perhaps Mrs. Trimple was one step ahead of me and knew I would need my coat. Maybe she knew she held the last card in the deck, which happened to be an ace.

On one hand, I am proud that as a six-year-old, I stood up against this "grave injustice" perpetrated against me by an authority figure. I held my ground as long as I could. But I was disappointed in myself too.

The record book shows that Mrs. Trimple won, and I lost. She ran the clock out on me, and in the end, she got me to cave and admit to a "crime" I did not commit.

If I had to do it over again, I would have just gotten on the bus without my coat and taken my chances at home. Or, I would have faked my abduction from the hallway and made Mrs. Trimple wonder if she was going to see my face on a milk carton.

She broke me. I acted against my will and compromised my integrity. The fact that I caved always stuck with me. (She did teach me to read and how to color within the lines, the latter reinforcing my viewpoint on coercion.)

Why is this story important?

While the event of first grade was insignificant on the one hand, it was significant on the other. It was my first exposure to "coercive authority," and I did not like it. Much of the COVID-19 pandemic was driven by coercive authority.

Many individuals who did not want to get vaccinated ultimately caved to the coercion they encountered and got vaccinated for good reasons, although unrelated to health. Some caved to keep their jobs. Some caved to see loved ones in assisted living and nursing home facilities. Some caved simply due to overwhelming pressures from family, friends, and doctors. Some were threatened with not seeing loved ones ever again if not vaccinated.

We can understand the reasons many caved. But in my opinion, none of that arm-twisting should have happened. It borders on being unethical and inhumane and was rooted in unfounded fear. Whatever happened to "All we have to fear is fear itself"?

Collective fear stimulates herd instinct and tends to produce ferocity toward those who are not regarded as members of the herd.

—Bertrand Russell

That is not to suggest that COVID-19 was not serious; it was serious and potentially deadly, but only for a small segment of the population. The pandemic was made to look worse than it was, and with the medical establishment and the media fomenting fear, in my eyes, that became more apparent to me by the time we got to the vaccinations.

When it came to the COVID-19 vaccines, I did not cave like I did in first grade. *I did not get vaccinated against COVID-19.* That does not mean that I believe no one should have been vaccinated, and I did recommend that my high-risk patients consider being vaccinated for COVID-19. Before some of you conclude that I am a horrible person, I had several reasons not to be vaccinated that I will soon share.

While vaccines in general might have a role in protecting health (especially the traditional childhood vaccines), I do not believe all patients should be indiscriminately vaccinated with every vaccine possible. I generally recommend vaccines only for high-risk patients (I do not see patients under 18 except for sports injuries) and any patient who asks to be vaccinated for a particular condition. The vaccine rate of my patients was typically 30–40 percent of our other physicians, so I have not been an anti-vaxxer, but have been selective with them, just as I have with medications.

While vaccines in general might have a role in protecting health (especially the traditional childhood vaccines), I do not believe all patients should be indiscriminately vaccinated with every vaccine possible.

Most of what I discussed regarding vaccines in "Does Medicine Matter?" was new information for me, which I did not learn until the summer of 2024. For me, being vaccinated is a personal choice, and I am not in favor of forced vaccinations, especially considering the data I presented earlier.

Also, I see a skewed population. Many of my patients are health-conscious and prefer not to be treated with medications, which also includes the use of adult vaccines.

My Reasons for Opposing the Vaccine

I opposed the vaccine based on

- my pre-existing distrust of the medical establishment, government, and media;
- several COVID-19 oddities;
- unproven vaccine method;
- I already had COVID-19 and had natural immunity;
- I had a cancer diagnosis shortly after the rollout of the vaccine; and
- I saw side effects in my vaccinated patients.

Those were my original reasons for not being vaccinated. Then came the icing on the cake. Pfizer's own study.

Pfizer's study showed that more people died in the vaccine group, which also had more adverse reactions than the placebo group. Plus, the vaccine was not nearly as efficacious as reported and perceived. I will save this for the next chapter.

Distrust

Based on most of what has been presented in this book, being distrustful of the medical establishment seems like a reasonable response. The same corruption in medicine goes on in government and its agencies and in mainstream media, both of which promote half-truths.

Much of what I've discussed thus far, specifically about the FDA and its incestuous relationship with the pharmaceutical industry, I already knew before researching for this book. Though I knew how drug companies misrepresented results of their drug studies, the depth of the data manipulation and the extent of infiltration of the medical infrastructure with Big Pharma money, especially the paying of medical editors, were new discoveries for me.

Just like medical journals are an extension of the marketing arms of pharmaceutical companies, the media are an extension of the powers that control the politicians and bureaucrats. We know from the Syracuse study that journalists have a political slant. One would hope that when it comes to matters of health, that would not be the case. What the media were reporting was not close, in some instances, to reality.

The goal of the media, like every other business, is to make money. They report the way they do to increase viewership.

I wasn't buying most of what the media were selling. The media specializes in sensationalizing everything, whether politics, medicine, sports, and so on. Rarely is anything as dramatic as the media portrays. They are trying to get ratings, clicks, and so on. Much of what the media reports isn't news; they are in the storytelling business.

The goal of the media, like every other business, is to make money. They report the way they do to increase viewership. I have had a couple of encounters with the media. My first one was as a senior in high school.

That year, we had three brother combinations on the varsity baseball team, including my brother and me. The local newspaper conducted phone interviews with the six of us. The reporter was trying to get me to say that there was an intense rivalry between my brother and me. Finally, I said, "Well, sure, I like to do better than my brother, but I like to do better than everyone. But I want my brother to do well."

That would be a true statement. But that's not what came out in the article. The article described this intense competitiveness and rivalry between the two of us as if there were a cut-throat relationship.

Subsequently, I have done a few medically related interviews. My conclusion is that the media has a predetermined slant to a story that it wants to report before it interviews anyone. Saying they spoke to an "expert" gives their stories the air of legitimacy.

They will take whatever you give them to write the story they want. They will misrepresent what you say, if necessary, to write the story because they will write it with you or without you. Their approach is the same as law enforcement: "Anything you say can and will be used against you." Some things are taken out of context or ignored to paint the picture that sells best.

COVID-19 Oddities

This could be an entire chapter. I will touch on just fourteen things I found odd about the origins and management of COVID-19.

As I write this, more is being revealed about the handling of the COVID-19 pandemic. On May 31, 2024, Dr. Fauci admitted the six-foot distancing was not based on any science, and he did not recall any evidence on the masking of children. (Dr. Fauci could not recall MSN's reporting?!) What more did he and his colleagues recommend that was not based on any meaningful science?

On January 12, 2017, eight days before the inauguration of President Trump, Dr. Anthony Fauci stated with confidence in a speech he delivered at George Washington University that the next administration (meaning President

Trump) would have to deal with a "surprise outbreak."[272] My first thought was, if you know it is going to happen, then it should not be a surprise, and part of your job is to be prepared for that.

His words may have been innocent. It may be that he said those words because we were "overdue" for an outbreak of something, but those words take on a new meaning when juxtaposed to comments he and others made at the Milken Future Health Summit held October 28–29, 2019, about two months before the official outbreak of COVID-19.

The main purpose of the summit was to change the perception of the seriousness of influenza, especially during pandemics. The discussion moved on to vaccine development and the slowness of the regulatory process that governs vaccine development. (You can view the video *Making Influenza History: The Quest for a Universal Vaccine* online.[273])

Dr. Fauci, Michael Specter, Richard Bright, Margaret Hamburg, MD (a former FDA Commissioner), Casey Wright, and Bruce Gellin, MD openly discussed the need to "blow up the system" regarding vaccine development and the regulatory process.

While all on the panel agreed that even though we get good and predictable results with the current technique of growing vaccines in eggs, "there must be a better way." They lamented the lengthy process of getting vaccine approval from the FDA.

Fauci said, "It is going to be difficult to change that unless you do it from within and, say, I don't care what your perception is, we are going to address the problem in a disruptive way and in an integrative way because you need both."

Richard Bright of HHS Biomedical Advanced Research and Development (BARDA) said this during that summit:

> To make it sexy, I think you have to, I like the concept "disrupting this field"... There might be a need or an urgent call for an entity of excitement out there that is completely disruptive, that is not beholden to bureaucratic strings and processes...But it is not too crazy to think an outbreak of a *novel avian virus could occur in China* [emphasis is mine] somewhere. We could get the RNA sequence from that, beam it to regional centers, if not local, if not even in your home, at some point, and print those vaccines on a patch and self-administer.

It seemed they were anxious for a pandemic to try a new method of vaccine development and bypass normal regulatory channels. They just needed the opportunity, which lo and behold, would come only a few months later.

COVID-19's Origins

There are two main theories on the origin of SARS-CoV-2. One is the lab leak hypothesis, and the other is the zoonosis hypothesis, where the virus naturally emerged in humans through naturally occurring animal-to-human transmission.[274] The zoonosis theory takes more steps to explain than the virus was the result of gain-of-function research and escaped the lab. If you apply Occam's razor for problem-solving, where the most obvious or smallest set of explanations is frequently the correct answer, you will lean towards favoring the lab leak hypothesis.

The immediate media response that the virus did not originate from the Wuhan lab in China, which was doing gain-of-function research, didn't seem trustworthy to me. It was as if a lab leak was not even a consideration. Anybody who brought up a possible leak of the virus from the Wuhan lab was labeled a "conspiracy theorist," even though that would be the most obvious and logical conclusion. One need not be a conspiracy theorist to conclude the virus came from the lab. Common sense tells you that is the most likely possibility; thus, the mere labeling of people as conspiracy theorists suggests a cover-up. It reeked of "doth protest too much."

Was there even time to conduct such an investigation to reach the conclusion that the virus arose spontaneously in nature and jumped from a couple of different animals, and, finally, to humans? Couple that with the remarks made at the Milken Future Health Summit, and that all seemed a little too coincidental for my comfort.

On May 4, 2020, Dr. Fauci said there was no scientific evidence the virus was *made* in a Chinese lab,[275] even though he was aware that the lab was engaged in gain-of-function since he was, in part, responsible for it. Made in a lab and leaking from a lab are two different things.

Follow the money. No one gains financially from favoring the lab leak hypothesis. Several virologists involved in gain-of-function research have a vested interest in favoring the zoonosis hypothesis to not limit or shut down such research.

Elusive Goalposts

The goalposts kept changing concerning the duration of the lockdown period and the number of people needed to achieve herd immunity with the vaccinations. Two weeks to flatten the curve never materialized. In September 2020, Dr. Fauci explained to *The New York Times* that vaccine coverage to ensure herd immunity went from 70 percent in March 2020 to 80 percent to 90 percent was not based on science but due to increasing acceptance of the public to the vaccines.[276]

This is from the man who said that an attack on him is an attack on science.[277] That is narcissism—a sociopathic characteristic. What is science? A tool to get to the truth. He is equating himself with the truth. That would be problematic for a significant part of the population.

Back to the ever-changing goalposts. In these cases, we saw more extreme measures being taken and touted. Why? Regardless, it did not instill a high enough level of confidence in me to trust whatever the experts might say in the future. Was it because the powers that be determined that two weeks and 70 percent were easier to sell, knowing in advance that neither was realistic?

The projected number of deaths in this country was not even close. Early projections were 2.2 million deaths in the first year. As of June 14, 2023, three-and-a-half years after the onset of the pandemic, there have been half that number (1,134,641).[278]

One can argue that the actual number was less due to the vaccines, but that would be a half-truth as it takes 22,000 individuals to be vaccinated to prevent one death from COVID per Pfizer's six-month study. I will get to that in more detail later.

At that rate, 22 billion people would need to be vaccinated to realize a reduction in deaths of 1 million. However, there are only eight billion people on the planet and 333 million in the US. In fact, at eight billion people and 22,000 needing to be vaccinated to prevent one COVID death, the best we could hope for is a death reduction of 363,363 worldwide from vaccination.

Basically, the experts were off on their projections for lockdowns, herd immunity, and deaths, and, in some cases, way off. COVID-19 was not the experts' "first rodeo." They had already dealt with HIV, Ebola, Zika, SARs, MERs, and H1N1.

Lockdowns

How successful could the lockdowns possibly be when 49 to 60 million essential workers were still working?[279] We did not have a lockdown. We had a *semi-lockdown.*

The semi-lockdown accomplished two things. It enabled the destruction of the economy while still allowing for the spread of the virus. If that was the goal, and I am not saying it was, it was the perfect plan. But if that were the plan, that speaks to another agenda.

With that many people traveling back and forth from work and interacting, did we really think that a semi-lockdown would contain the virus (assuming lockdowns are effective to begin with, which is debatable)? And the World Health Organization stated the lockdowns have profound negative impacts.[280]

I have a simple, no-nonsense definition of an essential worker: one who works and pays taxes. I am sure every employer considers his or her employees essential. The definition of e*ssential worker* during the pandemic was an idiotic term.

We abandoned all previous knowledge of natural immunity and infection control. For the first time in history, natural immunity was not considered good enough. Why? In the initial wave of COVID-19, which largely affected older individuals and those most feeble, why did we lock them down in facilities with other similar individuals (rather than isolate them), which only served to spread the infection like wildfire, making the pandemic look worse than it should have?

During the Spanish flu outbreak, those infected patients treated outdoors, in fresh air, and in sunlight fared better than those inside.[281] We did the opposite with COVID. Why?

We even made it seem the reason for *you* to get vaccinated is to protect others, not you. If the vaccine works and you are vaccinated, you are protected against the virus, whether you encounter someone vaccinated or unvaccinated. If the vaccine does not work, then it matters not who is vaccinated.

Questionable Vaccine Development

Why use a new method for vaccine development (other than it might be faster), never proven before, and in the middle of a pandemic that was billed as going to kill millions and millions? Why not use the tried-and-true method of vaccine development, so that predictable results could be realized?

Is there any evidence that you can vaccinate your way out of a pandemic once it starts? Not only that, but one of the COVID-19 vaccine makers, Moderna, had never made a vaccine before. But Moderna *was* on the forefront of mRNA technology.

Where was the solid evidence to support masking and social distancing? Even Scott Gottlieb, former FDA Commissioner, admitted in September 2021 that the six-foot distance was arbitrary and not backed by science.[282] Yet, people are still masking.

I found it odd that, best to my knowledge and recall, there was not one discussion by Dr. Anthony Fauci, Dr. Deborah Birx, or Dr. Rochelle Walensky on measures that people could take to enhance their own immune systems to better fight the virus and other measures to prevent infection, like taking vitamins D and C, zinc, quercetin, or even exercise or saunas. Why was the emphasis on vaccines and preventive measures like masks and social distancing only?

Beyond supportive care, they proposed no outpatient treatment protocols. You had to go to the Front Line COVID-19 Critical Care Alliance, Peter McCullough, MD, and Vladimir Zelenko, MD, and others to find preventive and early treatment protocols similar to one another.

Evidence on the C19early.org website shows that even lifestyle measures like exercise could reduce infection and severity.

Depending on the temperature, something as simple as one to five minutes in a sauna can deactivate viruses.[283] This raises the question of whether we should treat fever in viral infections. Below are the sauna temperature and duration requirements to deactivate viruses.

- One minute at a temperature of 80°C or 176°F;
- Three minutes at a temperature of 75°C or 167°F;
- Five minutes at a temperature of 65°C or 149°F; or
- 20 minutes at a temperature of 60°C or 140°F.

Of the things mentioned above to enhance immune function and fight infection, saunas would be by far the most expensive. I am not suggesting the government buy saunas, but to put the cost of saunas in perspective, consider this. We have 128 million households in the US.[284] At $2,000 (and even less) per sauna, we could have provided every household a sauna at a total cost of $256 billion, far less than the $3 to $5 trillion printed out of thin air during the pandemic, and we would have created jobs in the process. And saunas could be used repeatedly for other outbreaks. Plus, regular sauna usage may be the most beneficial passive modality to improve health. At the least, we could have provided every household with vitamins D and C, zinc, quercetin, and more for a fraction of the cost.

These are simple fixes. Too often, we look for complex solutions when simple ones suffice.

The Push Against Hydroxychloroquine and Ivermectin

A multi-faceted movement tried to dissuade physicians from using ivermectin and hydroxychloroquine because they were determined to be "unsafe" for COVID-19 despite proven safety and efficacy for parasitic infections over decades of use. Why were non-verifiable data used to make hydroxychloroquine look dangerous as a COVID-19 treatment?[285]

Drs. Pierre Kory and Peter McCullough estimated that using ivermectin and hydroxychloroquine would have prevented five hundred thousand deaths—and that's just through May 2020. It was felt that those drugs would have prevented 75–80 percent of deaths. At one point, there were 6 million COVID-19 hospitalizations with seven hundred thousand deaths. A 75 percent reduction using ivermectin and hydroxychloroquine equates to five hundred thousand deaths and billions of dollars.[286]

Both drugs are FDA-approved and have been around for decades. Ivermectin was FDA-approved in 1996. Its developers received the Nobel Prize, becoming the only infectious disease medication in sixty years to win the award. It has been described as a "wonder drug" by Japan's Kitasato Institute.[287]

Hydroxychloroquine (HCQ) was first synthesized in 1949 and is listed by the World Health Organization as an "essential medicine," as is ivermectin. It has been prescribed billions of times for malaria prevention and treatment and is used to treat some autoimmune diseases. It is the most used medication in India. In some countries, it is available over the counter.[288]

In 2012, ivermectin was shown to inhibit replication of a wide ranges of viruses in *in vitro* studies but, more importantly, a systematic review of *in vitro* and *in vivo* studies over fifty years showed ivermectin has antiviral effects for Zika, dengue, yellow fever, West Nile, Hendra, Newcastle, Venezuelan equine encephalitis, chikungunya, Semliki Forest, Sindbis, Avian influenza A, Porcine Reproductive and Respiratory Syndrome, HIV type 1, and SARS-CoV-2, which can lead to COVID-19.[289]

In April 2020, lab experiments showed that ivermectin eliminated SARS-CoV-2 in forty-eight hours.[290] A 2021 study showed that ivermectin binds to the SARS-CoV-2 spike protein and is not specific to any coronavirus variant. This suggested that it would be an effective agent against future variants.[291]

In a prophylaxis study out of Argentina, COVID-19 infections were found in 20 percent of 788 healthcare workers who took ivermectin weekly, whereas 58 percent of 407 controls became ill with. COVID-19.[292]

As early as 2004, hydroxychloroquine (HCQ) and its forerunner, chloroquine, were found to be effective against coronavirus.[293] As early as March 2, 2020, China published protocols for treating COVID-19 with chloroquine.[294]

Harvey Risch, MD, PhD, a highly esteemed epidemiologist from Yale University, published a meta-analysis of five outpatient studies affiliated with Johns Hopkins Bloomberg School of Public Health, concluding that the evidence is unequivocal for the early use of HCQ with azithromycin.[295]

In *Newsweek* magazine, he said this about hydroxychloroquine:

> As professor of epidemiology at Yale School of Public Health, I have authored over 300 peer-reviewed publications and currently hold senior positions on the editorial boards of several leading journals. I am usually reasons having nothing to do with a correct understanding of the science, has been pushed to the sidelines. As a result, tens of thousands of patients with COVID-19 are dying unnecessarily. Fortunately, the situation can be reversed easily and quickly.[296]

When hydroxychloroquine was studied, it was frequently used in excessive doses on some of the sickest COVID-19 patients, leading to excess deaths and complications. In her article, "COVID-19 Has Turned Public Health Into a Lethal, Patient-Killing Experimental Endeavor," Dr. Meryl Nass uncovered three studies where doses four times the recommended dosage for hydroxychloroquine were used on hospitalized COVID-19 patients.

These studies included Solidarity, Recovery, and REMAMP. In some studies, HCQ was not only given in high doses but also along with medications whose combinations are contraindicated. She discovered that the online protocols for the three studies were stamped "Not for IRB (Institutional Review Board) submission."[297]

Again, ivermectin and HCQ had to look dangerous and ineffective. Otherwise, the COVID-19 vaccines could not be tested under Emergency Use Authorization. They would have to go through the usual FDA approval process, which could take years.

Both drugs are on the World Health Organization's list of essential medications and were considered safe until COVID-19.

Dr. Fauci said he was open to hydroxychloroquine if it were shown effective in randomized, double-blind, placebo-controlled studies. However, in 2013, he allowed the use of ribavirin/interferon during the MERS outbreak despite the lack of its safety and effectiveness in randomized placebo-controlled studies.[298]

Such openness rings hollow. Who will fund double-blind, placebo-controlled studies using drugs for which there is little profit?

There are ethical issues in requiring randomized, double-blind, controlled studies during pandemics. It is one thing to test a vaccine in people *not yet infected* with a virus using such studies. I question the ethics of giving a placebo to someone fighting a potentially life-threatening infection when you think you have something that might help. As I believe it is cruel to demand a randomized, double-blind, placebo-controlled study in such situations.

In 2016, the 21st Century Cures Act recognized this scenario and directed the FDA to accept real-world evidence in lieu of controlled clinical trials. Now you know why the trials on hydroxychloroquine and ivermectin were designed and fabricated to look unsafe and ineffective.

Did Dr. Fauci "Mrs. Trimple" the country by running the clock out by suppressing the use of hydroxychloroquine and ivermectin long enough to give Big Pharma time to develop patented monoclonal antibodies, antivirals, and mRNA vaccines?

Remember what I said earlier about "hiding in the open" and acting as if you are doing good.

Why were patients with COVID-19 instructed to stay at home and only seek medical attention when their conditions were severe enough to warrant a trip to the hospital, where survival would be less certain? We knew of other potential interventions with low risk that could have been used early in the course of the infection, as noted on the C19early.org website.

The Push for Vaccination

Why the heavy push to vaccinate everyone with an experimental vaccine to protect against a virus associated with an average death rate of less than 1 percent?

We rushed things when the death rate was less than 1 percent for all age groups other than those over age 75, who made up 84 percent of the deaths.[299] Why not vaccinate only those at the highest risk level?

If you look at Pfizer's six-month data, 168 unvaccinated patients got COVID-19, and two patients, or 1.2 percent, died. But this figure is misleading as the death rate is likely much lower; many patients were suspected of having COVID-19 during the trial but were never tested for it. I will review that in the next chapter.

Why are illegal immigrants not required to be vaccinated? If we are genuinely humanitarians and believe in vaccinations, should we not be vaccinating them?

We have allowed millions of illegals to enter this country, and we provide them with many resources, which you and I pay for, and they do not require the COVID-19 vaccines. On top of that, we allow them to bring us other infectious diseases.[300]

I completed my undergraduate studies at Wittenberg University in Springfield, Ohio, the county seat of Clark County and center of the recent Haitian controversy. Haitians started to arrive in Springfield in 2018. From 2019 to 2023, there were 12 cases of TB in Clark County. In the five years preceding their arrival (2014 to 2018), there were only three cases.[301] Thus, TB cases in Clark County have quadrupled since the arrival of Haitians. It's important to note that more cases of TB are drug-resistant these days.

The Haitians in Springfield are there under temporary protective status and, based on my understanding, are not considered "illegal." Nonetheless, my point about disease remains valid.

In the early 1900s, immigrants coming from Europe to this country legally (including my ancestors) were processed and examined at Ellis Island and quarantined if they had a communicable disease. A scene in the movie *The Godfather: Part II* depicts these processing and quarantining procedures.

In my opinion, the tactics to market the vaccines met the definition of propaganda. Healthcare workers gave patients buttons and stickers to wear after vaccination to show others they were good citizens. Some states held lotteries to entice people to be vaccinated. And let's not forget the commercials promoting the COVID-19 vaccines and live TV segments showing politicians and celebrities being vaccinated—we knew these were placebos because the powers in charge could not chance anyone having a reaction on national television.

It all seemed over the top. None of this was done for other outbreaks, some of which have been more serious. Why the hard-core sales pitch?

Why did the CDC change the definition of a vaccine?[302] In 2018, *vaccination* was defined as a product that stimulates a person's immune system to produce immunity to a specific disease, protecting the person from that disease. Vaccines are usually administered through needle injections but can also be administered by mouth or sprayed into the nose.

The definition of *vaccination* as of September 1, 2021, was preparation [that is] used to stimulate the body's immune response against diseases. Vaccines are usually administered through needle injections but can also be administered by mouth or sprayed into the nose.

The definition has morphed from a product that protects against disease to a preparation that stimulates the body's immune response *without necessarily providing protection* against a specific disease.

For me, many things about COVID-19 and what we were doing were not adding up.

Since then, we have learned that on April 9, 2024, Congressman Rand Paul reported that as early as January 2018, the DEFUSE project informed fifteen federal agencies were informed of its intent to create a virus similar, if not identical, to COVID-19. EcoHealth Alliance and the Wuhan Institute of Virology were seeking federal funding for the project in 2018.[303]

Not one agency alerted the public that the Chinese lab was ready to move on such a project. The NIAID (National Institute for Allergy and Infectious Diseases), headed by Dr. Fauci, was listed as a participant in the initial DEFUSE pitch.

Unproven Vaccine Method

At the beginning of the pandemic, it was projected that 2 million Americans would die in the first year.[304]

While mRNA technology has been around for about thirty years, it had never been used before to make a vaccine. A pandemic of this projected magnitude hardly seemed like the time to try a new vaccine production method. Dr. Fauci told Congress on May 25, 2020, "There's no guarantee that the vaccine is actually going to be effective."[305] It would have made more sense to test the mRNA vaccine platform first against already existing vaccines to see how well the technology performed against a traditional flu vaccine, for example.

COVID-19 Risk Factors

People dying from COVID-19 had a specific profile—they were overweight, diabetic, suffered from hypertension, or were elderly and frail. Few without those comorbidities were dying, so why the push to vaccinate everyone? Doing so speaks to another agenda.

Little Data Available at Vaccine Rollout

We had only a two-month efficacy date on the vaccines as that data on approximately 44,000 subjects (22,000 vaccinated and 22,000 unvaccinated) when the mass vaccine rollout began, and that two-month data showed more adverse effects in the vaccine group. Six-month data would become available on September 15, 2021. To put that 22,000 vaccinated number in perspective, over 600,000 children received the polio vaccine when it was being studied.[306]

I consider two-month data on a vaccine using a new vaccine platform inadequate.

For nine months, we vaccinated people against a virus with a less than 1 percent average death rate. That did not seem right to me.

Though individuals with heart disease, cancer, autoimmune disease, neurodegenerative disease, and other chronic diseases were vaccinated, that two-month study did not report data on adverse effects related to these specific diseases.

The Pfizer-BioNTech vaccine did not gain FDA approval until August 23, 2021, and its six-month trial data was not released until September 15, 2021, about nine months after the mass experiment started.

mRNA Vaccine Rationale

The rationale behind using mRNA technology did not make sense to me. Here are a few of my thoughts on the mechanics of the mRNA vaccines.

There are 29 proteins in SARS-CoV-2.[307] When you become infected, you develop an immune response to all or, at least, most of those proteins. With the mRNA vaccines, your body is being primed to develop an immune response only to the spike protein.[308] How can that give you better immunity than an infection?

Let me rephrase it: The medical establishment claimed that immunity to 29 proteins was inadequate protection and that vaccination was still necessary. Yet, immunity to one protein alone via a vaccination would provide all the protection one would need. Does the medical establishment really believe that? Or are they being coerced? Either way, the profession has been hijacked.

Also, we know the spike protein is pathogenic, whether from natural infection or the vaccine. If I have already been infected with SARS-CoV-2 (which I was), have spike protein floating around my body, and it is pathogenic, why would I want my body to produce more spike protein via vaccination? We are still vaccinating people to trigger their bodies to make a protein that we now know is pathogenic. If that weren't enough, we know that the lipid nanoparticles that envelope the mRNA are inflammatory. This was six months before we started to vaccinate the masses. Yet, Dr. Fauci's whole game plan hinged on waiting until the vaccines were available.[309]

If you watch the Milken Health Summit video, it seems like those on the panel were eager to "disrupt the system" at the first chance they could and try a new vaccination method.

Imagine if we put astronauts on the first rocket we developed, sent them to the moon, and said, "Boy, we sure hope this works." We would all think that ludicrous. Yet we allowed the ludicrous with the vaccines. Yes, the mRNA may have allowed for faster development, but many people would prefer results to speed.

Finally, we have seen that the gene that encodes the spike protein mutates. In that case, how does the mRNA vaccine protect you?

Vaccines and Herpes Are Forever

Whether discussing medications, supplements, vaccines, or any other intervention, there must be a good enough reason to receive an intervention to offset any risk because everything has adverse effects. The benefits should far outweigh any potential risk. When assessing any risk, we should ask whether the risk is permanent or temporary, should it occur.

When it comes to risk, vaccines are different from medications. If you have an adverse reaction to a medication, you stop taking it, and the side effects typically resolve once the medicine clears your system.

How can you undo a vaccine's adverse effects should one occur outside the typical temporary arm soreness and fever?

The effects of vaccines can be forever, like herpes. Once that vaccine hits your body, you cannot easily undo anything bad it might do, and thus, like herpes, it can affect your body forever. So, you should have an excellent reason to get a vaccine, in my opinion, considering what "vaccine safety" means. It doesn't mean what you or doctors believe. In the case of

COVID-19, the vaccines' long-term adverse effects will be unknown for years, and then, it will be too late to do much about them.

Based on the vaccine charts from *Dissolving Illusions*, is there a good enough reason to get some of the vaccines? That's up to you to decide. My goal is to get you to look at the big picture and think and ask questions, rather than be vaccinated because you are told to. We have much experience with the original childhood vaccines, but no prior experience with mRNA vaccines. Consequently, I believe a more thoughtful approach should have been undertaken with the COVID-19 vaccines.

Vaccines stimulate the immune system, but they prime it into action when it has little reason to fight against a disease. We are tricking the immune system into action. I wonder whether doing that is wise. I compare it to sounding a false fire alarm, which we repeat up to one hundred times over a person's lifetime. This seems like a potential recipe for system failure.

How many times can you "trick the immune system into action" before problems occur? Maybe, at some point, the body says, "Oh, another false alarm," when you really do have an infection or cancer cells floating around. And then it fails to react. Or vice versa, when the immune system is called into action and has nothing to fight, it begins to fight and attack itself. Though never definitively proven, there have long been concerns with the potential role of vaccines triggering autoimmune diseases.

Some groups, like Public Citizen, recommend that you not take a new medication or vaccine until it has been on the market for *seven years* unless it is a real blockbuster in terms of its effects, not sales. Few drugs have lived up to their hype despite doing well in the marketplace. There are blockbuster drugs in terms of sales, but not as many in terms of results.

One drug that has been a blockbuster that I reviewed in "The Pharmaceutical Funded FDA" is ivermectin, but we were "forbidden" to use it for COVID-19.

I will not go into it here, but there may be some ways to "neutralize" the spike protein, whether it be from infection or the COVID-19 vaccine. I recommend following Dr. Peter McCullough's recommendations.[310]

In the next chapter, I will show the actual data from Pfizer's six-month trial. When you see that data, you will wonder how Pfizer's vaccine gained approval. It all goes back to medicine's half-truths and corruption.

I Had COVID-19 Already

I got COVID-19 in December 2020, right around the vaccine rollouts. My body ached, and I had occasional fevers but no respiratory symptoms. I felt well enough to continue my exercise program. My symptoms largely diminished by day 4 and were entirely resolved by day 7.

Over 160 studies showed little to no benefit from the COVID-19 vaccines in those already infected with the SARS-CoV-2, the virus that causes COVID-19.[311]

Pandemics typically pick off the low-hanging fruit (the frailest and those with comorbidities) during the first wave. If you get infected and survive that first wave, you will probably be fine moving forward due to long-lasting immunity. Thus, while death rates may seem high at first, they eventually fall and stabilize as those who are going to die have already died.

I survived COVID.

I had natural immunity, which historically has been felt to last a lifetime, though it may wane with age and time. Dr. Fauci, in 2004, even stated that the best "vaccination" for viruses is being infected with the virus. He restated that during the Milken Future Health Summit in October 2019.[312]

So, I saw no need for an unproven vaccine using unproven technology related to vaccine development (mRNA technology has been used with success for other purposes) to prevent a viral infection with a high survival rate of 99 percent-plus.

Before the vaccine rollout, I came across a study published in *Nature* that looked at the immunity of individuals infected with SARS-CoV-1 in 2003. The study found that they still had T-cell immunity seventeen years later and showed cross-reactivity to SARS-CoV-2, which causes COVID. This supports the notion that immunity from infection is long-term.[313]

Cancer Diagnosis

After the vaccines' rollout, I was diagnosed with prostate cancer. It had spread beyond the prostate, raising the possibility of metastatic disease, for which I would need further testing to see whether it had spread to my bones and lymph glands. At the same time, we discovered that women vaccinated for COVID-19 were having abnormal mammograms and enlarged lymph glands. These symptoms were, eventually, attributed to the COVID-19 vaccines.

I did not want anything that might affect the results of the tests I would need, plus I already had COVID-19. Though patients with cancer were vaccinated in the Pfizer trial, there were no safety data on how cancer patients fared compared to cancer-free patients.

Side Effects in Patients

Because I had natural immunity, I decided to sit back and see how this new vaccine method worked while I did more research.

So, I watched how others, including my patients, responded to the vaccinations. I had front-row seats at the show—an advantage those not in healthcare did not have.

I used that time to read the literature and news reports from the US and other countries. Many times, what was reported in the US differed from what other countries reported.

Why?

I began to keep files of studies and reports I found legitimate that contradicted the mainstream narrative here in the US. These came in handy later, in 2021 and 2022, when I saw the need to write two letters, parts of which I will share later in this chapter.

Treatments being suppressed here, like ivermectin, were successful in other countries. In New Delhi, India, physicians used ivermectin to obliterate 97 percent of COVID cases as reported in April 2021.[314]

The C19early.org website reported that other non-vaccine success stories showed the success of using repurposed medications and over-the-counter supplements. The site provides up-to-date information on every intervention being tried for COVID-19, including ivermectin and hydroxychloroquine.

Studies showed that some of these non-vaccine alternatives outperformed the drugs being used in our hospitals, and some were available without a prescription. Supplements like vitamin D, melatonin, curcumin, quercetin, and lifestyle habits like exercise were shown to be reasonably effective in preventing and treating COVID-19.

This is *not* misinformation.

Earlier, I discussed the issue of coercion and the medical establishment. I found it interesting that I could easily access the C19early.org website from home. Using my cellphone, I could easily access it in my medical office using our Wi-Fi. However, I could not access it from my office when I used my office computer. I was blocked. I tried, over several weeks, to see if I could access the website using my office computer, but I was always blocked.

Why was this information being blocked or suppressed, and who was suppressing it?

My Own Patient Experience

The real-time data from my own patients proved invaluable.

I'm uncertain how many of my patients were vaccinated, as most who were vaccinated did so outside of our office. Also, patients avoided coming to the office, so getting accurate data was impossible. Given that my practice is somewhat skewed, though, I would estimate that the number of my vaccinated patients was probably 10–15 percent less than the national average. I do know of only one patient of mine who died from COVID-19, which suggests COVID-19 was not as deadly as advertised.

Everything I noticed in my practice and related to you is purely anecdotal. And because of my doubts about the pandemic, I may have been on high alert looking for issues with the vaccines. Although I cannot prove the vaccines caused what I saw, I will share what I did see.

The most common thing I noticed was breakthrough infections of COVID. Why should that be? Vaccines are supposed to prevent infections.

Interestingly, without fail, patients would say, "It's a good thing I was vaccinated, or it may have been worse."

Apparently, they did not know they should not be infected if the vaccines were effective. Outside the annual flu vaccine, I have not seen a vaccine fail this often in doing what it was supposed to—prevent infection.

Another thing I saw then and still see is that those vaccinated seem to be getting more upper respiratory infections than normal, and the infections seem to last longer.

I had about eight vaccinated male patients aged 28 to 52 develop chest pain. Some I sent to cardiologists, who could not explain it. Except for one, they all had normal EKGs. These tests were done before the link to the vaccines and myocarditis was firmly established. Eventually, the chest pain resolved in all of them without any definitive diagnosis being made.

The most frequent *significant* adverse effect I saw was an uptick in blood clots in the legs and lungs. What was unusual is that I saw more clots or DVTs (deep vein thromboses) in the thigh, which are more dangerous than those in the calf, and some measured up to fifteen inches long.

I had two patients with vague abdominal pain. One ended up having a blood clot in his celiac artery; the other had a clot in his superior mesenteric artery. I don't ever recall seeing these before in my time in medicine.

Both COVID-19 infections and vaccines have been associated with increased occurrence of blood clots, with a higher rate of blood clots shown in those infected rather than vaccinated. That seems to confer some benefit to the vaccines.

[315]But why should vaccinated patients get blood clots if they are "protected" against infection with the SARS-Co-2 virus that causes COVID-19? Protection should mean no infection, and no infection should mean no blood clots.

What's the most dangerous part of the SARS-CoV-2 virus? The spike protein and the COVID-19 vaccines stimulate your body to make the spike protein. That is my "guess" for the reason for blood clots in vaccinated individuals.

Can anyone name another vaccine linked to blood clots? I can't think of one, though I am sure there might be a few isolated cases. That would seem to suggest that the mRNA platform and its concept are lacking, or that priming the body against the only spike protein was a mistake.

Yale researchers have discovered that the spike protein can persist for two years in the body. Thus, those who receive boosters accumulate spike protein with each booster.

I saw an uptick of shingles and Bell's palsy more than I would say is normal for my practice. One patient suffered acute memory loss.[316]

I also had two vaccinated patients with advanced cancer in cancers I rarely see; one being stage 4 ovarian cancer and the other stage 4 pancreatic cancer, both in previously very healthy individuals.

All these cases may have been coincidental and not linked to the vaccine, but all occurred within weeks and a few months of their vaccinations. I did not see such events in my non-vaccinated patients, especially the unusual number of blood clots, and I did not see aggressive cancers in my unvaccinated patients during this time.

The CDC and American Cancer Society state that the COVID-19 vaccines do not increase the cancer risk. Some patients might disagree with that, as will some oncologists off the record.

After reviewing Pfizer's six-month data, which became available online in September 2021, I concluded the evidence for the safety and efficacy of the vaccines was lacking. This lack of evidence became my main personal objection moving forward, which I will review in the next chapter.

Vaccine Mandate

Our medical group's administration told me that I was one of three out of 506 physicians in our medical practice who were not vaccinated by the fall of 2021, when our group mandated everyone be vaccinated. If not vaccinated, I would be tested weekly for COVID-19. Whether the other two physicians, subsequently, were vaccinated, I do not know.

Our medical group mandated COVID-19 vaccines, coinciding with the then-recent FDA approval of Pfizer's vaccine and the release of Pfizer's six-month data. The Centers for Medicare and Medicaid Services (CMS) mandated healthcare professionals be vaccinated as a condition of Medicare and Medicaid participation. All hospital systems in Central Ohio and, likely, most throughout the country, adopted the mandate because they treat Medicare and Medicaid patients.

My first COVID-19 test was scheduled for September 17, 2021. On September 10, my wife and I saw Sebastian Maniscalco perform his stand-up comedy act with three thousand other people. The following day, I went to the Ohio State–University of Oregon football game, sitting in a crowd of 102,000 people with another 150,000-plus milling around the stadium.

Obviously, I was exposed to many people that weekend.

What happened with my first COVID-19 test results? On Monday, September 20, I got to the office, booted up my computer, and received a call from our medical director saying I tested positive for COVID-19 and needed to leave the office immediately. I am sure many had a good laugh at the fact that I tested positive, given my refusal to be vaccinated.

I had zero symptoms.

I have no doubt that I may have been exposed to the SARS-CoV-2 virus given my exposure to thousands the previous week, but I had absolutely no symptoms, and this is another important point. Testing positive does not mean you have been infected, and if I were infected, then my immune system, triggered by the earlier COVID-19 infection, was doing what it was supposed to.

Kary Mullis, who developed the polymerase chain reaction (PCR) test that detects genetic material from a virus, said that if you run forty cycles on a PCR test, you can detect as little as one molecule for anything for which you are testing. He says, "PCR does not tell you if you are sick, and it does not tell you that thing you ended up with is really going to hurt you."[317] This does not necessarily mean infection. Even Dr. Fauci stated that positive tests with cycles of thirty-five or more likely represent "dead DNA material." That means you are not infectious.[318]

Testing positive for COVID-19 that first week was a blessing in disguise because I was exempt from testing for the next ninety days (it was known that a person could test positive for that time). It also acknowledges that there is some degree of natural immunity.

Dealing with Our Group and Hospital

I am going to share parts of two letters that I wrote; one I sent to our medical group, and the second to the hospital where I was on staff and in jeopardy of losing my hospital privileges unless it approved my medical exemption to the vaccinations.

Both letters are filled with medical references that supported my position and views. I sent the letter to the medical practice in early September 2021, before the mandate would take effect; the letter to the hospital was sent in April 2022, when much more was known about the vaccinations.

The medical group's letter focused on natural immunity, concerns about an unproven vaccine production method, and cited data that death from COVID-19 was being over-reported. Because CMS was driving the mandate for healthcare workers, I did not expect the letter to have any influence. I sent it to provide data because I didn't think many physicians knew, considering that 503 of 506 were vaccinated before the mandate.

The letter to the hospital provided evidence about the actual efficacy and safety of vaccines, showing some of the numbers behind the numbers that were obscured by sleight-of-hand reporting to physicians and the public.

The Two Letters

I will now share parts of two letters, primarily parts not discussed elsewhere in this book.

This letter was sent seven to ten days before *The New England Journal of Medicine* published Pfizer's six-month vaccine trial results (September 15, 2021).

I left the group in December 2022 of my own accord. My decision to leave had nothing to do with the circumstances surrounding COVID-19 and the mandate, though it may have confirmed it was time for a change. I had found myself wandering too far away from the type of medicine I wanted to practice. I had an opportunity to join another physician in a preventive medicine practice focusing on nutrition, exercise, and hormone replacement in a model that does not accept health insurance.

At the group's request, I stayed longer than planned until the group recruited my replacement. I emailed and addressed it to the 15 members of our board of directors, the CEO of the group, and one of our medical directors. All are physicians.

> In discussing COVID-19 and vaccine mandates, the emphasis should be on immunity rather than vaccination. The purpose of the vaccine is to achieve immunity, but it is not the only way to achieve immunity. Mounting evidence shows that individuals infected with COVID-19 have superior immunity to those who have received one of the COVID-19 vaccines.
>
> I recall no time in history where immunity from vaccination was found, or felt, to be superior to natural immunity from actual infection, but that seems to be the opinion as it relates to COVID-19.
>
> Individuals who have contracted COVID-19 have been infected with the entire live virus, enabling the development of a more robust immune response than simply producing a spike protein in response to a vaccine and triggering an immune response.
>
> Martin Kulldorf, MD, a professor of medicine at Harvard University and Brigham and Women's Hospital, says the following:
>
>> Since you have recovered from COVID, you have very good immunity, and we know that it's long-lasting, and we have more evidence of immunity from having recovered from COVID-19 than we have from vaccines because millions of people have had COVID-19.

> Now, you can still be reinfected. That's what is expected. But, having had COVID-19 already prevents you from having severe disease or death, so people who had COVID-19 do not need the vaccine.[319]

Recent studies from highly reputable institutions, including the Cleveland Clinic, Emory University, Washington University School of Medicine St. Louis, and Rockefeller University report long-term robust immune response in individuals infected with the coronavirus with little additional benefit to be gained by vaccination in those already infected.[320]

A summary of these studies' conclusions are below.

- The Cleveland Clinic study involved over 52,000 of its employees and concluded that "individuals who have laboratory-confirmed symptomatic SARS-CoV-2 infection are unlikely to benefit from COVID-19 vaccination, and vaccines can be safely prioritized to those who have not been infected before."
- Not one Cleveland Clinic employee who had COVID-19 was reinfected during the study period.
- Rockefeller University: "We conclude that memory antibodies selected over time by natural infection have greater potency and

breadth than antibodies elicited by vaccination.

- Emory University: "The study suggests that patients who survived COVID-19 are likely to also possess protective immunity even against some SARS-CoV2 variants.

SARS and SARS-2 have a genetic overlap of 75–80 percent. A study from Duke University and the National University of Singapore showed long-term T-cell immunity after infection with SARS in 2003 concludes: "SARS-recovered patients (n=23) still possess long-lasting memory T-cells reactive to SARS-NP 17 years after the 2003 outbreak, which displayed robust cross-reactivity to SARS-CoV-2."[321]

In the United States, we hear that it is the unvaccinated who are being hospitalized and the cause of the resurgence, but that is not what is being reported in other countries.

Israel (whose data are felt to be most reliable of all countries) reports that 85–90 percent of hospitalizations are in VACCINATED with 95 percent of the severe cases occurring in the VACCINATED.[322]

In Singapore, 75 percent of COVID-19 cases were in the VACCINATED.[323]

In Great Britain, there were higher death and hospitalization rates for the VACCINATED, who were 6.6 times more likely to die than the unvaccinated.[324]

There was a recent outbreak of COVID-19 on a Carnival Cruise ship. On the ship were 1,441 crew, of whom 99.98 percent were vaccinated, and 2,895 passengers of whom 96.5 percent were vaccinated. There were 27 cases of COVID-19 all occurring in vaccinated individuals.[325]

Vaccines are not the only way to prevent/reduce death in COVID-19 patients. Prevent or reduce the cytokine storm, and lives will be saved. Something as simple as vitamin D appears to be a potent inhibitor of the cytokine storm.[326]

Outdoor hospitals, fresh air, and sunlight (vitamin D) have been used during prior pandemics with good results.[327] We have done the complete opposite with COVID-19. Why?

The COVID-19 vaccines may not be as safe as advertised. As of 8/6/2021 there have been 12,791 deaths linked to COVID-19 vaccines reported to the VAERs data base. Thus, in eight months of vaccine use, there have been more COVID-19 vaccine deaths than deaths from all vaccines administered over the preceding 15-year pre-COVID-19 period.

French virologist, Luc Montagnier, who was awarded the Nobel Prize in 2008 for his discovery of HIV, fears COVID-19 vaccines could lead to neurodegenerative diseases and may be causing the COVID-19 variants through Antibody-Dependent Enhancement.[328]

At the beginning of the pandemic, we were led to believe that this would be a pandemic to end humanity (2,200,000 were projected to die in the US in the first year alone). We closed schools and businesses and advised people not to leave their homes. And then, we came up with a brilliant idea. Let's combat this pandemic with a technology never employed before in humans.

Does it not seem odd and disconcerting that we would rely heavily on a vaccination method that has never been tried before in humans?

Does that not concern any of you?

mRNA technology started in the 1990s. It is not new, but it certainly represents an ongoing development. Would it not have made more sense to use this technology first to make a flu vaccine and compare its safety and efficacy to the traditional flu vaccine, or a shingles vaccine, or hepatitis vaccine, and compare to the existing traditional vaccines?

I trained during the early to late 1980s (medical school and residency). when HIV was a certain death sentence. When you have that situation, that's when you try a new technology without testing it beforehand and out of desperation, not when there is a 99 percent survival rate like we have with COVID-19.

The potential risks of the new technology outweigh the benefits. And one risk is that the vaccines may be triggering the variants or are weakening the immune system in ways we do not yet understand, allowing for breakthrough infections to occur.

Twenty months into the pandemic, here is what we know. Two million plus did not die the first year. If we count January 2020 as the first month of the pandemic, there have now been 600,000 deaths in 20 months, or 360,000 annually. Much less than those who die from heart disease and cancer, each of which kills 600,000 annually.

The overall death rate in 2020 is similar to prior years. In most states, the median age of COVID-19 death is equal to or exceeds the life expectancy in most states.

To put this into further perspective. Consider that 1.6 million, including 500,000 children, die annually from infectious diarrhea.

To put this into even more perspective. Only 6 percent of those 600,000 who have died with COVID-19 had no comorbidities. That translates to only 36,000 deaths or 21,600 annually solely related to the disease. This is half the number who die from MVAs [motor vehicle accidents] every year.

It is only in the over-70 age group that the infection fatality rate exceeds 0.5 percent.

We are engaged in the largest human experiment in history, and I prefer not to be one of its subject participants.

Joe Jacko, MD

The letter was mainly a protest vote but also an opportunity to share information that I believe many of them had never seen and did not know.

Review the sources I referenced regarding natural immunity. These are highly reputable medical centers. These studies do not represent drug studies by pharmaceutical companies designed to encourage use of a drug. These are independent studies, with no financial gain in the background, concluding that, if you already had COVID-19 and natural immunity, there was little to be gained by being vaccinated; that is, a vaccine (drug) was not indicated.

Yet, the government via CMS still wanted all healthcare professionals vaccinated (allowing for some exemptions). What happened to evidence-based medicine?

Now for the second letter. In the next chapter, I will cover much of the information included in the second letter, sent to the hospital where I had privileges. Primarily, it deals with the safety and efficacy of the Pfizer-BioNTech vaccine plus some additional information.

April 13, 2022

RE: COVID-19 Vaccine Mandate

Dear Dr. ________:

I am in receipt of your letter dated 3/23/2022 regarding the COVID-19 Vaccine Mandate.

I have no intention of being vaccinated based on my review of the science and the fact that I have natural immunity against COVID-19. I consider my history of prostate cancer a medical exemption.

I learned early in my medical career (40 years including medical school) that one must go to the original source of information as much as possible. The CDC, FDA, and Dr. Fauci are not the original source of information on COVID-19.

It is quite clear that most physicians have not read thoroughly enough of Pfizer's 6-Month Trial Study published in *The New England Journal of Medicine* and instead have been relying on secondary sources; otherwise more would object to the vaccines and vaccine mandates.

- The best available evidence on the efficacy of COVID-19 vaccines is Pfizer's 6-Month Trial which demonstrated that more patients in the vaccine arm died than in the placebo group.[329]
- The number to treat in that study to prevent a single COVID-19 death was 22,000. Preventing death—the main reason people seek vaccination. There were **just** two COVID-19 deaths in the control group of 22,000 over six months and one COVID-19 death of 22,000 in the vaccine group.[330]
- The **absolute risk reduction** to prevent a single COVID-19 infection in Pfizer's study was 0.84 percent (protection of which we now know is very short-lived). This does represent a 95 percent **relative risk reduction.** But 95 percent of a small number is even a smaller number. The risk of infection in the unvaccinated was 0.88 and was 0.4 in the vaccinated, which gives us a 95 percent relative risk reduction, but it borders on being meaningless. Thus, there is not even a 1 percent absolute risk reduction

from **experimental vaccines** with unknown side effects yet to come. There is a difference between statistical significance and clinical relevance. Physicians are swayed by pharmaceutical companies, which couch results by stating them in terms of relative risk, but absolute risk is the more important number. Absolute risk addresses clinical relevance.

- The chance of survival of COVID-19 is on average 99 percent if not higher. Getting vaccinated, therefore, seems to represent a long run for a short slide. A recent study out of Israel showed that a second Pfizer booster only provided protection for 4 to 7 weeks.[331] At some point, one should question if these are really vaccines. The median age of COVID-19 death in the US is higher than the life expectancy. The virus is largely killing people who are "playing with house money."
- I was infected with COVID-19 in December 2020, showing only minimal symptoms. SARS (now SARS-1) shares an 80 percent genetic overlap with SARS-2. A 2020 study showed that individuals infected with SARS-1 in 2003 still had humoral and T-cell immunity 17 years later.[332] COVID-19 infected individuals develop immunity to 29 proteins on the virus. Vaccinated individuals only mount a response to the spike protein. To think COVID-19 vaccines provide

better protection than natural immunity contradicts all prior knowledge/evidence of the superiority of the natural immunity over vaccination. Recently, a video of Dr. Fauci has resurfaced where, in 2004, he said the best vaccination against a virus is to be infected with the virus.

- The NCAA now recognizes natural immunity and considers athletes infected with COVID-19 as fully vaccinated.[333]
- I have a history of prostate cancer (with possible recurrence based on recent uptick in my PSA—workup in progress) and some studies are showing recurrences of previous cancers in those vaccinated.
- VAERS data over 30 years, show more people have died from the COVID-19 vaccines in a single year than from all vaccine over the previous 29 years.[334] Thus, their safety is highly questionable.
- Vaccine studies in the past have been halted when 25 deaths have occurred. There have been at least 25,000 deaths from COVID-19 vaccines reported in VAERS, which is felt to underestimate reality by a factor of 10- to 41-fold. The COVID-19 vaccines are the least efficacious and most dangerous vaccines ever approved by the FDA. Thus, whatever VAERs shows, it is only a fraction of the truth.

- OneAmerica, an Indianapolis insurance company, reported a **40 percent increase in deaths** among working age people ages 18-64 (the very population subjected to work vaccine mandates) in the third quarter and into fourth quarter, 2021. The company provides group insurance to employers and their employees. The insurance industry typically only sees a 10 percent increase in deaths when there is a one in 200-years catastrophe. Why so many deaths in the working age group in less than a one-year period coinciding with the administration of COVID-19 vaccines? Not all these excess deaths are from COVID-19 or delays in medical care related to the lockdowns. Other insurance companies report similar findings to OneAmerica.[335]

This recent article from the *British Medical Journal* titled "The Illusion of Evidence-Based Medicine" discusses how evidence-based medicine has been corrupted by corporate interests, failed regulation, and the commercialization of academia.[336] Our profession has become increasingly corrupt in my forty years.

Three former FDA Commissioners are now on the board of directors or medical directors for the companies making COVID-19 vaccines. This includes Scott Gottlieb (Pfizer), Mark McClellan (J&J), Stephen Hahn (Moderna). Might there be a conflict of interest?

Pfizer has a long history of criminal activity including bribing 5,000 physicians and scientists and fined $2.3 billion dollars in 2009 for committing the largest healthcare fraud in history.[337] Why should Pfizer be trusted when it comes to its vaccine?

I don't have confidence in the safety and efficacy of the COVID vaccines as it relates to me personally.

Respectfully,
Joseph Jacko, MD

Not-So-Wacko Jacko Rule of Medicine:

Regarding health data, data from an insurance company is likely more accurate than that from a government health agency. Insurance companies go out of business if they have poor data, health agencies do not.

If a health agency is stating that the vaccines are "perfectly safe" and the insurance industry is reporting up to a 40 percent increase in deaths in the population being subjected to the vaccine mandate, it is probably wiser to believe the insurance data.

Abandoning Ethical Standards

Perhaps the most disturbing part of the COVID-19 pandemic was the way the medical profession turned its back on ethical standards.

Previously established ethical standards were abandoned during the COVID-19 pandemic, and other ethical concerns were raised. These include:

- Vaccinating the masses instead of those at high risk for a virus for which there was a high survival rate.
- Physicians not being "neutral" with experimental treatment.
- FDA and pharmacies encroaching on the practice of medicine.
- Coercive tactics and financial incentives to boost vaccine rates.
- Questionable informed consent for experimental treatment.

Let's examine these concerns in depth.

Vaccinating Masses

In my view, the purpose of a vaccine is to prevent death or a serious life-altering complication. If you are not a high-risk patient, getting vaccinated to reduce the symptoms should you be infected, in my opinion, is a poor reason to get a vaccination. Remember, you cannot undo a vaccine. Once that vaccine hits your body, you are not reversing any of its effects. That's why I am selective in who gets vaccinated.

Many people get vaccinated nowadays for shingles. Do you know how many people die from shingles annually? Less than 100.[338]

Drugs and vaccines are studied and approved in isolation, and while each drug and vaccine may be safe and effective in isolation, they may not be safe and effective when prescribed in clusters (like medications) or piggybacked on top of each other over the years (like vaccines). We don't know the simultaneous effects of multiple drugs being used at once or the cumulative effects of vaccines because those simultaneous and cumulative effects have never been studied.

Also, when an infection has a 99 percent survival rate, what is to be gained with a vaccine by subjecting the entire population to a vaccine? In that case, the vaccine should be reserved for those most at risk of death or life-altering complications should they be infected.

Side effects of vaccines and even drugs may not become evident for years. Some recommend that patients wait for a drug or vaccine to be on the market for seven years before trying it.

"Unneutral" or Biased Physicians

Pfizer's six-month study was published on September 15, 2021, nine months after we began vaccinating a mass of humanity without any reliable data and without the vaccine being properly tested by previous standards.

This was made possible because Pfizer was granted to *test* its vaccine under Emergency Use Authorization. You may not realize this, but if you were vaccinated prior to August 23, 2021 (when the FDA approved Pfizer's vaccine), you were part of an experiment—the largest in human history.

Until a drug or vaccine is approved by the FDA, it is considered experimental.

When a treatment is still experimental, a physician should be neutral and not encourage or discourage someone from the experimental treatment because you have little data to support a decision either way.

We did know that the bulk of the deaths (85 percent) were occurring in those over 75 years old and that individuals with obesity, diabetes, and hypertension were at more risk.[339] Those were the few things we knew that we could hang our hat on.

Many physicians were largely encouraging, to the extent of badgering, their patients to be vaccinated. Some physicians dumped patients from their practices if they were not vaccinated against COVID-19. Those physicians claimed things that were not true or yet known, such as the vaccine was perfectly safe for pregnant women.

Everything I learned from my research, I did not learn all at once. My knowledge grew in a stepwise fashion, so I was continually adjusting my conversation with patients, but I stayed as neutral as possible.

Also, remember that the results of Pfizer's six-month study were not yet known during the period from December 2020 to August 2021. During this nine-month window, I had no reason to think the vaccine was not effective. I concluded only later that it was not nearly as effective as being reported.

Probably 90 percent of my vaccinated patients did so on their own at one of the many vaccination centers. Most of those were Medicare patients, many over the age of 70, the very group most likely to die from COVID-19 and, possibly, the group most likely to benefit from the vaccines.

If I were asked for my opinion, I simply stated something like, "Well, you are in a high-risk group, and the group who has the most to gain from the vaccine if it does what it is supposed to do. You are over 70 and have diabetes and high blood pressure, so you may want to consider the vaccine."

Or I might have responded, "You are young and in good health without risk factors that would raise your odds of dying from COVID-19. Your chance of dying from COVID-19, should you get it, is less than 0.5 percent. We can vaccinate if you want, but we don't have any short-term or long-term data on adverse reactions. We can vaccinate you today, but I don't think it is unreasonable if you take a wait-and-see approach."

Coercive Tactics and Financial Enticements

There are other ways the medical profession has abandoned ethical standards. Below is a small portion of the Nuremberg Code.[340] The Code is an outbirth of the Nuremberg Trials following World War II, providing a set of ethical principles for human experimentation.

I am including all ten principles for completeness' sake in the Appendix, but for our purposes, I will focus only on the first and second principles. The bolded section in principle 1 is my doing.

The Nuremberg Code

1. The voluntary consent of the human subject is absolutely essential.

   This means that the person involved should have legal capacity to give consent; should be so situated as to **be able to exercise free power of choice, without the intervention of any element of force, fraud,**

deceit, duress, overreaching, or other ulterior form of constraint or coercion; and should have sufficient knowledge and comprehension of the elements of the subject matter involved as to enable him to make an understanding and enlightened decision. This latter element requires that before the acceptance of an affirmative decision by the experimental subject there should be made known to him the nature, duration, and purpose of the experiment; the method and means by which it is to be conducted; all inconveniences and hazards reasonably to be expected; and the effects upon his health or person which may possibly come from his participation in the experiment.

2. The duty and responsibility for ascertaining the quality of the consent rests upon each individual who initiates, directs, or engages in the experiment. It is a personal duty and responsibility which may not be delegated to another with impunity.

The experiment should be such as to yield fruitful results for the good of society, unprocurable by other methods or means of study, and not random and unnecessary in nature.

Principle 1

It is my opinion that the section in bold type was violated with the mRNA vaccines. The results of Pfizer's six-month study misrepresented the efficacy of its vaccines and downplayed the adverse reactions that were seen. Although I am not a lawyer, that seems to constitute fraud.

Some patients were coerced into being vaccinated out of fear of losing their jobs and were vaccinated under duress.

Remember the earlier quote of Dr. Fauci, "it's been proven that when you *make it difficult* for people in their lives, they lose their ideological bullshit, and they get vaccinated."[341]

Some individuals were enticed with monetary rewards. The State of Ohio offered a vaccine lottery called Ohio Vax-a-Million. The lottery offered a series of five weekly drawings with a chance to win one million dollars per week if vaccinated.

Some medical practices in Ohio paid their employees up to $1,000 if they were vaccinated.

Enticing people with monetary rewards to receive something that has undergone limited testing and is of questionable value is unethical. Things that truly bring value and live up to hype do not require a sales pitch.

Part of the vaccine sales pitch was shaming people to be vaccinated to protect their loved ones. You do not get vaccinated to protect your neighbor. And you don't get vaccinated to protect yourself from your neighbor. You get vaccinated to protect *yourself* against a bug, like a virus or bacteria. Somehow, that concept became twisted, and people were made to feel guilty that they were putting others at risk by not being vaccinated.

I have never heard a patient say that they want to be vaccinated for shingles, or hepatitis, or pneumococcus to protect a family member from those diseases, but people were getting vaccinated for COVID-19 primarily to protect their loved ones.

Why should I demand you to be vaccinated to protect me, when I can simply get vaccinated myself and cut *you*, the middleman, out of the equation?

If a vaccine does what it is supposed to do and you received it, it should not matter whether your neighbor is vaccinated or not—you are protected. And, if the vaccine fails to live up to its expectations, then it matters not whether you and your neighbor are vaccinated, as it will not help either of you.

This is just one example of the media protecting Big Pharma's financial interest with an outright lie. It demonstrates how little regard the media has for its viewers and readers. And many readers fell for the deceit.

Who you listen to matters.

If you were vaccinated, do you think you received adequate informed consent based on principle 1 of the Nuremberg Code?

Principle 2

There were other effective treatments available, notably ivermectin, hydroxychloroquine, azithromycin, and many others. Some are available without a prescription. I refer you to C19early.org website for other beneficial treatments for COVID-19.

Pharmacists and the FDA Playing Doctor

One of the hot topics and controversies with COVID-19 surrounded the use of anti-parasitic drugs to treat COVID-19. These include ivermectin and hydroxychloroquine.

I asked a pharmacist whether he was seeing a lot of ivermectin prescriptions. He was and said, "But I refuse to fill them."

In effect, he was practicing medicine without a medical license as he was making patient care decisions. Later, he shared, "Our pharmacy made $80,000 last month giving COVID vaccines. We get it free and get paid $100 per vaccine."

If you do the math, they gave eight hundred vaccinations that month, about 26 or 27 a day, which certainly seems plausible.

The pharmacy probably makes only a few dollars for an ivermectin prescription.

I have tremendous respect for pharmacists. They are the most underutilized professionals in healthcare. They know far more than we do as physicians about pharmacology. I have learned much from them, especially compounding pharmacists. But…

Regardless of a physician's view on the use of ivermectin and hydroxychloroquine, *every physician* should be upset that pharmacists were picking and choosing which prescriptions they would fill. In doing so, they are making patient care decisions, which falls under the umbrella of practicing medicine. And patients should be upset too.

The FDA itself was playing doctor. The FDA's job is to evaluate the safety and efficacy of drugs. That's it. The agency oversteps its role when it tells doctors how to diagnose a particular condition and what they should and should not prescribe. And it is stepping out of its lane when it tells patients what to do and not do.

The FDA played doctor by discouraging ivermectin's use. Drugs are approved for certain conditions. Ivermectin is approved for the treatment of parasitic infections, but a physician does not have to limit his or her prescribing it to parasitic infections.

Physicians Not Protecting Their Turf

I found it particularly bothersome that many physicians seemed to have no problem with the pharmacists' and FDA's actions. Many physicians thought they were doing society a favor with these actions.

It's an example of how bamboozled, duped, and hoodwinked physicians have become.

It is no wonder we have lost control of our profession. We don't protect our turf; we blindly do what we are told; and we blindly trust our health agencies, which are corrupt and under regulatory capture.

The FDA-approved condition does not limit how a doctor can prescribe a medication. The approved condition limits how the pharmaceutical company can market a medication. This is a huge difference.

When a doctor prescribes a medication for a non-FDA-approved condition, that is called writing the medication off-label. Depending on the source, anywhere from 30–40 percent of prescriptions are written off-label. The physician should inform the patient a medication is being used off-label because insurance may not cover the medication's cost if used off-label.

The FDA was out of line when it said that ivermectin should not be used to treat COVID-19, and it did so, intentionally, to protect the vaccine makers. Regulatory capture was at play. The FDA knows full well that physicians can write prescriptions for ivermectin or hydroxychloroquine off-label. The FDA is Big Pharma's heavy muscle in times of need.

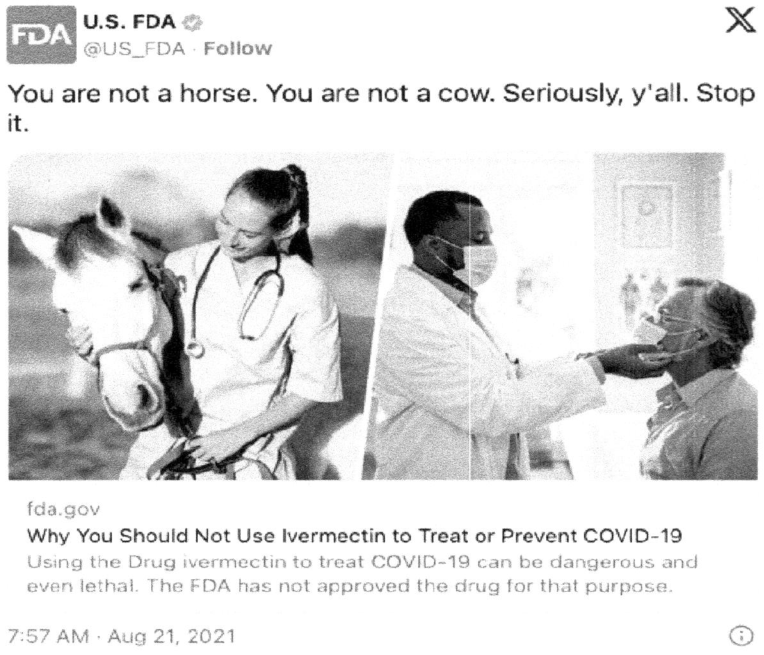
FDA
U.S. FDA
@US_FDA · Follow
You are not a horse. You are not a cow. Seriously, y'all. Stop it.
fda.gov
Why You Should Not Use Ivermectin to Treat or Prevent COVID-19
Using the Drug ivermectin to treat COVID-19 can be dangerous and even lethal. The FDA has not approved the drug for that purpose.
7:57 AM · Aug 21, 2021

The above ad is a classic example of the half-truths and misinformation coming from within medicine. Individuals fell for a half-truth because of the perceived credibility of the source of information. It also highlights how poorly educated doctors are about the FDA's role and how the agency is funded. It matters who you listen to. Our health agencies are corrupt, like many other federal agencies.

Hospitals Overwhelmed with COVID-19

You likely heard that hospitals were overrun with COVID-19 patients. That, too, is a half-truth. Regardless of the number of beds a hospital physically has, they only count the beds available based on the number of staff they have available to manage those beds.

If a hospital has nine hundred beds but only enough staff to man six hundred of them, then it only has "six hundred beds." For several reasons, hospitals were short-staffed during much of the pandemic. Some of that was related to the vaccine mandates that may have served their purposes in getting people vaccinated but also triggered people who didn't want to be vaccinated to quit working. Some staff, close to retirement, simply retired a little sooner than planned. Others quit out of fear of contracting COVID-19 and dying from it.

In October 2022, a patient of mine experiencing chest pains went to the ER and spent his entire two-day hospitalization in the hallway outside the ER department, along with thirty other patients, because the hospital had "no beds," that is, they did not have the staff.

If a hospital has nine hundred beds but only enough staff to man six hundred of them, then it only has "six hundred beds."

Shortly after that, another of my patients, a nurse at the same hospital, which is part of one of the larger health systems in Ohio, told me her hospital system was short 954 nurses.

This is second-hand information that I cannot verify, but I have no reason to disbelieve either of my patients. The patient-nurse did corroborate what my chest pain patient said about being in the hallway as likely. Plus, one of my physician partners heard the same thing about patients in the ER hallways.

The entire healthcare system has not recovered from this staffing shortage. It is not uncommon today to have weeks of delays in getting patients scheduled for tests or to see a specialist for a consultation. We have turned into a developing country in some respects.

Hospitals started to rely on travel nurses, who are paid at higher rates, which only made nursing shortages worse because more nurses quit, realizing they could make more money working for a travel nurse agency. It was not unusual for a nurse to quit the hospital, sign up as a travel nurse, and be assigned to the same hospital but now making more money. Earning more means one does not need to work as many hours, which also contributed to nursing shortages.

The vaccine mandate of hospital employees, to some degree, backfired on the system.

This is what happens when ethics are abandoned and ulterior motives prevail.

Not to minimize the seriousness of COVID-19 cases and deaths from it, but to put COVID-19 numbers and hospitalizations in perspective, consider this. The State of Ohio has some thirty-four thousand hospital beds within a state of a population of 11,800,000. If every one of those beds is filled with patients with COVID-19, it represents 0.29 percent of the population of the State of Ohio.

Numbers need to be put into proper perspective. It is the number behind the numbers that matters.

Acute Renal Failure Related to COVID-19 Treatment

On August 26, 2024, two researchers studying acute renal failure independent of one another, utilizing two different databases, concluded that there has been an *excess* of 150,000-plus deaths from acute renal (kidney failure) since late 2020.

Using state death records, John Beaudoin reported 155,000 excess deaths from acute kidney failure since 2021, coinciding with a decline in COVID-19 cases. (President Biden considered the pandemic over in September of 2022.) Thus, it is felt the excess deaths are related to mostly COVID-19 vaccines and possibly some from COVID-19 hospital protocols. (Remdesivir, given to hospitalized COVID patients, is known to cause kidney failure.)

Ed Dowd, using CDC data, came to similar conclusions, reporting 153,000 excess deaths from acute renal failure during the same time.

Beaudoin reported a 200 percent increase in deaths from acute kidney failure in 2021 and a 300 percent increase in 2022. Despite the decline in COVID-19 cases in 2023, the cases of renal failure continued to rise, likely related to the vaccines. Many of the deaths occurred in the younger population. Beaudoin calculated the life years lost from these deaths exceed life years lost from COVID-19, smallpox, polio, H1N1, and Hong Kong flu, and anything else in the past one hundred years, except for life years lost stemming from World War II.[342]

For the latest information on COVID-19 and the COVID-19 vaccines, please go to my website www.JackoMD180.com.

Pfizer's Deceptive COVID-19 Vaccine Trial

If there were an epidemic, that would definitely make people accept vaccines.
—Bill Gates

Doctors will have more lives to answer for in the next world than even we generals.
—Napoleon Bonaparte

In the opening scene of the movie *The Princess Bride*, the sick grandson asks his grandfather whether the story he is about to read contains sports. The grandfather replies, "Are you kidding? Fencing. Fighting. Torture. Revenge. Giants. Monsters. Chases. Escapes. True love. Miracles."

In one book was nearly everything a young boy could want, except maybe true love.

The same is true with Pfizer's six-month study of its COVID-19 vaccine. In a single study, we see nearly everything wrong with medicine and medical research. We see half-truths of every persuasion. We see manipulation and misrepresentation of data. We see falsification of data. We see conflicts of interest, greed, and deception. We see more harm than good. We see the powers of medicine protecting each other. We see the ultimate in being bamboozled, duped, and hoodwinked.

And nearly everyone in medicine and beyond fell for it or turned their eyes.

But before we get to the study: On November 9, 2021, in a conversation with Frederick Kempe, CEO of Atlantic Council, a think tank, Pfizer CEO Albert Bourla said there is a small group of people who "circulate, on purpose, misinformation so that they will mislead those that they have concerns (with the vaccine)." He further stated, "Those people are criminals. They are not bad people. They're criminals because they have literally cost millions of lives."[343] Those are strong words from a CEO who oversees a company with a laundry list of crimes committed and fines and lawsuits levied against it over decades.

He made those comments just fifty-five days after Pfizer's study was published online on September 15, 2021. What is remarkable about his comments is that the mRNA vaccine study showed that *more* people in the vaccine group died than in the placebo group and that the vaccine group had *more* adverse reactions.[344]

Dr. Bourla labeled individuals as "criminals" those who do not want his company's product and share vaccine information with others. We all should find that disconcerting and unbecoming of a Fortune 500 CEO. Two months later, he admitted the Pfizer-BioNTech vaccine offered limited protection.

Have you heard of more deaths and adverse effects in the vaccinated group in Pfizer's study? If not, you might want to review where you get your information. It matters.

Keeping Dr. Bourla's comment in mind, remember what I said earlier about listening to advice from those who have little to profit from it. No one profits by suggesting people not be vaccinated. Such people may, ultimately, be proven wrong with their advice, but they probably believe they have your best interests in mind.

We do know Pfizer has about $63.2 billion worth of reasons you should get vaccinated regardless of any side effects, complications, or deaths its vaccine causes, especially when it has been indemnified against any of these events. It made $33.5 billion on the vaccine in 2021 and projected a revenue of $29.7 billion for 2022.[345]

What a sweet deal: Make a product that does not do well what it is supposed to do (prevent infection). Make billions of dollars from it. Accuse others of the same tactics you are engaged in (sharing misleading information). And assume no liability for any problem your product causes.

You likely heard that Pfizer's mRNA vaccine for COVID-19 was 100 percent effective in preventing death and 91.3–95 percent effective in preventing infection. If you heard that you would be silly not to be vaccinated. Right?

Those numbers are correct. But those numbers don't mean what you think. In fact, those numbers may represent the biggest half-truths and greatest deception in medical history.

Remember the Not-So-Wacko Jacko Rule to Live By:

The numbers do not tell the story. The numbers *behind* the numbers tell the real story.

Those numbers relate to *relative* risk reduction. The numbers you really want to know are the *absolute* risk reductions, which were dismal at best when it comes to the Pfizer-BioNTech vaccine.

First, let's get some background information.

Pfizer's Phase I/II study of its COVID-19 RNA vaccine BNT162b1 in adults was published on August 12, 2020, about eight months into the pandemic.[346] The RNA platform allows for rapid vaccine development, which is why it was likely used over the tried-and-true platform of growing vaccines in eggs.

Between May 4, 2020, and June 19, 2020, forty-five participants were screened and enrolled in the Phase I/II trial. Participant ages ranged from 19 to 54 years, with a median age of 35, 51 percent males and 49 percent females.

These were *healthy* individuals. No one in the study had heart disease, cancer, diabetes, or was pregnant. Three different doses were tested: 10μ, 30μ, and 100μ.

The purpose of this study was to document reactions and side effects; the study concluded these to be minimal and assessed the immune response to the vaccine. The 30μ dose was determined to be the "sweet spot" in terms of safety and immune response and was used in the phase 3 trial.

Phase 3 Trial

Pfizer's phase 3 trial began on July 23, 2020.

Recall what I said in "How Pure Is the Evidence?" about designing a study to yield the results you want. We see a classic example of this with Pfizer's study on its mRNA vaccine.

A primary endpoint of the study was to test the vaccine's efficacy against confirmed COVID-19 with onset at least seven days after the second dose. I will come back to this later in the chapter when discussing the CDC (Centers for Disease Control and Prevention.

Data on adverse effects through fourteen weeks after the second dose were included in the reported study, although data up to six months were collected. Deaths from all causes were not an endpoint. Why is this important? A drug or vaccine may be effective in treating/preventing the condition being studied, yet may be causing more harm and deaths in other ways. Avandia and Vioxx were effective for the conditions for which they were approved, yet caused excess heart attacks.

The study included participants who already had COVID-19, but vaccine safety in those subjects was not an endpoint, so there was no attempt to determine if the vaccine was safe in that subset who already harbored spike protein from prior infection.

Safety data was provided on all participants who provided informed consent and received at least one dose of the vaccine. Because not all participants received both doses, this has the potential to make the vaccine appear safer since some adverse reactions may be cumulative with a second dose.

I will shortly go over more issues with the study design.

Pfizer published two-month safety and efficacy data from the phase 3 trial on December 10, 2020, and six-month safety and efficacy data on September 15, 2021. The outcome of the two-month publication was that Pfizer was able to show that the Pfizer-BioNTech mRNA vaccine was efficacious enough to receive emergency use authorization (EUA). Pfizer then unblinded the study, which was to be a three-year study, and offered the vaccine to those in the placebo group while simultaneously conducting its trial, mostly without a control group.

EUA does not mean FDA-approved. During the EUA period, the mRNA vaccine was still experimental.

At the time of the two-month publication, 21,720 patients were in the vaccine group and 21,728 in the placebo group. At the time of the six-month publication, 21,926 patients were in the vaccine group and 21,921 in the placebo group. *The New England Journal of Medicine* published data from both the two-month and six-month studies.

In summation, the Canadian COVID Care Alliance determined that Pfizer's study had several problems in how it was designed and executed:

1. Not everyone in the vaccine group or placebo group was tested for COVID-19. Thus, they made no attempt to detect asymptomatic cases.
2. Only suspected cases were tested, and *not even all of them were tested.* In fact, there were more suspected but unconfirmed cases in both arms of the studies than suspected and confirmed cases.
3. The study was unblinded after only two months in what was supposed to be a three-year study, and ended at six months. Thus, after two months, there was not a control group for comparison.
4. The vaccine was tested on a healthier population than is representative of the general population.
5. All-cause mortality was not an endpoint.

These issues will be discussed below. I am going to see if I can pull this off as a multimedia discussion through a book.

Pfizer's Two-Month and Six-Month Studies

As I go through this discussion, it may be helpful for you to access three documents or sources online. One is Pfizer's two-month study, "Safety and Efficacy of the BNT162b 2mRNA Covid-19 Vaccine," published in *The New England Journal of Medicine*.[347]

The second is the 6-month study, "Safety and Efficacy of the BNT162b2m mRNA COVID-19 Vaccine through 6 Months," also published in *The New England Journal of Medicine*.[348]

You will want to access the Supplementary Appendix of both studies. The Supplementary Appendix in the two-month study can be found under "Efficacy" under the "Methods" heading (https://bit.ly/41FhS9G).

The Supplementary Appendix for the six-month study (online at https://bit.ly/43horAh) can be found under "Methods," but not the "Methods" listed under "Abstract." Scroll down to next subheading called "Methods."

The tables of interest that I will go over are the S3 and S4 tables in the two-month study (page 9 of the Supplementary Appendix) and the S3 and S4 (pages 10 and 11 of the Supplementary Appendix) tables in the six-month study.

I have condensed those tables below, including only the information I will discuss here.

I have included the tables, but you should know how to access the studies and familiarize yourself with published medical studies, as you may find a need to conduct your own research moving forward.

Canadian COVID Care Alliance

The third source of information to access comes from the Canadian COVID Care Alliance (CCCA), which produced an excellent slide and video presentation that breaks down the Pfizer study in understandable terms. You can download the presentation, "The Pfizer Inoculations for COVID-19: More HARM Than Good," online.[349]

I am, primarily, going to review its presentation. There are fifty pages to the presentation, and page numbers are found on the bottom left on each page. Don't worry, I will not review all fifty. I will refer to specific page numbers throughout this discussion.

On page 5 of CCCA's presentation, you will find an Overview of the Presentation. The links are active and will take you to the topic of interest. I encourage you to spend time looking at the information beyond what I cover here.

The CCCA presentation contains the complete tables found in the Supplementary Appendices of *The New England Journal of Medicine* articles, in case you have issues accessing them on your own.

Relative Risk vs. Absolute Risk Reduction

The presentation provides a video (p. 8) providing a very nice explanation for relative risk reduction versus absolute risk reduction, which I have discussed earlier in this book. The video specifically addresses relative and absolute risk reduction as it relates to the Pfizer-BioNTech COVID-19 vaccine, however.

It is important to understand the difference between these two risk measurements. The numbers behind the numbers are what provide the difference between relative and absolute risk reduction. Absolute risk reduction is the more important number.

Vaccine Efficacy

The Pfizer study showed a relative risk of reduction of 95 percent of getting COVID-19 with its vaccine, but the absolute risk reduction was just 0.84 percent. Thus, there was a less than 1 percent absolute risk reduction in getting COVID-19 by being vaccinated (p. 7 of the CCCA presentation).

That data comes from the two-month safety and efficacy study (table S4 of the two-month study). The 95 percent represents the vaccine efficacy. The top line of table S4 shows eight people in the vaccine group had confirmed COVID-19 (the efficacy endpoint) and 162 had confirmed COVID-19 in the placebo group. There were 18,198 people in the vaccine group and 18,325 in the unvaccinated or placebo group. Thus, there were 170 confirmed cases of COVID-19 in both arms of the study out of 36,000 participants, which equates to 0.47 percent of the study population

How do we get to 0.84 percent absolute risk reduction?

Eight divided by 18,118 equals 0.04 percent, the percentage of vaccinated individuals who contracted COVID-19 during the study. One hundred sixty-two divided by 18,325 is 0.88 percent, the percentage of the unvaccinated who got COVID-19 during the same time period.

A simplified table from the S4 table in the two-month study is below.

	Vaccine Group	Placebo Group
Efficacy Endpoint	**18198**	**18325**
COVID-19 infections	8	162
Infection rate	8/18198 = 0.04%	162/18325 = 0.88%

Therefore, 0.88 percent, or not even 1 percent, of the unvaccinated got COVID-19. The 95 percent vaccine efficacy refers to the relative difference from 0.88 percent to 0.04 percent. To calculate vaccine efficacy, subtract 8 from 162 and divide by 162. The result is 95 percent. This is impressive on relative terms but only represents a 0.84 percent absolute reduction in getting COVID-19 in the vaccine.

The number that jumps out to me is the 0.88 percent (162 subjects out of 18,325) of the unvaccinated getting COVID-19. That seems to suggest that COVID-19 was not spreading as rampantly as advertised.

Note: Not every participant was enrolled in the study at the same time. The cut-off for analyzing the two-month data was October 9, 2020. Thus, the numbers included in the two-month study are less than the actual number of participants. The data on those participants not included in the two-month study would be included in the six-month study.

Ninety-five percent vaccine efficiency does not mean 95 percent of those vaccinated will not get infected. Many people received an *experimental* vaccine with unknown side effects for a less than a 1 percent absolute risk reduction for an infection most would survive if not vaccinated.

I will come back to these numbers because COVID-19 probably occurred in more individuals in both the vaccinated and unvaccinated than Pfizer reported in the study, but you must go to an FDA document from December 2020 to discover that.

You would think that all participants, vaccinated and unvaccinated, would be periodically tested for COVID-19 during the study. That did not happen. Only *suspected cases* were tested, and not even all of those, and that testing was left up to the discretion of each site's principal investigator.

And it turns out not all suspected cases in either arm of the study were tested for COVID-19. So, right off the bat, the study is misleading. And, since not everyone was tested for COVID-19, there was no attempt to detect asymptomatic cases.

I will come back to these suspected but unconfirmed cases later.

Adverse Reactions Two-Month Data

Now, look at Table S3 and the adverse events. There were more adverse events in the vaccine group, more than twice as many at the two-month mark, with nearly identical life-threatening adverse effects slightly favoring the vaccine group, but about 50 percent more serious effects in the vaccine group. The difference in the number of adverse reactions between both groups becomes more noticeable when looking at the six-month data.

Adverse Events	Vaccine Group N= 21621	Placebo Group N= 21631
Any Event	5770	2638
Related	4484	1095
Severe	240	139
Life-threatening	21	24

A related event is an event that the researchers felt was related to the vaccine or the saline (placebo) injection in the placebo group.

Let's move on to the six-month data on adverse events. I have summarized the pertinent data in the table below from Table S3 found in the six-month study.

Adverse Events	Vaccine Group N= 219326	Placebo Group N= 21921
Any event	6617	3048
Related	5241	1311
Severe	262	150
Life-threatening	21	26

Again, we see more adverse events in the vaccinated group, with nearly four times as many related events compared to the placebo group, with about 75 percent more severe reactions but less life-threatening.

Study Design

On page 9, the Canadian COVID Care Alliance shows how Pfizer's study was to be conducted and how it was conducted. The study was originally designed to be a three-year study but was unblinded at two months and ended at six months.

A common trial strategy is stopping the trial early if results are trending in the wrong direction.

Two studies published on October 6, 2021, one from Israel and the other from Qatar, showed that protection from the Pfizer-BioNTech vaccine began to wane as early as *two months* after the second vaccination.[350]

In its six-month study, Pfizer does admit to "a gradual decline in vaccine efficacy." Should there be a decline in efficacy within six months? How many other vaccines lose efficacy within six months outside the annual flu vaccine? That efficacy declined so soon seemed to telegraph that boosters would be needed in the future, which we now know to be true.

Perhaps to offset the decline in efficacy, Pfizer included data from the 12- to 15-year-old cohort even though the trial in that age group did not start until four months after the trial on adults. This would make the efficacy numbers look better by offsetting the decline in efficacy being seen in adults (see p. 32 of the CCCA presentation). This is another example of muddying the waters.

Pfizer also unblinded the study prematurely, enabling those who had received the placebo to receive the actual vaccination. In doing so, Pfizer eliminated the control group, making long-term safety data unavailable for comparison. One of the problems in determining long-term safety regarding any vaccine is that a majority of the US population is vaccinated, so we do not have an unvaccinated, or control, group for comparison.

Pfizer can justify the decision to unblind the study early because it received the EUA based on that two-month data. Thus, we can argue it would be unethical to withhold the vaccine from those who originally received the placebo, given the "impressive" 95 percent vaccine efficacy.

Increased Risk of Illness

Page 11 of the CCCA presentation shows that vaccinated individuals demonstrated more illness and side effects than those who received the placebo. This slide corresponds to page 10 of the Supplementary Appendix (Table S3).

Those vaccinated witnessed a 300 percent increase in any adverse reaction compared to the placebo group, with a 75 percent increase in severe reactions (anything that interferes with normal function) and a 10 percent increase in serious reactions (those requiring a visit to ER or hospitalization).

On page 11 of the CCCA presentation, we see the vaccine efficacy had dropped from 95 percent to 91 percent.

Increased Risk of Death

Page 12 mentions an increased risk of death in the vaccinated. The slide shows table S4 of the Supplementary Appendix (p. 11 of the Supplementary Appendix in Pfizer's published study). That table shows that fifteen in the vaccinated and fourteen in the unvaccinated group died. These deaths are from all causes, not just COVID-19. More people died in the vaccinated group.

But those numbers are misleading, too. The number of deaths among the vaccinated was really higher.

If you look at that page on the CCCA presentation and compare it to information from the Supplementary Appendix, there appears to be a discrepancy. The CCCA presentation shows *20 vaccinated patients* dying during the study, compared to fourteen of the unvaccinated dying. But the supplementary appendix shows only fifteen vaccinated dying. Where did the other five deaths come from?

Those five extra deaths occurred after the study was unblinded, which is mentioned only in passing within the study's text. Pfizer only reported in the Supplementary Appendix events up to the unblinding period.

You must go to "Adverse Events" in the actual text of the study and the third paragraph to see that "3 participants in the BNT162b2 group and 2 in the original placebo group who received the BNT162b2 after unblinding died."

I have summarized the total deaths in the table below without listing all the specific causes of death, but those that are most concerning; thus, the numbers for specific causes of death do not equal the total deaths.

In the end, after the study was unblinded, there were 20 total deaths in the vaccine group and 14 in the placebo group (unvaccinated).

Because heart disease is the number one killer in our country, historically, any intervention that leads to more cardiac deaths is not approved or is withdrawn from the market once the excess cardiac deaths become evident, as in the cases of Avandia and Vioxx.

There were more cardiac deaths in the vaccine group than the placebo group, yet the mRNA vaccines received FDA approval while only preventing one COVID death per 22,000 vaccinated subjects.

Reported Causes of Death	Vaccine Group N = 21,926	Placebo Group N = 21,921
Total Deaths before unblinding	15	14
COVID-19/COVID pneumonia	1	2
Cardiac arrest	4	1
Other cardiopulmonary events	2	1
Deaths during unblinding	5	0
Total Deaths after unblinding	20	14

On the same slide, on the bottom right of the CCCA presentation, you see "Concerning Causes of Death." Two patients who received the placebo died of COVID-19, and just one who was vaccinated with the mRNA vaccine died. That is where we get the 100 percent vaccine efficacy in prevention of COVID-19 deaths. Two deaths compared to one death are a 100 percent relative risk reduction. See the above table's "COVID-19/COVID pneumonia" cell.

This does not mean, as we were led to believe, that there were no deaths among the vaccinated group. Saying

100 percent efficacy in preventing deaths seems to imply no deaths in the vaccinated group. That is not what it means, though.

Were you informed of that as well?

The two deaths in the unvaccinated in a six-month trial call into question the veracity of media reports that made it sound like unvaccinated people were being hospitalized, dropping like flies, and dying from COVID-19. Remember, 41 percent of Democrats thought that over 50 percent of the unvaccinated were hospitalized with COVID-19.

It took 22,000 (more specifically 21,926) patients to be vaccinated to prevent that one COVID-19 death. One divided by 22,000 is 0.000045 or a 0.0045 percent absolute risk reduction in COVID-19 deaths in those vaccinated with the mRNA vaccine. Preventing death is the main purpose behind most vaccines.

If the entire eight billion on the planet were vaccinated for COVID-19, then 360,000 COVID-19 deaths would have been prevented, but there would be 2,160,000 more total deaths based on six more deaths (20 to 14) occurring per 22,000 in the vaccine group.

It took 22,000 (more specifically 21,926) patients to be vaccinated to prevent that one COVID-19 death.

If you knew this before you were vaccinated, would you have been vaccinated? Many of you would probably say "no." You were bamboozled, duped, and hoodwinked.

You also see, on that same slide, that nine deaths occurred relating to cardiovascular disease in the *vaccinated* group and five in the placebo group, a difference of four. Overall, there were six more deaths in the vaccinated (20 to 14). So, 67 percent of the increased deaths (from four to six) seen in the vaccinated group came from cardiovascular disease.

What Went Wrong (CCCA Presentation)

The data is even more misleading than that. In the real world, 85 percent of COVID-19 deaths occurred in the over-75 age group, yet that age group only represented 4.4 percent of those in Pfizer's study (p. 15 of the CCCA presentation). The over-75 age group makes up about 7.3 percent of the US population;[351] at the very least, the trial should have reflected that.

Of those who died from COVID-19 in the real world, 95 percent had at least one comorbidity (high blood pressure, diabetes, obesity, etc.) listed as a cause of death, with the average being four comorbidities. In Pfizer's study, only 21 percent had a coexisting condition.

Thus, the vaccine was tested in a healthier population in the phase 3 trial than those who received it in the real world (p. 16 of the CCCA presentation).

Remember the tricks researchers use to get the results they want that we reviewed in the chapter in "How Pure Is the Medical Evidence?"

The vaccine was not studied in those who had already recovered from COVID-19 to determine whether the vaccine was safe and effective (p.17).

Illness and death from *all causes,* not just COVID-19, were not endpoints of the study. A drug/vaccine might be effective in preventing the studied condition but may be causing more illness and death from other causes. That is something Pfizer's study bears out, though it was not terribly effective at doing so (p. 18).

The study was not designed to look for a spread reduction of COVID-19 (p. 19). How many times did we hear that COVID-19 was a "pandemic of the unvaccinated," yet there was no verification that the vaccinated were spreaders and no attempt made to detect asymptomatic cases?

Confirmed vs. Suspected but Unconfirmed Cases

This may be the biggest issue with the study.

Emergency use authorization was based on the relative risk reduction of 95 percent (review the video on p. 8), in which there were eight confirmed COVID-19 cases in the vaccinated and 162 confirmed cases in the placebo group.

However, an additional 1,594 suspected COVID-19 cases were in the vaccinated groups, and an additional 1,816 suspected COVID-19 cases in the placebo group. *None of these suspected cases were tested for COVID-19 for confirmation.* One of the primary endpoints was to test the efficacy of the vaccine against laboratory confirmation; the study did not do what it said it was to do, that is, confirm *all* suspected cases against laboratory testing.

Thus, there were far greater numbers of suspected but unconfirmed cases than confirmed cases in both arms of the trial, which makes the *data completely unreliable* (p. 22). If all those suspected cases turned out to be confirmed, the relative risk reduction of the vaccine would have dropped from 95 percent to 19 percent, leading to a much lower probability that emergency use authorization would have been approved (p. 23).

Also, only symptomatic individuals in both arms of the study were tested, which was left up to the investigators at each location (p. 21, CCCA). To know if there were asymptomatic cases, everyone enrolled in the study should have been periodically tested for COVID-19.

The data on suspected but unconfirmed cases does not come from Pfizer's six-month study but rather from page 42 of an FDA Briefing Document on the Pfizer-BioNTech COVID-19 Vaccine titled "Vaccines and Related Biological Products Advisory Committee Meeting, December 10, 2020."

This is an observation or wonder on my part. Ninety-five percent is a key landmark to reach in drug approval studies. When you look at the numbers used in the Pfizer-BioNTech month study used to determine vaccine efficacy and to obtain EUA, they almost come out perfectly to 95 percent. Were just enough suspected but unconfirmed cases "ignored" to achieve this near "perfect percentage"? Is that observation coincidental or intentional? I will discuss those two words more in the final chapter.

Conflict of Interest

Dr. Eric Rubin, a pediatrician, is editor-in-chief of *The New England Journal of Medicine,* which published Pfizer's study. He is also a member of the FDA Advisory Council, and as a member of the council, he voted to approve the rollout of the Pfizer-BioNTech vaccine in the 5 to 11 age group (p. 28).

Remember the relationships I discussed between journal editors and Big Pharma and the FDA and Big Pharma. Dr. Rubin is a classic example of having ties to both Big Pharma and the FDA while serving as editor-in-chief of one of the most prestigious medical journals. Many would consider that a major conflict of interest. His journal received revenue by publishing Pfizer's study.

On November 2, 2021, the *British Medical Journal* published an article about its investigation of Ventavia Research Group, one of the research groups Pfizer hired to conduct the trial.[352] A regional director of the company turned whistleblower and reported to the FDA that the company falsified data, unblinded participants, employed inadequately trained vaccinators, and did not follow up on patients reporting symptoms. Again, several suspected cases of COVID-19 in both the vaccinated and the placebo groups were never tested for confirmation.

Pages 37–38 discuss the increase in deaths among young athletes vaccinated for COVID-19 who died during physical exertion. Athletes dying during sports participation *increased fivefold* in the International Football Association (FIFA) compared to the average number of deaths annually over the preceding 20 years. If these deaths are not vaccine-related, then what did those athletes die from? What other possibility or event could lead to a fivefold increase in exercise-related deaths in such a short period of time?

Page 43 lists the crimes and fines that Pfizer has committed over the years.

Page 44 lists the conflicts of interest among the Pfizer report authors. Eighty-four percent had conflicts of interest, with most being employed either by Pfizer or its partner BioNTech and several owning Pfizer stock.

In the Supplementary Appendix of Pfizer's six-month study, you will find a section where you can download "Disclosures" and see the names of all authors and any conflicts of interest.

Pfizer has been indemnified for damages its vaccine may cause (p. 47). It cannot be held responsible for the harm its vaccine has caused and will cause. And we can be most certain there is more harm to be revealed in the next few years.

One thing I find interesting is that it did not take very long to report the two-month data to get EUA but seemed to take longer than necessary to report the six-month data. The two-month data were reported two months after the cut-off date, March 13, 2021, and it took six months to report the data that included only three hundred or so additional participants in both arms.

It makes me wonder if the reporting of the data was delayed until after half the population was vaccinated. In my mind, it should not take an extra four months to analyze the data on these additional numbers, especially since the six-month study was basically a continuation of the two-month study.

There is only one winner in this game as it relates to COVID-19—the vaccine makers.

In "The Power of the Half-Truth," I mentioned how the game was played—how all the dots connected and interrelated. Some of you were probably skeptical about my description of that game. You now see a real-life case of how the game is played, and some of you have been, or will be, directly and negatively affected by that game.

There is only one winner in this game as it relates to COVID-19—the vaccine makers. The FDA and CDC, which ran interference for the pharmaceutical companies, will come under scrutiny for being complicit by protecting Big Pharma and spreading many half-truths. This will happen once more people are awakened and demand changes.

CDC's Role in the Cover-Up

Much, if not all, you need to know about the safety and efficacy of the Pfizer-BioNTech vaccine can be discerned from

Pfizer's study. It was a double-blind placebo (until the company unblinded it prematurely), representing the strongest form of evidence. It is all in black and white.

These numbers are Pfizer's numbers, and it has painted those numbers in the best possible light using nearly every research gimmick available. Still, it comes up short on "proving" that its product does what it is supposed to do because the product does *not* do what it is supposed to do. Researchers did their best to dress up the data, but you can only make it look so pretty.

What anybody else says to justify the safety and efficacy of the vaccines is an attempt to mislead you. The bigger question is, for what reason?

I have not said much about the CDC in this book. You likely heard from the CDC how safe and effective the COVID-19 vaccines are. How did the CDC reach that conclusion, and how did it support that? Did it not read Pfizer's six-month trial data?

The CDC engaged in its own statistical manipulation of the data and deception, including using a definition of "fully vaccinated," which greatly skewed results.

Frequently, we heard we had a pandemic of the unvaccinated. Before going into that answer, we need to understand how the CDC defined unvaccinated. People were not considered fully vaccinated against COVID-19 until two weeks after they received their second dose of Moderna or Pfizer-BioNTech vaccines, or two weeks after Johnson & Johnson's single-dose vaccine.

It was recommended that the two doses of the Pfizer-BioNTech vaccine be given three weeks apart and four weeks apart for the Moderna vaccine. Add another two weeks to each schedule, and you have a five-to-six-week window before someone is considered fully vaccinated.

Many vaccine-related adverse reactions, regardless of the vaccine, occur during the first six weeks. But with the COVID-19 vaccines, any adverse reaction occurring within that five-to-six-week window is attributed to the "unvaccinated." *Any* death that occurred within that window is attributed to the "unvaccinated," plus some of those deaths the CDC counts as COVID-19 deaths, further skewing the data in favor of the vaccines.

Another trick used by the CDC was to include hospitalizations and deaths from January to June 2021 in its calculations. It admitted doing so in August of 2021.[12,13]

Remember, this was a period when *less than half* of Americans were vaccinated. By mid-June 2021, only 48.7 percent of the population was vaccinated. Going backwards, in April 2021, it was 31 percent, and on January 1, 2021, only 0.5 percent.[353]

Apples were not being compared to apples. Like denominators were not being used to compare both groups. You do not have an equal number of vaccinated versus unvaccinated to make direct comparisons without first correcting for the imbalance in raw numbers between both groups.

Nearly all COVID-19 deaths in January 2021 would occur in the unvaccinated since nearly everyone was still unvaccinated. So, to say we had an epidemic of unvaccinated was misleading.

Let's look at April, when 31 percent of the US population was vaccinated. Suppose we have a population of 1,000, and 31 percent or 310 are vaccinated, leaving 690 unvaccinated.

Suppose there were 20 COVID-19 deaths among the 690 unvaccinated and ten COVID-19 deaths among the 310 vaccinated. You cannot directly compare 20 deaths in the unvaccinated to ten deaths in the vaccinated and conclude that the unvaccinated are dying at twice the rate because you do not have equal denominators. Nonetheless, the CDC took that approach. The CDC misled us.

Twenty deaths per 690 in the unvaccinated is 2.9 percent, and ten deaths per 310 vaccinated is 3.2 percent. Those two percentages are close, with a lower death rate in the unvaccinated in this illustration, and if you adjust the numbers to reflect 310 in both groups, we will have 9.0 deaths in the unvaccinated (0.029 x 310). Or, if you adjust the other way so that the denominator is 690, you will have 22 deaths (0.032 x 690) in the vaccinated. Now, you can compare the numbers because they are based on the same denominator.

Using that illustration, even though the raw numbers show more deaths in the unvaccinated, when you adjust for the denominator, the death rates in the unvaccinated are lower. Again, these are made-up numbers to illustrate the importance of adjusting the raw data to equal denominators.

Not-So-Wacko Jacko Rule to Live By:

The numbers do not tell the story.
The numbers behind the numbers tell the real story.

Here is another deception. In countries that kept better data than the US, a disproportionately higher number of *vaccinated* patients with the Delta variant required hospitalization. The CDC omitted hospitalizations from the Delta variant in its calculations. The Delta variant was associated with twice the hospitalization rate and, in some areas, was 80–90 percent more transmissible than other variants.[354]

The CDC owns over two hundred patents, with approximately 57 tied to vaccines.[355] Logically, the CDC would seem to be motivated to promote vaccines, even on ones it does not have patent rights.

VAERS Data

Let's look at VAERS (vaccine adverse event reporting system) data and compare the COVID-19 vaccines to previous vaccines. VAERS is, largely, a voluntary reporting system, though pharmaceutical companies are obligated to report any adverse reactions for which they are aware (how that is enforced, I am unsure). So, whatever numbers show up in VAERS are likely to underrepresent actuality given its volunteer nature.

According to VAERS, less than 1 percent of adverse effects are reported.[356]

VAERS is co-managed by the FDA and CDC, and it first started collecting data on all vaccines in 1990. They are responsible for the data and verifying it.[357]

The adage that a picture is worth a thousand words has never been truer than when looking at data on COVID-19 vaccines compared to all other vaccines, as depicted in the upcoming table and graphs.

VAERS Summary for COVID-19 Vaccines through 12/27/2024

All charts and tables below reflect the data release on 1/5/2025 from the VAERS website, which includes U.S and foreign data, and is updated through: **12/27/2024**.

High-Level Summary	COVID19 vaccines (Dec'2020 - present)	All other vaccines 1990-present	US Data Only COVID19 vaccines (Dec'2020 - present)	US Data Only All other vaccines 1990-present
Number of Adverse Reactions	1,658,332	1,016,331	1,022,223	871,410
Number of Life-Threatening Events	40,778	16,233	15,437	10,770
Number of Hospitalizations	219,594	95,315	90,793	42,471
Number of Deaths	38,264*	11,104*	19,176	5,833
# of Permanent Disabilities after vaccination	72,721	23,688	18,686	14,465
Number of Office Visits	246,649	71,836	201,379	68,011
# of Emergency Room/Department Visits	156,157	222,499	119,875	211,721
# of Birth Defects after vaccination	1,394	267	625	141

*Note that the total number of deaths associated with the COVID-19 vaccines is more than TRIPLE the number of deaths associated with all other vaccines combined since the year 1990.

From VAERS Analysis. https://vaersanalysis.info/.

Look at the table above: VAERS Summary of COVID-19 Vaccines through 12/27/2024. Look at the US data represented by the two right columns of the table. The COVID-19 vaccines have caused 1,022,223 adverse reactions since their inception. All other vaccines **combined** since 1990 have caused 871,410. COVID-19 vaccines are linked to 19,176 deaths since their inception, while all other vaccines **combined** since 1990 are linked to 5,883 deaths.

Now, look at the graph below, which is called: Cumulative Reported Deaths After Vaccinations – 4 Year Summary. COVID-19 deaths are in the blue. Deaths from COVID-19 vaccines have leveled off as fewer and fewer vaccines are being administered.

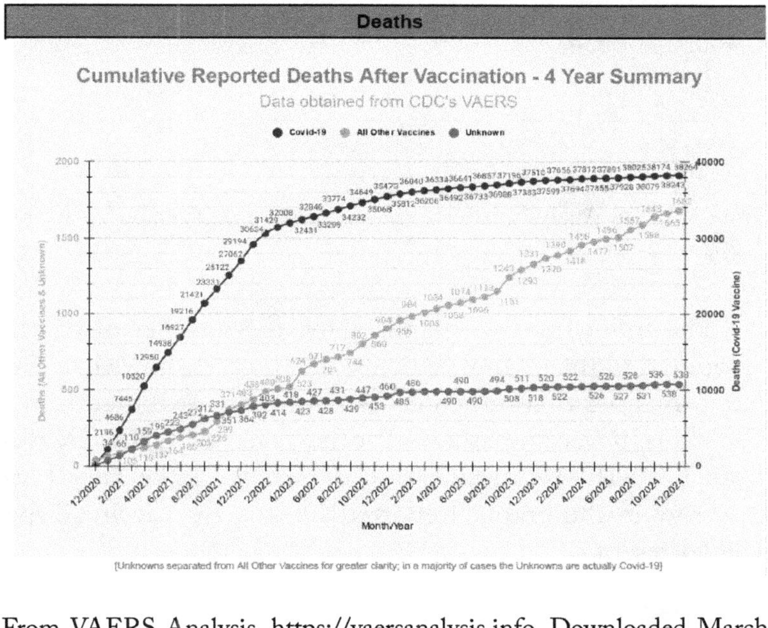

From VAERS Analysis. https://vaersanalysis.info. Downloaded March 1, 2025.

The graph below shows the cumulative deaths caused by all other vaccines versus the COVID-19 vaccines and shows that deaths attributed to COVID-19 vaccines exceed the cumulative deaths of all other vaccines over 30-plus years. COVID-19 vaccines are represented by the blue line.

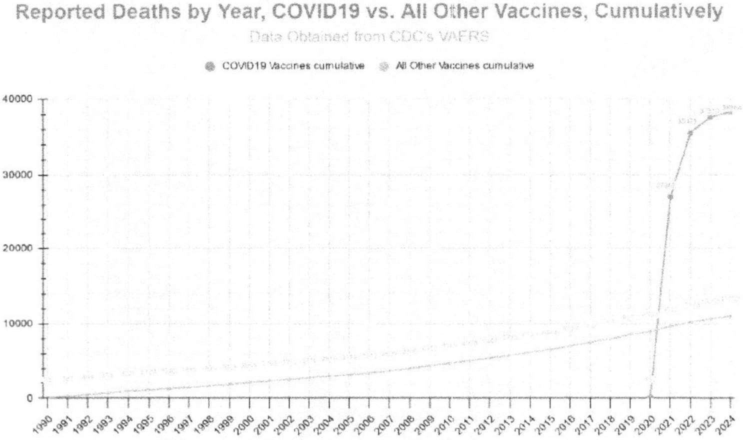

From VAERS Analysis. https://vaersanalysis.info. Downloaded March 1, 2025.

The following two graphs show the number of deaths attributed to the various available vaccines. It shows in a different manner that more deaths have been attributed to the COVID-19 vaccines than all other vaccine types. Deaths from COVID-19 vaccines are depicted on the very bottom row in the graph: Reported Deaths By Vaccine Type, 1990-Present.

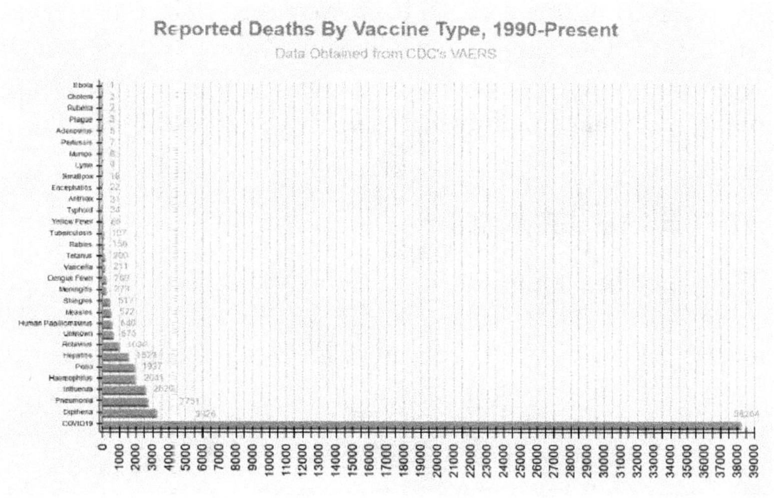

From VAERS Analysis. https://vaersanalysis.info.

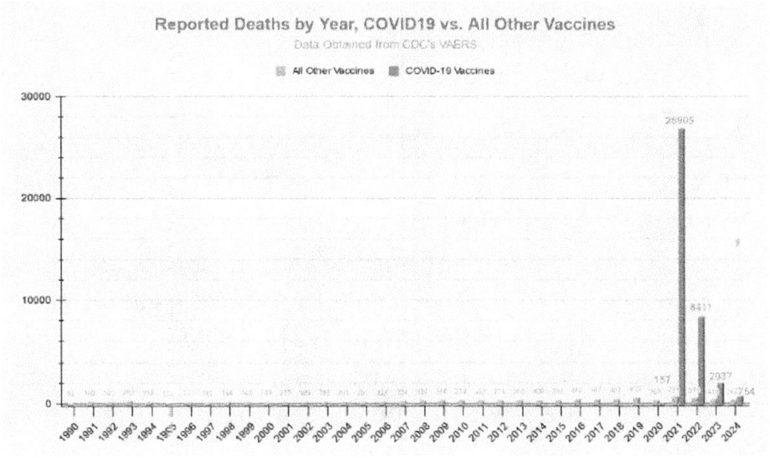

From VAERS Analysis. https://vaersanalysis.info.

Keep in mind, VAERS is co-managed by the FDA and the CDC. They are responsible for these numbers, which seem to strongly contradict what the CDC has been saying publicly about the safety of the COVID-19 vaccines.

International Databases

The following countries with high vaccinations rates found more hospitalizations and more severe cases and deaths among the vaccinated: Gibraltar, England, Wales, Scotland, Israel, Ireland, Portugal, Thailand, Malaysia, Uganda, Nepal, Namibia, Mongolia, Zambia, Bahrain, Paraguay, Uruguay, Taiwan, Vietnam, The Bahamas, Sri Lanka, Afghanistan, Tunisia, Bangladesh, Burma, Fiji, and Cambodia.[358]

These countries reported not just higher numbers but higher hospitalization and death rates in their vaccinated population versus the unvaccinated population. In other words, they adjusted for the imbalance in numbers between vaccinated and unvaccinated.

Let me walk through the numbers for some of these countries.

In Wales, in October 2021, 80 percent of the Welsh were fully vaccinated, with 87 percent of the COVID-19 hospitalizations occurring in the fully vaccinated. Again, the purpose of the vaccine is to prevent hospitalizations and death.

That same month, 70 percent of the Scots were fully vaccinated, with 87 percent of the COVID-19 deaths occurring in the vaccinated. In Israel, 61 percent were fully vaccinated by July 2021, with 71 percent of the critically ill from COVID-19 being fully vaccinated.

Nearly 75 percent of the Belgians had received one jab of the vaccines, and 65 percent were fully vaccinated by June 2021. By the end of June, new cases of COVID-19 infections rose from five hundred daily infections to two thousand daily infections.

In Singapore, COVID-19 daily cases rose from ten in June to 150 in July, to 1,246 towards the end of September 2021, despite 80 percent of the population having received at least one dose of a vaccine by the end of July 2021.

Great Britain reported negative vaccine effectiveness in its over-40 population, where the COVID-19 cases were 53 percent higher in the vaccinated than the unvaccinated, with higher infection rates in the double-vaccinated.

Gibraltar achieved a 115 percent vaccine rate by July 2021 (it vaccinated tourists too). In December 2020 (before the vaccine rollouts), Gibraltar had only 1,040 confirmed cases of COVID with five deaths. Following the vaccination success, new infections increased fivefold to 5,314, but deaths from COVID-19 increased nineteenfold.

It seems clear that the mRNA vaccines were not preventing infection or reducing hospitalizations or deaths, despite everything you heard.

Dr. Bourla's About-Face

In an interview with *Yahoo Finance* on January 12, 2022, Dr. Bourla said, "We know that the two doses of the vaccine offer very limited protection, if any."[359] What happened to cause this turnaround from two months earlier? Was he guilty of peddling misinformation in November 2021 when he called people criminals who were against the vaccine?

Here's one thing to keep in mind about vaccines: They are more lucrative the less effective they are because ineffectiveness leads to the need for boosters. I'm sure Pfizer would love it if patients had to get two to three COVID-19 boosters a year.

I Got the Vaccine, Now What?

I have some patients who received the mRNA COVID vaccines and now regret it. Some of them had a reaction or complication, most likely related to the vaccine. Others just regret getting it because they "caved" to the pressure. These patients feel they have been bamboozled, duped, and hoodwinked, and are disappointed in themselves for not resisting more.

If you're like those patients, don't "beat yourself up" over that decision. The full force of federal health agencies, the medical establishment, the pharmaceutical companies, and the media worked together in a coordinated plan to scare and instill fear, and they were successful. Consider using Dr. Peter McCullough's COVID-19 detoxification protocol if you feel you have had some harmful effects from the vaccine.

Learn from your experience. You will have more opportunities to "say no." COVID-19 will not be the last push to scare you into being vaccinated for something. We are already seeing a vaccine push for RSV and, likely, the bird flu.

Pfizer's Crimes, Fines, and Lawsuits

Many of you have entrusted your health to the makers of the COVID-19 vaccines. Below is a profile of one of those companies in whose hands you have placed your health—Pfizer, founded in 1849. Pfizer had the lowest reputational score among pharmaceutical companies in 2018.[360] Perhaps its executives viewed COVID-19 as an opportunity to change the company's image.

The entire pharmaceutical industry scores poorly in reputational surveys. In 2021, RepTrak reported the pharmaceutical industry ranked eighth (an improvement) and listed five companies in the top 100.[361]

- Sanofi at 64
- Novo Nordisk at 71
- Eli Lilly at 82
- Roche at 87
- Bristol Myers Squibb at 94

Back to Pfizer. The CCCA presentation, on page 43, provides "Links to the Public Record of Pfizer's Culture," without going into the details and lawsuits and settlements that Pfizer has been involved in.

Pfizer's Trail of Misconduct

What follows is a table of 18 of Pfizer's lawsuits, settlements, and misconduct since 1992. For a more detailed description of each case, I refer you to *Kanekoa News*. Some of these cases are also found in the CCCA's listing of Pfizer's lawsuits. Each case has a reference should you desire even more detail.

Miscon-duct #	Year	Drug or Device	Amount of Fine or Settlement	Description of Offense
1	1992	Heart valve	$165 million to $215 million	Fracturing of Bjork-Shipley Heart Valve.[362]
2	1994	Heart valve	$10.75 million plus $9.25 million to monitor patients	Lied to get federal approval of valve.[363]

3	1996	Experimental drug trial to 200 Nigerian children		Lack of consent and "illegal trial of an unregistered drug," which caused 11 deaths and brain damage in others.[364]
4	2002	Lipitor	$49 million	Defrauded government.[365]
5	2004	Neurontin	$430 million	2 felonies involving fraudulent promotion of Neurontin for unapproved uses. Planted company operatives in audience to bribe doctors with trips.[366]
6	2008	Neurontin	See #5	Manipulated studies, suppressed negative studies, controlled flow of research.[367]
7	2009	Bextra	$2.3 billion – largest fine at the time	"Intent to defraud or mislead". Kickbacks to doctors.[368]
8	2009	Rezulin	$750 million	Settled 35,000 claims related to 63 deaths and dozens of cases of liver failure.[369]
9	2010	Neurontin	$142.1 million	Violation of federal antiracketeering law by fraudulent marketing of Neurontin.[370]
10	2010	Signed disclosures to settle federal investigation …	… related to illegal promotion of drugs for off-label use.	Admission of payments to 4.500 doctors and 250 academic medical centers and research groups.[371]
11	2010	Bextra. See #7	Suit filed by Blue Cross Blue Shield	Bribing 5,000 doctors with Caribbean vacations.[372]

12	2010	Experimental drug in Nigerian children. See #3.		Leaked cables between Pfizer and a US official in Nigeria showing attempt by Pfizer to blackmail Nigerian attorney general.[373]
13	2012	Bribing doctors in foreign countries	Bulgaria, China, Croatia, Czech Republic, Italy Kazakhstan, Russia, and Serbia	Charged by the SEC for violating Foreign Corrupt Practices Act. Cash given to bribe government doctors in these countries to Pfizer products.[374]
14	2012	Prempro	$1.2 billion in settlement to nearly 10,000 women.	Caused breast cancer. Millions of dollars also paid for punitive damages.[375]
15	2013	Protonix	$55 million	Criminal charges for failing to warn patients and doctors about risks of kidney disease/ injury/failure and interstitial nephritis.[376]
16	2013	Chantix	$288 million	Settle claims that Chantix caused suicidal thoughts and severe psychological disorders. Drug possibly also linked to higher risk of heart attack.[377]
17	2014	Rapamune	$35 million	Bribing doctors to use Rapamune for unapproved use, utilizing "misleading presentations of data".[378]
18	2016	Phenytoin	£84.2 million	Overcharged NHS (UK) by 2,600%, increasing cost to UK taxpayers from £2 million to £50 million.[379]

These are just the fines, lawsuits, and criminal activity since 1992. In fairness to Pfizer, it inherited some of these judgments from subsidiaries that it had acquired, including the Prempro and Rapamune suits.

Paying such fines for a pharmaceutical company is simply the "cost of doing business" and is built into its medications' pricing. The revenue from the Pfizer-BioNTech COVID-19 alone more covers all the above fines.

I mention these legal issues to show that one does not need a gun to harm or kill people. One does not need to perpetrate a Ponzi scheme to deceive people. You just need bad products and unethical behavior mixed in with bad healthcare policy.

More people have died from the COVID-19 vaccines than did on 9/11 or at Pearl Harbor and all other vaccines combined, based on VAERS data. More people died from the poor COVID-19 response led by our federal health agencies. Just the number of unnecessary COVID-19 deaths (500,000-plus just through May 2020) is nearly comparable to the US deaths in World War I, World War II, and the Vietnam War *combined.*

Those 500,000-plus patients were parents, grandparents, siblings, children, aunts, and uncles, and they did not just die. They were *allowed to die* because we did very little until it was too late, and we could have done more much sooner. What may have started off as deception to give Big Pharma time to develop drugs/vaccines for COVID-19 turned into true evil.

Not-So-Wacko Jacko Rule to Live By:

The people who control medicine are willing to risk your health in their quest for money, power, and control.

If you are someone intent on harming and deceiving people for your own benefit with a high probability of getting away with it, then business, politics, and medicine are where you want to be. It is where you can hide in the open. But there is a chance you will get caught. The bigger question is, will anything be done about it?

Summary of COVID-19

COVID-19 was real, but our country's response to it was unreal, as in something poorly planned and not based on much science or with the welfare of people in mind. We cast aside common sense. Too many things still do not add up. For nine months in 2020, from March to December, we did nothing of any beneficial consequence.

The shutdowns in 2020 led to a delay in diagnoses and treatment of non-COVID-19 conditions, leading to preventable deaths and disability. Individuals lost jobs and faced financial ruin, which led to an increase in suicides and mental health disorders. Loneliness and social isolation increased during COVID-19, with severe loneliness going from 6 percent pre-COVID-19 to 21 percent during the pandemic. Loneliness, in general, was 28.6 percent during COVID-19. Loneliness is associated with an increased risk of premature mortality of 26 percent. Fear-mongering created riffs among families and friends. All for a virus with a death rate of less than 1 percent. No doubt the virus was potentially lethal, but only to a small subset of the population.

The strategy of lockdowns, masking, and social distancing was not nearly as effective as being touted.

During the pandemic, I attended a party (after lockdowns lifted) with medical and non-medical people in attendance. One was a doctor, a hospitalist. He told a story of a family that was upset with him because he would not give ivermectin to their loved one (father and husband), who was on a ventilator with COVID-19. The hospitalist told the family that their loved one only had a 2 percent chance of surviving based on his overall condition.

Patients *were allowed to die* during the height of the COVID-19 pandemic because treatments were withheld.

I was thinking the same as a non-medical person. She asked, "If the situation is that hopeless, what do you have to lose by giving him ivermectin? You will, at least, make the family feel like you are trying something."

He did not respond.

Chances are, though, even if he had wanted to give him ivermectin, the hospital probably would have prevented it, or it may have taken any ivermectin in stock off the shelves of its pharmacy.

"Trying something" seems like common sense and a better strategy than lockdowns, masks, and distancing.

I cannot say it more simply or strongly. Patients *were allowed to die* during the height of the COVID-19 pandemic because treatments were withheld. Why more people are not upset about how the pandemic was managed, I find both baffling and troubling. Maybe they only know the half-truth—until now.

But once more people wake up, we will see how the management of COVID-19 created even greater distrust in the medical system, which is already higher than the establishment realizes. More people are being turned off by today's medicine, and the medical establishment had better come up with some answers. Medicine needs to take a close look at itself and decide who it wants to serve.

I shall restate the words of Devin Pendas, PhD, on evil men substituting *deceptive* for *evil*:

> It's not that a handful of deceptive men can do deceptive things. It's that a handful of deceptive men can convince a large majority of ordinary men to help them do deceptive things.

We will, eventually, see some of the ordinary men (and women) who were convinced to do deceptive things come into the open. They will save their skin once they know where this outcry is heading.

But the "handful of deceptive men" who convinced them will go down with the ship.

History repeats itself. Repeatedly.

CONCLUSION

Becoming Unbamboozled, Unduped, and Dehoodwinked

Now that you realize that you have been bamboozled, duped, and hoodwinked and see how deceptive and corrupt medicine is, what can you do to protect yourself?

I will address this from both a patient's and a physician's perspective.

Patients First

The most important thing you can do as a patient is to be as informed and knowledgeable as you can about your health. Do your own research, no matter what your doctor may say. Because of how the medical system is currently structured, you have little medical freedom. Physicians who have limited knowledge due to a tightly controlled and narrowly focused medical education system provide limited options to you. To gain more freedom and more choices, you need to conduct your own research here and abroad.

Prior to the Internet, the medical establishment had a monopoly on medical information. That is no longer true. You, as a patient, have access to all the information that I do as a physician, or at least, close enough. Take advantage of that opportunity.

You can become an "expert" on any health issue that may plague you. In fact, it should be easier for you to become more knowledgeable about the one or two medical conditions you may have than your physician, who must be more "expert" on many more problems and has many more patients to worry about. You need to worry only about yourself.

We have seen an example of this with users of anabolic steroids spending far more time researching anabolic steroids and being more knowledgeable than most physicians. Take the same approach.

Do Your Own Research

So, do your own research. Some of what you read may sound like a foreign language for a while, but like a foreign language, you will gradually make sense of it. If you can read, you can learn. Ask for help from medical professionals if you need assistance interpreting information.

Research topics on PubMed (National Library of Medicine) and Cochrane Reviews, and see what clinical trials are going on at Clinicatrials.gov. Read what the CDC says. Information on its website is reliable when it comes to symptoms, diagnoses, and data/information, though its treatment recommendations, in my opinion, serve the pharmaceutical-medical complex. Scour social media and the internet for podcasts on medical topics that interest you. Research the medical professionals behind these podcasts to know their credentials and experience. Practicing physicians are likely to give you better practical information than someone who does not, or has not, engaged in much clinical practice.

Some doctors don't like you to do your own research. My advice? Find another doctor. I don't mind when patients come in and say, "I know I am not supposed to say this, but I checked with Dr. Google, and he says I might have such-and-such disorder."

Many times, I learn something from the patient's research. I find some of their research interesting and, occasionally, there are possible diagnoses that I think are unlikely to be the cause of their problem, but something that should be considered. Sometimes, I get new ideas from a patient's research.

I learn much about a patient who has done their own research. It tells me something about their thought process. It tells me about their concerns too. I understand them better as a person.

Be careful getting information from patient advocacy groups when it comes to *treatment*. They fall into the same camp as medical journals. Such advocacy groups get millions of dollars from pharmaceutical companies and other sponsors, and frequently, from the food and agriculture industries. The information on these sites is good, though, when it comes to signs, symptoms, and diagnosis.

What else can you do to better protect yourself as a patient from the half-truths of medicine?

- Stay healthy.
- Align yourself with like-minded physicians.
- Be willing to pay out of pocket.

- Get second opinions.
- Research your doctors on OpenPayments.CMS.gov.

Stay Healthy

There are a lot of wonderful innovations going on in medicine, which make the future exciting for both doctors and patients. Surgeries are becoming less invasive. We see game-changing treatments in the field of regenerative medicine. Medications are being repurposed that may extend longevity.

The challenge and shortcomings will be in the model of delivery of care. The following are my opinions, and I may be completely wrong.

I think more primary care will be delivered by mid-level providers like nurse practitioners and physician assistants—that trend is already occurring. Because most providers are employed, this is an economic decision being driven by large employers like hospital systems as well as insurance companies, who can reimburse less for personnel of less skill.

Recognize that your care will come from lesser-trained individuals, many of whom do a good job for their level of training, but their training is not, and will not, be enough in every case. Many of them do a very good job, but their training is about half that of a physician.

So, you need to be vigilant with your health.

Much specialty care will be delivered by physicians, but even in specialty and subspecialty areas, we are seeing more and more mid-level providers. There are now cardiology nurse practitioners, hospitalist nurse practitioners, infectious disease nurse practitioners, and so on. The same holds true for physician assistants.

Like physicians who recognize the corrupt nature of medicine, you will want to minimize how often you interact with the healthcare system. Adopt a "use it only if you have to" mindset. The fewer the encounters, the less likely you will be bamboozled, duped, and hoodwinked. Staying healthy will enable you to minimize your encounters with the system. That said, don't avoid the system purely for the sake of avoiding the system. If you have a problem, be sure to address it.

Adopt a "use it only if you have to" mindset.

You will want to focus on lifestyle, especially nutrition and exercise. This book is not meant to address those topics or give medical advice. Many individuals are stressed these days for multiple reasons. Stress magnifies and uncovers many health issues. Find ways to manage stress in a healthy manner.

Align Yourself with Like-Minded Physicians

In the past, physicians had different views and approaches to medicine, and patients gravitated to those doctors who shared similar mindsets. That relationship does not exist like it used to.

For the most part, if you see a physician who takes insurance or is employed, you will likely receive the same care regardless of who you see. The providers are all practicing from the same playbook. The only thing that might differ is the provider's personality.

You will likely need to go outside the insurance world to find a doctor not married to the half-truths of medicine or someone closely aligned with your goals. All physicians are conventionally trained, but a small number do not stop there. They will seek out additional training to provide more options for their patients.

Physicians who see the dark side of medicine have gravitated to fields like longevity medicine, functional medicine, anti-aging medicine, age management medicine, lifestyle medicine, and integrative medicine. Mainstream medicine frequently downplays these fields and physicians, but you should not.

Though the names are different, many of the goals of these disciplines are similar. The emphasis is on a more comprehensive and holistic approach to medicine. This includes focusing on a healthier lifestyle (nutrition and exercise), hormonal balance, gut balance, stress management, use of nutritional supplements, and incorporating forms of complementary and alternative therapies.

The examination and testing these physicians do is far more detailed than you will get from an insurance-based model physician. They place more emphasis on prevention, catching and addressing problems sooner in the process, and treating problems at their root cause, which prescription medicines rarely do.

These doctors will spend much more time with you. Some of these providers may push supplements they sell through their office and offer expensive diagnostic testing that is not always necessary. That is one potential downside. Supplements can be helpful, but if you feel like you are being sold everything under the sun, I suggest finding another doctor.

I recommend going to the websites of professional organizations tied to longevity medicine, functional medicine, anti-aging medicine, age management medicine, lifestyle medicine, and integrative medicine. Some of them have physician directories enabling you to locate a physician in your area.

Pay Out of Pocket

If you want more medical freedom, you will have to pay out of pocket. Many of the physicians who go beyond conventional medicine do not take insurance for their professional services. However, typically, use your health insurance for lab tests, diagnostic studies, and prescription medications. You may also be able to use your HSA or health savings account for such physicians.

No one wants to pay more than necessary if they can avoid it, but there is a lot of truth to "you get what you pay for." If you want to use your health insurance and are only willing to pay an office co-pay, you will only get so much in return. If that is the case, you will have a hard time getting away from the bamboozled, duped, and hoodwinked version of medicine.

If your finances do not allow for many of these expenses, use your health insurance to see a hospital-employed physician and go outside the system for care for select problems. Your choice does not have to be all or none.

No one wants to pay more than necessary if they can avoid it, but there is a lot of truth to "you get what you pay for."

Some patients see me for hormone replacement only and use their health insurance to see a different physician for any other medical problems they may have. Or I have patients who come in for a second opinion regarding a particular problem to see how our practice may address it.

A growing model is the Direct Patient Care or Direct Primary Care model. Many of these physicians practice medicine like they did in the insurance model, but they no longer take insurance. Some offer a monthly membership fee, and some you pay a la carte when you have a medical need. These doctors usually won't have the additional training that those in functional medicine, integrative medicine, longevity medicine, anti-aging medicine, and others have, but they are less restricted by insurance.

In this model, you will be getting a doctor who will likely spend more time with you. That's another point. To practice medicine well requires an investment in time and education on the doctor's end, and the insurance-based model does not allow for that. It is difficult to fully address a patient's concern in 15 or 20 minutes if you are lucky.

If your budget is tight, it may be helpful to seek out one of these non-insurance-based physicians in your area for a one-time evaluation and consultation while keeping your insurance-based doctor.

Below is the business model for our practice, The Armory (wearethearmory.com). Patients pay $195 a month, which gives them

- unlimited doctor visits for the year;
- exercise treadmill test and VO2 max annually;
- body composition and bone density study;
- resting metabolic rate;
- pulmonary function testing;
- consult with a dietician;
- fitness membership to three gyms;
- unlimited physical therapy; and
- consult with an exercise physiologist.

Patients can use their HSAs. Some people in my area pay $200 a month to join a CrossFit gym without all the added benefits that our combined medical/fitness model provides.

As a patient, you are geared to thinking you must use your health insurance for everything. You are partially paying for it, so you want to use it. But you still have a deductible to meet, so you will be spending X amount of dollars out of pocket every year. It may be wise to spend those dollars on a cash-based practice, especially one that offers an annual membership. Our annual membership fee is less than $2,400. Most of you have deductibles higher than that.

Second Opinion

It is *your* health. If you feel uncomfortable with a diagnosis or advice, then seek out a second opinion.

To get a true second opinion, you will want to go outside the practice or health system that gave you the first opinion. Doctors within the same practice or health system are less likely to give an opinion that might contradict that of their colleague.

Also, share all your information with the second opinion doctor that the first doctor used to formulate his opinion. However, to avoid any potential bias, do not tell the second doctor the diagnosis that was made earlier, nor the treatment plan recommended by the first doctor. Let the second doctor formulate his or her own diagnosis and treatment recommendations based on the records provided and the exam performed. Doing all of this will better ensure a legitimate second opinion. That is why you are going to them.

Go outside your health system to get a true second opinion.

Open Payments

Earlier, I talked about pharmaceutical companies paying physicians. You can verify whether any of your physicians has received any money from industry sources by going to OpenPaymentsData.CMS.gov.

The site breaks down payments into four categories:

1. general payments like food and beverages
2. research payments
3. associated research payments
4. ownership and investment

Many doctors will receive some general payments, typically in the form of lunches or dinners, like I received.

Payments that might trigger some concern for you will be the research payments and the ownership and investment payments, as these might influence a doctor's treatment recommendations for you.

If You Are a Physician

I trust that I have convinced you that our profession is unethical and corrupt in many ways and probably nowhere near the profession that you anticipated when you entered the field. I hope you now realize that the system is using doctors. In many ways, the system has pitted doctors against patients.

Physicians must take two steps, not twelve, to unbamboozle themselves.

1. Realize and admit you have been bamboozled, duped, and hoodwinked.

2. Do not let it happen again.

Our education has been carefully scripted and crafted to serve the needs of the pharmaceutical-medical complex, not necessarily patients.

If you have any doubts about some or most of this book, feel free to do your own research to verify or disprove what is printed.

Medicine can still be very rewarding when physicians and patients are aligned in reaching mutual health goals. The insurance and employment-based models do not allow for partnering with the patients easily. You are there for the patient's benefit. To ensure your medical career is rewarding for you and your patients, you may want to

- develop a strong identity;
- stop relying on health agencies for information. Go beyond them;
- do your research by going to the source of information if possible;
- go to meetings not affiliated with your specialty boards;
- avoid being employed; and
- have more than one state medical license.

Develop a Strong Identity

Even if you are hospital-employed, you need a strong identity or reputation that supersedes that of your hospital system. Hospitals make that difficult to do, however. I never worked at the Cleveland Clinic but was born there (my first exposure to medicine occurred there while *in utero*) and did a medical school rotation there. But let's say I work there.

Even though the Cleveland Clinic has a great reputation, I would not want to rely on that alone as a physician. I would want patients to say, "I see Dr. Joe Jacko. He's fantastic. By the way, he is at the Cleveland Clinic." I don't want them to say. "I see a doc at the Cleveland Clinic. He's pretty good. His name is Joe Jac….Jacoby…Jackowiz…Jablonsky… something like that." I would not want the reputation of the Cleveland Clinic to overshadow mine.

To develop a strong reputation, you must develop strong relationships with patients. If you are a primary care physician with no other skills, you are increasingly replaceable by mid-level providers and AI, especially if you are hospital-employed. You need a Plan B, like a cash-based practice, and will want a strong enough reputation so that a critical number of patients will follow YOU and not remain patients of the *hospital system*. You want to be so good and so well-liked that patients will pay out of pocket to see you.

Work on making the doctor-patient relationship more of a partnership. Create your own patient education website, give talks geared towards patient education, and so on. One of my former colleagues said that the only legitimate way for physicians to market themselves is through patient education. Any marketing piece should have an educational message.

Go Beyond Health Agencies

Do not rely solely on health agencies, like the CDC and FDA, for guidance on how to practice medicine. The CDC has something like 3,400 corporate sponsors trying to buy its influence, including school boards. Why else are they giving it money? It is not an unbiased organization. Hopefully, I have convinced you that the FDA is in the hip pocket of the pharmaceutical companies.

Research

Whenever possible, go to the original source and not rely on secondary outlets of medical information. Review the references and articles that health agencies cite. Sometimes, they give guidance without references. Go beyond and view studies done in other countries as well as those in the US.

Learn more about the FDA and pharmaceutical industry relationship. Talk to a compounding pharmacist to better understand their role in patient care and how they differ from retail pharmacies. Many of you have been misled on this topic and have unfounded fears or concerns about compounding pharmacies.

Search for podcasts relevant to your field of medicine or your own health interests.

Meetings

Start going to medical meetings *in person* sponsored by some of these other disciplines in the following fields: longevity medicine, functional medicine, anti-aging medicine, age management medicine, lifestyle medicine, and integrative medicine.

Go in person, not online. You will experience a whole other level of energy and excitement when you attend such meetings in person, and you will quickly learn there is more to practicing medicine than reaching for the prescription pad.

Getting Continuing Medical Education (CME) online, which became the routine during the pandemic, has taken away much enthusiasm from the learning process that occurs with in-person conferences. The network of contacts you make when attending CME meetings in person can enhance your career and even save it.

Consider doing a fellowship or obtaining a certification in one of the following areas: longevity medicine, functional medicine, anti-aging medicine, age management medicine, lifestyle medicine, and integrative medicine.

Look at the Direct Primary Care model and free yourself of the insurance hassles. You may find telemedicine on the side as a way to bridge the financial gap when you begin to transition to a cash-based practice. MDVIP, SignatureMD, and PartnerMD are companies that help physicians transition out of the insurance-based model to cash-based models.

There is a group of patients who will always prefer to see a doctor over a mid-level provider. You will want to capture them before another physician does, so you should evaluate your situation with some urgency.

I may be entirely wrong, but I think we will drift to an insurance-based model dominated by mid-level providers and a cash-based alternative dominated by physicians looking for medical freedom. With time, more patients who want to use their insurance will realize they may be better off using their own money to see a physician. I have experienced that, having switched from insurance to cash-based practice two years ago. Some patients who were resistant to the change in my practice model have gradually come on board.

Talk to Physicians Who Have Left the Insurance World

Talk and meet with other physicians who have taken steps to distance themselves from the insurance-based practice model. Learn about the challenges they faced and how a cash-based practice affects their revenue. Ask about their overall professional gratification.

The transition is not easy. You will want to live well within your means prior to making a change to a cash-based practice, as you are likely to see a drop in income initially. Many physicians are trapped in their practice situations due to student loans or living too high a lifestyle that enslaves them. If you are a younger physician, I recommend not entrapping yourself with more debt. I understand this is difficult when you have already delayed gratification by getting through training and want to enjoy the fruits of your labor.

You attract that which you are. Decide what type of patient you want to see and design your practice to see that type of patient.

Our medical practice has gone from a medical practice with a gym to a state-of-the-art fitness facility with a medical office. We started as a medical practice with a 5,000-square-foot gym. We now have a 60,000-square-foot complex providing fitness, athletic development, sports recovery, physical therapy, and medical.

Morphing from medical to more fitness has provided unintended benefits. We now attract individuals who are more interested in our fitness, athletic, and performance recovery features, so they sign up as members. Some don't care if they ever use us for medical issues, though they do when they have problems.

Our main fitness center is on par with NFL training rooms and is directed by a former professional football player and former NFL head strength and conditioning coach. We have some of the latest technology to improve fitness, athletic performance, and recovery. Fitness is more important than drugs, and we attract patients with a similar mindset.

That is another important point. You attract that which you are. Decide what type of patient you want to see and design your practice to see that type of patient.

Because of our membership model, I have a predictable income floor that is not tied to the number of patients I may see in a month. Offering a membership model only for medical will be more challenging and a harder sell to patients. To capture more patients, you will want to offer other services (aesthetics is a common one) that do not consume as much of your professional time. We have fitness centers.

If you move to a cash-based model, the transition is easier if you do it during your prime practice years when your patient panel is at its peak. One challenge I have encountered at my age is this question: "How much longer do you plan on practicing?" Patients are hesitant about the cash-based model to begin with, and more so if they don't think you will be practicing long enough to care for them.

The challenge is that patients have been bamboozled, duped, and hoodwinked into believing that they should use their health insurance for everything. Many balk at the cash-based model, not realizing that our annual membership is less than the deductibles that many of them must meet. It's an educational problem.

Avoid Being Hospital-Employed

If you are a primary care physician and do not have technical skills, you are at risk of being replaced by mid-level providers and AI. This is truer if you are employed, especially by a hospital system. Plan now for the inevitability.

If you value freedom, avoid hospital employment. As you know, that is not always easy, especially for physicians in certain fields or those coming out of residency training. If you are employed, you are someone else's property. Not only that, but you have the full weight of the medical establishment on you. Let's explore that further.

Because I no longer accept insurance, I no longer need hospital privileges. Because I do not need hospital privileges, I do not need to maintain board certification, though I remain board-certified. One of the potential problems for me during COVID-19 was that hospital privileges were linked to being on health insurance plans.

Because I was planning to move to a cash-based practice, I did not initially bother to apply for a vaccine exemption because I would not need hospital privileges. But because I delayed my departure date, not getting an exemption would complicate things for me in the large group practice I was in. If I did not apply for a medical exemption and received it, I risked losing my hospital privileges. Losing hospital privileges would mean being removed from health insurance plans, which would have affected my practice and patient volume during my remaining time with the old practice.

It is an example of how the establishment entities work together to control physicians.

In my current practice, no one tells me how many patients I need to see. No one tells me how to practice medicine. No one tells me that I am not ordering enough flu shots. No one tells me that I am not ordering enough MRI scans. No one gives me a difficult time if I deviate from clinical guidelines. No one monitors how many antibiotics I am prescribing or how much vacation time I have, and when I can take it. No one tells me I must see a particular patient.

I don't have a non-compete. I don't even have a contract. For about one-third of my career, I have operated without a contract and have had no issues. Just handshake deals. Many will feel that's unwise, but it has worked out well for me. If you deal with quality people, handshake deals work well. My diverse training and multiple state medical licenses give me a lot of freedom. In some ways, I am a free agent.

I value freedom above all else. If someone does not live up to the handshake or contract (which has not happened), I am confident I can find something better or similar.

More Than One State Medical License

Be sure to have a medical license in more than one state before you need it. In 2005, I was practicing in Dallas when Hurricane Katrina hit Louisiana. Overnight, nearly six thousand doctors were out of work. If you are a surgeon or an anesthesiologist, you likely experienced something similar during the peak of COVID-19 when elective surgery was on hold and your ability to make a living was compromised.

Many of those Hurricane Katrina-displaced doctors sought licensure in Texas. In most states, it takes three months to get a medical license, and that is required before you can apply to get on most health insurance plans as a provider, which is, not uncommonly, another three months. Those hurricane-displaced doctors were looking at six months of little or no income.

An event like Katrina is unlikely to come into play for most doctors, but we now live in uncertain times, and you may want to uproot for any number of reasons and go to another state. You want to have another license before you need it.

Though the non-compete laws may be improving, making it easier to make a local change in practice, simply having another medical license opens more opportunities for you. Even if you have no intention of ever leaving your current state, I recommend you have at least one other state's medical license.

The Interstate Medical Licensure Compact now makes getting multiple state medical licenses easier. Keeping up with all the different CME requirements can be challenging and probably represents the biggest hassle. Once you have a license, I recommend keeping it active. The renewal fees are nominal compared to all that you invested in your education, training, and career.

There are companies you can pay that will do the grunt work to help you obtain another state license. These companies will gather all the necessary documents on your behalf and forward them to the state's medical board where you are applying for licensure.

Another thing about moving is that medicine is practiced somewhat geographically. You may find a move to another state energizing or more in line with your thinking or approach. Study how medicine is practiced within your specialty based on geography.

I am currently in Columbus, Ohio, which I describe as being a calcified or static medical community. Many doctors here are home-grown and, when that happens, innovation and new approaches are not readily accepted. There is a bit of a stale mindset in Columbus compared to other places I have been, but I have been able to work around that.

Greenville-Spartanburg, South Carolina, was more open to new ideas, and there appeared to be more collaboration among specialties than I see in Columbus. Dallas was far more receptive to new ideas and innovation. I am convinced that any idea or concept, medical or otherwise, can be made to work in Dallas.

Physicians Are the Key to the Profession

Physicians are the key to the medical profession, not administrators, not hospitals, not insurance companies. Not even Big Pharma. Remember, nearly everything in medicine flows through physicians. We have the power; we just don't think we do. One reason for the gravitation to mid-level providers is to neutralize our potential power (should we wake up and realize that power).

Without physicians, hospitals have little to survive on. And yet, we have been made to believe we are insignificant. We are not.

We can control things if we choose. It is time to start using our power and influence. And it is time to stop believing everything we are taught.

Uncommon Common Sense

In politics, nothing happens by accident.
If it happens, you can bet it was planned that way.
—Franklin Delano Roosevelt

Regardless of the topic, I have found you can typically pigeon-hole people into one of three categories.

When it comes to approaching the day, we have those who

1. get through the day;
2. get from the day; and
3. make the day.

There are three types of medical students. Those who

1. claim they are always studying, and in fact, are always studying;

2. claim they never study, but in fact, are always studying; and
3. study just enough.

When it comes to sports. We have

1. spectators;
2. officials and refs; and
3. players and coaches.

There are people who

1. attempt and win;
2. try but lose; and
3. don't even try.

When it comes to current events we have

1. conspiracy theorists;
2. coincidental believers; and
3. common-sense disciples.[IP]

Conspiracy Theorist

The term "conspiracy theorist" is used these days to describe or label anyone who disagrees with the mainstream narrative, regardless of the topic. We heard the term repeatedly used during the COVID-19 pandemic to deride anyone who would not submit to the medical establishment's narrative or be accused of spreading "misinformation."

As far as I can tell, those physicians that the medical establishment came down hard on have done nothing more than cite the medical literature and describe their own experiences dealing with COVID-19. How can either be construed as misinformation?

If a group of physicians says, "In our experience, 80 percent of those with COVID-19 treated early with ivermectin improved in forty-eight-to-seventy-two hours," how is that statement misinformation or conspiratorial?

The medical literature is replete with studies that contradict each other, so this would seem to suggest that the medical profession is responsible for creating confusion and, thus, opening the door for what may be perceived as misinformation by sending conflicting messages through medical publications. But that is unavoidable because medical science is not so pure as to provide a universal answer to all questions.

Labeling someone a conspiracy theorist discredits the person. It is a tactic to silence people and discourage others from listening to them. It is a power play foisted on society by those trying to maintain their control, especially when they sense they are beginning to lose it.

Often, it is used by those whose positions are not supported by fact. When you cannot win on facts, you attack the messenger. The medical establishment, controlled by Big Pharma, is losing control of the monopoly it once enjoyed on medical information.

Revoked Board Certifications

As I put some of the finishing touches on this book, the American Board of Internal Medicine (ABIM) revoked the board certifications of Pierre Kory, MD, and Paul Marik, MD, both of whom were strong proponents of ivermectin and critical of the mRNA COVID-19 vaccines.[380]

Dr. Marik is probably the most published intensivist (critical care doctor) in the country. His COVID-19 patients' survival rate was 90 percent with ivermectin. When he was forced to follow the CDC protocol and stop using it, that survival rate dropped to 50 percent.[381]

Historically, one method to gain control of society has been via medicine. It looks like our country's plan is to facilitate this control is to censure those physicians who do not toe the line. That is consistent with one of the messages of this book: If you control physicians, you control medicine. We should add: If you control medicine, you have more control over people. That leads to: If you control physicians, you have more control over people.

Ultimately, such a plan will backfire once more physicians wake up to what is occurring. And when that happens, there will be more distrust of the system. At that point, being board-certified will simply mean a physician has been sufficiently indoctrinated, conditioned, and groomed. It will become a warning label alerting awakened patients to avoid those physicians.

We find ourselves living in a bizarro world where up is down, down is up, good is bad, and bad is good. The real misinformation that *is most damaging* comes from the medical establishment, making much of the profession illegitimate. Again, spend time on the C19early.org website, which provides several meta-analyses of treatments used in COVID-19, and compare the results of the "forbidden" treatments to the "politically" favored ones. And you have already seen, with your own eyes, Pfizer's own numbers about the real safety and efficacy of its vaccine. By now, you should realize that the published medical literature is not as trustworthy as we have been led to believe.

The ABIM has access to all the data on ivermectin. Drs. Kory and Marik provided the ABIM with over 170 references defending their positions. When the ABIM chooses to ignore the evidence, allows only one point of view, and revokes board certifications, that means the organization and its stated mission have been compromised or another agenda is in play.[382]

All of that simply reinforces that medicine is built on half-truths. Medicine has been hijacked and is slipping into a totalitarian state where discussion or disagreement is not allowed.

I thank ABIM for making my case for me. Its actions are an example of attacking the messenger.

In response to losing his board certification, Dr. Marik responded:[383]

> The bottom line is we're disappointed because we stand up for the truth. To censor science is to censor progress. Science is based on dialogue, and people can have different points of view. That is the principle of science: it's people having different points of view.

He further referred to the ABIM as part of the medical-industrial complex, stating:

> They seem more interested in making money than in protecting physicians. There have been a number of lawsuits against ABIM, so they don't have the best of reputations. But, unfortunately, they are the main certifying organization in the U.S., so they have enormous power and leverage.

GlaxoSmithKline tried to destroy Dr. John Buse for reporting that Avandia caused an increase in heart attacks. Dr. Buse reported the truth. Drs. Kory and Marik have done the same. History repeats itself.

I have found that when things do not make sense, it is because they are beyond logic and explanation based on what is known. That typically speaks to another agenda at play, and one that is hidden.

I have kidded with some of my patients that, the way medicine is going, patients may get better care from a veterinarian. We may be closer to that date than I previously thought.

Coincidental Believer

Are events coincidental, mere happenings that come about without cause or purpose? I suspect that we can probably safely extrapolate President Roosevelt's words and apply them to medicine and other things beyond politics. Few things are coincidental.

Have you ever considered what the opposite of a conspiracy theorist is? To me, it is a "coincidental believer," that is, someone who believes that much of what happens, including their very existence, is purely coincidental. They believe things occur without a particular cause or reason and without purpose—like a virus that materializes *de novo* rather than from a lab engaged in gain-of-function research.

If things are not coincidental, then maybe they are the result of incompetence. Sometimes, we confuse intentionality with incompetency, though they can coexist, especially in government. What appears as incompetency may be intentional. Intentional is not coincidental. Intentional is deliberate.

As I write this paragraph, it is July 20, 2024, one week after the assassination attempt on former President Donald Trump. In a span of sixty-two minutes, at least nine Secret Service mistakes occurred that have been identified. Do these mistakes represent incompetency or intentionality? There is a third possibility. Neither. It could be pure coincidence—coincidence that nine mistakes were made in a short period of time—by supposedly some of the best trained in the business.

Likewise, was our country's government-led poor response to COVID-19 due to incompetency, intentionality, or pure coincidence, and led, supposedly, by some of the brightest minds in the country?

At some point, you need to answer that question for yourself. You need to weigh all the evidence, inject some common sense, and ask more questions so you can answer that one question with a degree of confidence.

By now, you have a better idea of how medicine works behind the scenes. You have seen its corrupt nature. You now know that some of the science that fuels medicine is manipulated and even fabricated. You have seen the power of Big Pharma to get what it wants and how it controls the overall practice of medicine.

In case of both the assassination attempt and COVID-19 response, we probably have a good idea of how President Roosevelt would respond.

If the cause and management of COVID-19 were not the result of coincidence, then the remaining two options are not acceptable, with one being more egregious than the other. Neither is acceptable, nor should it happen. There is no excuse for our country's poor performance. We allowed patients to die because we did far less than we could and with what we had available.

Think about what the more likely scenario is. Was COVID-19 management the mere result of coincidence, was it driven by incompetence, or was it intentionally intentional? And if intentional, why? And by whom? I will leave you to search for the answer. Everyone needs to do some of their own thinking and research.

Common-Sense Disciple

There are some crazy conspiracy ideas out there, and they typically come from crazy people who are easy to identify. But others called "crazy" have been labeled as "conspiracy theorists," but these individuals have done their research, engaged in critical thought, and made compelling arguments for their views. They will keep asking "why" as long as it takes for things to make sense and come together.

They make up a third category of people, and they are disciples of common sense. These folks tend to be rare or uncommon. They engage in critical thinking, ponder facts, use logic where data are absent, consider the role of human motivation, verify what others say, and more.

They come to their own conclusions and are not easily swayed by public opinion or majority thought. I believe these are the "conspiracy theorists" to which Zuby referred and whom he says are ahead of the mainstream narrative.

Common Sense Says or Asks

- The likely origin of the SARS-CoV-2 was the Wuhan lab engaged in gain-of-function research.
- We should repurpose existing FDA-approved drugs (of which there are many), while waiting for antivirals and vaccines to be developed.

- We should instruct people on steps they can take to enhance and fortify their immune systems.
- We should employ strategies effective during prior pandemics.
- We should be careful using an untested vaccine platform.
- Should we vaccinate everyone, or just those at high risk?
- There is so much about COVID-19 that does not add up. Is there more to the story?
- Is there another reason for the ongoing push of the COVID-19 vaccines given the weak data that they are safe and effective in the true sense of what those words mean?
- Do federal health agencies and media truly have my best interest in mind?
- Does Big Pharma have my best interest in mind?
- How well can we believe medical data and research?
- Is medicine the only area where some of the science is tainted?
- Do we need all these drugs?
- Surely there are things safer and more effective than drugs.
- Be careful following advice from people motivated by money.
- I should do my own research and use my own brain.

- I have access to all the world's information due to my own research.
- Does medicine really do much good?
- I am tired of being bamboozled, duped, and hoodwinked.
- I won't allow it anymore.

Moving forward, you have a choice of which category you wish to belong to. Which do you choose?

History will repeat itself. More accurately, perhaps I should say, man repeats history. There will be more pandemics. They are becoming like elections and the Olympics, coming around every four years or so. In fact, we are averaging a pandemic every 3.3 years in this era of gain-of-function research.

More attempts will be made to strip you of your freedoms using medicine and public health as a reason and supported by bogus science. There will be multiple opportunities and attempts to misrepresent science and medical literature to misguide you, so others can profit. Expect an onslaught of attempts to feed you a daily cocktail of drugs.

The medical establishment will attempt to persuade you not to think for yourself or do your own medical research. They will say that all you need to do is listen to your doctor or, better yet, the experts—those sitting behind desks playing a game of chess in which you are nothing more than a pawn.

You have been bamboozled, duped, and hoodwinked. We all have. It is time for a wake-up call.

Not-So-Wacko Jacko Rule of Medicine:

Many people have a plan for their life, including their health. Some people want to control you and will

attempt to do so whatever the cost. You would be wise to have a plan of your own. You are the only one that has your best interest in mind.

The Game in a Nutshell

Medicine lacks scientific integrity. Much of medicine is inauthentic as it is based on half-truths tied to questionable and misrepresented science and faulty precepts. Some of medicine is based on science fiction, making that part of the profession an actual farce.

Physician education and training is carefully crafted to serve the pharmaceutical-medical complex, which does not always have the full and complete interest of the patient in mind.

Patients are being misled by the political-media complex. And both patients and physicians are being misled by the pharmaceutical-medical complex. And neither one knows it—maybe until now. That is the purpose of this book. To. Wake. You. Up.

Time to Wake Up!

Patients, physicians, and all the entities that comprise medicine need to wake up. Many have been sleepwalking. The medical profession needs to examine itself closely and decide who it wants to represent and protect—patients or industry? I am not confident the medical establishment will make the right choice. It has little courage. Therefore, we must awaken patients and physicians to demand changes.

Much of the practice of medicine, especially in non-surgical fields, needs to be re-examined and challenged.

The drug-first approach to lifestyle-related chronic disease falls short in providing meaningful results. More emphasis should be placed on lifestyle changes with programs directed to improving nutrition and physical activity. When it comes to vaccines, the conversation should move beyond safety and efficacy and should question whether some of the vaccines are still needed or can they be reserved for high-risk populations with little risk to the general population during this modern era of sanitation and water filtration.

Existing FDA-approved drugs should be evaluated for repurposing. Patient care decisions should be between patients and their doctors. Assuming legitimate science to support its use and with proper monitoring, should we concern ourselves if a patient wants to try a fifty-five-cent antiparasitic drug (already proven to be safe) as an adjunct to their cancer therapy or to prevent an infectious disease? Should that not be their choice? This does not mean health insurance needs to pay for such treatments, but should patients be denied such options?

This also applies to areas like neurodegenerative diseases like Parkinson's and dementia, where current treatments are minimally effective. Peptides show promise in treating some of these conditions but their use is prohibited by the FDA because they compete with patented pharmaceutical drugs. Patients do not have time on their side to wait for new drugs to be developed.

Health insurance companies need to more closely examine scientific studies that they base their decisions on as some of their decisions are likely based on misrepresented science.

The partial funding of the FDA by pharmaceutical companies should cease. Savings from wasteful government spending elsewhere can be redirected to fully fund the FDA, precluding the need for industry assistance. Independent groups should perform the drug studies for FDA approval, not the pharmaceutical companies. Finally, the benchmark for determining drug effectiveness should be more demanding than simply besting a placebo.

Go back and look at Zuby's 21 observations (pp. 57-58). How much do you agree or disagree with each of his observations now? Some of his observations may not seem as outrageous to you as they may have appeared at the beginning of the book.

Keep President Roosevelt's words in mind. Things are usually planned or intentional. Few things are coincidental. Do not confuse intentionality for incompetency, although they frequently co-exist. In fact, it might be wise to assume things are intentional until proven otherwise.

Not-So-Wacko Jacko Rule for Life:

Stop being a coincidental believer.
Few things happen by chance.[IP]

Some individuals have malicious and perverse intentions and occupy leadership positions throughout our institutions, including medicine. Keep Zuby's 21st observation in mind, and you are less likely to be bamboozled, duped, or hoodwinked. His observation is real, and it is ever present in medicine and beyond.

When the whole world is running headlong towards the precipice, one who walks in the opposite direction is looked at as being crazy.

—T. S. Eliot

The goal of this book was to find something absent, frequently, in medicine—the truth—and to prompt you into critical thinking and research. Be the crazy but uncommon common-sense one ahead of the mainstream narrative. Have the courage not to follow the masses. Go through the narrow gate and find that truth.

Engage in critical thought and do not believe all that you hear from "credible sources." Remember: Who you listen to matters. Educate yourself well enough so you can confidently trust to listen to yourself...and maybe the God you don't think you need. Science alone is not trustworthy enough to get many to where they want to go in this life and the one hereafter.

I wish you well.

Joseph G. Jacko, MD

APPENDICES

The Nuremberg Code

1. The voluntary consent of the human subject is absolutely essential.

2. The experiment should be such as to yield fruitful results for the good of society, unprocurable by other methods or means of study, and not random and unnecessary in nature.

3. The experiment should be so designed and based on the results of animal experimentation and a knowledge of the natural history of the disease or other problem under study that the anticipated results will justify the performance of the experiment.

4. The experiment should be so conducted as to avoid all unnecessary physical and mental suffering and injury.

5. No experiment should be conducted where there is an *a priori* reason to believe that death or disabling injury will occur, except, perhaps, in those

experiments where the experimental physicians also serve as subjects.

6. The degree of risk to be taken should never exceed that determined by the humanitarian importance of the problem to be solved by the experiment.
7. Proper preparations should be made and adequate facilities provided to protect the experimental subject against even remote possibilities of injury, disability, or death.
8. The experiment should be conducted only by scientifically qualified persons. The highest degree of skill and care should be required through all stages of the experiment of those who conduct or engage in the experiment.
9. During the course of the experiment, the human subject should be at liberty to bring the experiment to an end if he has reached the physical or mental state where continuation of the experiment seems to him to be impossible.
10. During the course of the experiment the scientist in charge must be prepared to terminate the experiment at any stage, if he has probable cause to believe, in the exercise of the good faith, superior skill and careful judgment required of him that a continuation of the experiment is likely to result in injury, disability, or death to the experimental subject.

mRNA and Cancer

The CDC and American Cancer Society state that the mRNA vaccines do not increase the risk of cancer or exacerbate existing cancers. Some patients and doctors will likely disagree with that based on their personal experience.

Should you believe the CDC and the American Cancer Society? Consider this:

Despite the CDC and American Cancer Society stating that the mRNA vaccines do not cause cancer, deaths from cancer have risen since 2020, particularly in the 15–44 age group. In 2020, death rates rose 1.7 percent; in 2021, they rose 5.6 percent; and in 2022, 7.9 percent.

Because cancer is primarily a disease of the aged, the increase in cancer deaths in this younger cohort is alarming. Case reports and social media reports have reported that the exposure to the spike protein, especially following mRNA vaccination for COVID-19, is associated with "turbo cancers," that is, rapidly progressive cancers.

Sources:

Marik, Paul E. *Cancer Care: The Role of Repurposed Drugs and Metabolic Interventions in Treating Cancer.* Second ed. Paul Marik Publishing: Norfolk, VA, 2014.

Goldman, Serge, Dominique Bron, Thomas Tousseyn, Irina Vierasu, Laurent Dewispelaere, Pierre Heimann, Elie Cogan, et al. "Rapid Progression of Angioimmunoblastic T Cell Lymphoma Following BNT162b2 mRNA Vaccine Booster Shot: A Case Report." *Frontiers in Medicine,* 8, no 798095 (2021). DOI: 10.3389/fmed.2021.79809.

Mizutani, M., H. Mitsui, T. Amano, Y. Ogawa, N. Deguchi, S. Shimada, et al. (2022). "Two Cases of Axillary Lymphadenopathy Diagnosed as Diffuse Large B-Cell Lymphoma Developed Shortly after BNT162b2 COVID-19 Vaccination." *Journal of the European Academy of Dermatology and Venereology,* 36, no. 8 (2022): e613-e5. DOI: 10.1111/jdv.18136.

Sekizawa, Akinori, Kenichi Hashimoto, Shinichi Kobayashi, Sawako Kozono, Takahiro Kobayashi, Yusuke Kawamura, Motohiro Kimata, et al. "Rapid Progression of Marginal Zone B-cell Lymphoma after COVID-19 Vaccination (BNT162b2): A Case Report." *Frontiers in Medicine,* 9 (2022): 963393. DOI: 10.3389/fmed.2022.963393.

Tachita, Takuto, Takenori Takahata, Satoru Yamashita, Toru Ebina, Kosuke Kamata, Kazufumi Yamagata, Yoshiko Tamai, et al. Newly diagnosed extranodal NK/T-cell lymphoma, nasal type, at the injected left arm after BNT162b2 mRNA COVID-19 vaccination. *International Journal of Hematology*, 118, no. 4 (2023): 503-7. DOI: 10.1007/s12185-023-03607-w.

Bharathidasan, Kavya, Vivie Tran, Sayed Reshad Ghafouri, Shabnam Rehman, and Luis Brandi. "Metastatic prostatic adenocarcinoma presenting as generalized lymphadenopathy unmasked by a COVID booster vaccine." *Clinical case reports*, 11, no. 12 (2023): e8278. https://doi.org/10.1002/ccr3.8278.

Barnett, Christopher, Nishi Mehta, William S. Towne, Kemi Babagbemi, and Rachel Marcus Sales. (2022). "Metastatic melanoma in the breast and axilla: A case report." (2022). *Clinical Imaging*, 85 (2022): 78-82. https://doi.org/10.1016/j.clinimag.2022.02.014.

White Emily, Nicholas Fazio, Konstantinos Tourmouzis, Samuel Ryu, Paul T. Finger, Jodi Sassoon, Roger Keresztes, et al. "Unilateral Conjunctival Classic Kaposi Sarcoma following a COVID 19 Booster." *American Journal of Ophthalmology Case Reports*, 34, no. 101986 (2024). https://doi.org/10.1016/j.ajoc.2023.101986.

Panou, E., V. Nikolaou, L. Marinos, S. Kallambou, P. Sidiropoulou, M. Gerochristou, and A. Stratigos. Recurrence of Cutaneous T-Cell Lymphoma Post Viral Vector COVID-19 Vaccination. *Journal of the European Academy of Dermatology and Venereology*, 36, no. 2 (2021): e91–e93. https://doi.org/10.1111/jdv.17736.

Cavanna, Luigi, Sergio Ottavio Grassi, Livia Ruffini, Emanuele Michieletti, Egidio Carella, Dane Palli, Adriano Zangrandi, et al. (2023). "Non-Hodgkin Lymphoma Developed Shortly after mRNA COVID-19 Vaccination: Report of a Case and Review of the Literature." *Medicina (Kaunas, Lithuania), 59*(1), 157. https://doi.org/10.3390/medicina59010157.

Bae, Edward, Suhwoo Bae, Michael Vaysblat, Mohammed Abdelwahed, Kumar Sarkar, and Stewart Bae. "Development of High-Grade Sarcoma After Second Dose of Moderna Vaccine." *Cureus*, 15, no. 4 (2023): e37612. https://doi.org/10.7759/cureus.37612.

Costanzo, Michele, Maria Anna Rachele De Giglio, and Giovanni Nicola Roviello. "Deciphering the Relationship between SARS-CoV-2 and Cancer." *International Journal of Molecular Sciences,* 24, (2023): 7803. https://doi.org/10.3390/ijms24097803.

Alegria, Carlos, David M. Wiseman, and Yuri Nunes. "US-Death Trends for Neoplasms ICD codes: C00-D48, Ages 15-44." *Research Gate.* (2024). DOI: 10.13140/RG.2.2.16068.64645.

Dr. Fauci's Patents

Anthony S. Fauci has filed for patents to protect the following inventions. This listing includes patent applications that are pending as well as patents that have already been granted by the United States Patent and Trademark Office (USPTO).

Use of Antagonists of the Interaction between HIV GP120 and A4B7 Integrin
Publication number: 20110086024
Abstract: Methods are provided for the treatment of an HIV infection. The methods can include administering to a subject with an HIV infection a therapeutically effective amount of an agent that interferes with the interaction of gp120 and ?4 integrin, such as a ?4?1 or ?4?7 integrin antagonist, thereby treating the HIV infection. In several examples, the ?4 integrin antagonist is a monoclonal antibody that specifically binds to a ?4, ?1 or ?7 integrin subunit or a cyclic hexapeptide with the amino acid sequence of CWLDVC. Methods are also provided to reduce HIV replication or infection. The methods include contacting a cell with an effective amount of an agent that interferes with the interaction of gp120

and ?4 integrin, such as a ?4?1 or ?4?7 integrin antagonist. Moreover, methods are provided for determining if an agent is useful to treat HIV.
Type: Application
Filed: December 6, 2007
Publication date: April 14, 2011
Inventors: James Arthos, Diana James, Claudia Cicala, Anthony Fauci

Use of antagonists of the interaction between HIV GP120 and A4B7 integrin
Patent number: 9193790
Abstract: Methods are provided for the treatment of an HIV infection. The methods can include administering to a subject with an HIV infection a therapeutically effective amount of an agent that interferes with the interaction of gp120 and ?4 integrin, such as a ?4?1 or ?4?7 integrin antagonist, thereby treating the HIV infection. In several examples, the ?4 integrin antagonist is a monoclonal antibody that specifically binds to a ?4, ?1 or ?7 integrin subunit or a cyclic hexapeptide with the amino acid sequence of CWLDVC. Methods are also provided to reduce HIV replication or infection. The methods include contacting a cell with an effective amount of an agent that interferes with the interaction of gp120 and ?4 integrin, such as a ?4?1 or ?4?7 integrin antagonist. Moreover, methods are provided for determining if an agent is useful to treat HIV.
Type: Grant
Filed: December 6, 2007
Date of Patent: November 24, 2015
Assignee: The United States of America, as Represented by the Secretary, Department of Health and Human Services
Inventors: James Arthos, Diana Goode, Claudia Cicala, Anthony Fauci

HIV related peptides
Patent number: 6911527
Abstract: This invention is the discovery of novel specific epitopes and antibodies associated with long-term survival of HIV-1 infections. These epitopes and antibodies have use in preparing vaccines for preventing HIV-1 infection or for controlling progression to AIDS.
Type: Grant
Filed: January 7, 2000
Date of Patent: June 28, 2005
Assignee: The United States of America as represented by the Secretary of the Department of Health and Human Services
Inventors: Giuseppe Scala, Xueni Chen, Oren J. Cohen, Anthony S. Fauci

Efficient inhibition of hiv-1 viral entry through a novel fusion protein including of cd4
Publication number: 20040265306
Abstract: Novel recombinant polypeptides are disclosed herein that include a CD4 polypeptide ligated at its C-terminus with a portion of an immunoglobulin comprising a hinge region and a constant domain of a mammalian immunoglobulin heavy chain. The portion of the IgG is fused at its C-terminus with a polypeptide comprising a tailpiece from the C-terminus of the heavy chain of an IgA antibody or a tailpiece from a C-terminus of the heavy chain of an IgM antibody. Also disclosed herein are methods for using these CD4-fusion proteins.
Type: Application
Filed: July 27, 2004
Publication date: December 30, 2004
Inventors: James Arthos, Claudia Cicala, Anthony S. Fauci

Immunoconjugates Comprising CD4 and Immunoglobin Molecules for the Treatment of HIV Infection
Publication number: 20090285815
Abstract: Nucleic acids encoding recombinant CD4-fusion proteins are disclosed herein that include a CD4 polypeptide ligated at its C-terminus with a portion of an immunoglobulin comprising a hinge region and a constant domain of a mammalian immunoglobulin heavy chain. The portion of the IgG is fused at its C-terminus with a polypeptide comprising a tailpiece from the C terminus of the heavy chain of an IgA antibody or a tailpiece from a C terminus of the heavy chain of an IgM antibody. Also disclosed herein are methods for using these CD4-fusion proteins.
Type: Application
Filed: March 21, 2008
Publication date: November 19, 2009
Inventors: James Arthos, Claudia Cicala, Anthony S. Fauci

Fusion Protein Including of CD4
Patent number: 7368114
Abstract: Novel recombinant polypeptides are disclosed herein that include a CD4 polypeptide ligated at its C-terminus with a portion of an immunoglobulin comprising a hinge region and a constant domain of a mammalian immunoglobulin heavy chain. The portion or the IgG is fused at its C-terminus with a polypeptide comprising a tailpiece from the C-terminus of the heavy chain of an IgA antibody ara tailpiece from a C-terminus of the heavy chain of an IgM antibody. Also disclosed herein are methods for using these CD4 fusion proteins.
Type: Grant
Filed: October 24, 2002
Date of Patent: May 6, 2008

Assignee: The United States of America as represented by the Department of Health and Human Services
Inventors: James Arthos, Claudia Cicala, Anthony S. Fauci

Use of Antagonists of the Interaction between HIV GP120 and A4B7 Integrin
Publication number: 20160333097
Abstract: Methods are provided for the treatment of a HIV infection. The methods can include administering to a subject with an HIV infection a therapeutically effective amount of an agent that interferes with the interaction of gp120 and ?4 integrin, such as a ?4?1 or ?4?7 integrin antagonist, thereby treating the HIV infection. In several examples, the ?4 integrin antagonist is a monoclonal antibody that specifically binds to a ?4, ?1 or ?7 integrin subunit or a cyclic hexapeptide with the amino acid sequence of CWLDVC. Methods are also provided to reduce HIV replication or infection. The methods include contacting a cell with an effective amount of an agent that interferes with the interaction of gp120 and ?4 integrin, such as a ?4?1 or ?4?7 integrin antagonist. Moreover, methods are provided for determining if an agent is useful to treat HIV.
Type: Application
Filed: August 3, 2016
Publication date: November 17, 2016
Applicant: THE UNITED STATES OF AMERICA, as represented by the Secretary, Department of Health and Human Serv
Inventors: James Arthos, Diana Goode, Claudia Cicala, Anthony S. Fauci

Use of Antagonists of the Interaction between HIV GP120 and A4B7 Integrin
Publication number: 20160075786
Abstract: Methods are provided for the treatment of a HIV infection. The methods can include administering to a subject with an HIV infection a therapeutically effective amount of an agent that interferes with the interaction of gp120 and ?4 integrin, such as a ?4?1 or ?4?7 integrin antagonist, thereby treating the HIV infection. In several examples, the ?4 integrin antagonist is a monoclonal antibody that specifically binds to a ?4, ?1 or ?7 integrin subunit or a cyclic hexapeptide with the amino acid sequence of CWLDVC. Methods are also provided to reduce HIV replication or infection. The methods include contacting a cell with an effective amount of an agent that interferes with the interaction of gp120 and ?4 integrin, such as a ?4?1 or ?4?7 integrin antagonist. Moreover, methods are provided for determining if an agent is useful to treat HIV.
Type: Application
Filed: September 21, 2015
Publication date: March 17, 2016
Applicant: The United States of America, as Represented by the Secretary, Department of Health and Human Serv
Inventors: James Arthos, Diana Goode, Claudia Cicala, Anthony S. Fauci

Use of Antagonists of the Interaction between HIV GP120 and ?4?7 Integrin
Patent number: 9896509
Abstract: Methods are provided for the treatment of a HIV infection. The methods can include administering to a subject with an HIV infection a therapeutically effective amount of an agent that interferes with the interaction of gp120 and

?4 integrin, such as a ?4?1 or ?4?7 integrin antagonist, thereby treating the HIV infection. In several examples, the ?4 integrin antagonist is a monoclonal antibody that specifically binds to a ?4, ?1 or ?7 integrin subunit or a cyclic hexapeptide with the amino acid sequence of CWLDVC. Methods are also provided to reduce HIV replication or infection. The methods include contacting a cell with an effective amount of an agent that interferes with the interaction of gp120 and ?4 integrin, such as a ?4?1 or ?4?7 integrin antagonist. Moreover, methods are provided for determining if an agent is useful to treat HIV.
Type: Grant
Filed: August 3, 2016
Date of Patent: February 20, 2018
Assignee: The United States of America, as Represented by the Secretary, Department of Health and Human Services
Inventors: James Arthos, Diana Goode, Claudia Cicala, Anthony S. Fauci

Use of Antagonists of the Interaction between HIV GP120 and ?4?7 Integrin
Patent number: 9441041
Abstract: Methods are provided for the treatment of a HIV infection. The methods can include administering to a subject with an HIV infection a therapeutically effective amount of an agent that interferes with the interaction of gp120 and ?4 integrin, such as a ?4?1 or ?4?7 integrin antagonist, thereby treating the HIV infection. In several examples, the ?4 integrin antagonist is a monoclonal antibody that specifically binds to a ?4, ?1 or ?7 integrin subunit or a cyclic hexapeptide with the amino acid sequence of CWLDVC. Methods are also provided to reduce HIV replication or infection. The methods include contacting a cell with an effective amount

of an agent that interferes with the interaction of gp120 and ?4 integrin, such as a ?4?1 or ?4?7 integrin antagonist. Moreover, methods are provided for determining if an agent is useful to treat HIV.
Type: Grant
Filed: September 21, 2015
Date of Patent: September 13, 2016
Assignee: The United States of America, as Represented by the Secretary, Department of Health and Human Services
Inventors: James Arthos, Diana Goode, Claudia Cicala, Anthony S. Fauci

Immunologic Enhancement with Intermittent Interleukin-2 Therapy
Publication number: 20030180254
Abstract: A method for activating a mammalian immune system entails a series of IL-2 administrations that are effected intermittently over an extended period. Each administration of IL-2 is sufficient to allow spontaneous DNA synthesis in peripheral blood or lymph node cells of the patient to increase and peak, and each subsequent administration follows the preceding administration in the series by a period of time that is sufficient to allow IL-2 receptor expression in peripheral or lymph node blood of the patient to increase, peak and then decrease to 50% of peak value. This intermittent IL-2 therapy can be combined with another therapy which targets a specific disease state, such as an anti-retroviral therapy comprising, for example, the administration of AZT, ddI or interferon alpha. In addition, IL-2 administration can be employed to facilitate in situ transduction of T cells in the context of gene therapy.
Type: Application
Filed: January 23, 2003

Publication date: September 25, 2003
Applicant: The Govt. of the USA as represented by the Secretary of the Dept. of Health & Human Services
Inventors: H. Clifford Lane, Joseph A. Kovacs, Anthony S. Fauci

Immunologic Enhancement with Intermittent Interleukin-2 Therapy
Patent number: 5696079
Abstract: A method for activating a mammalian immune system entails a series of IL-2 administrations that are effected intermittently over an extended period. Each administration of IL-2 is sufficient to allow spontaneous DNA synthesis in peripheral blood or lymph node cells of the patient to increase and peak, and each subsequent administration follows the preceding administration in the series by a period of time that is sufficient to allow IL-2 receptor expression in peripheral or lymph node blood of the patient to increase, peak and then decrease to 50% of peak value. This intermittent IL-2 therapy can be combined with another therapy which targets a specific disease state, such as an anti-retroviral therapy comprising, for example, the administration of AZT, ddI or interferon alpha. In addition, IL-2 administration can be employed to facilitate in situ transduction of T cells in the context of gene therapy.
Type: Grant
Filed: May 26, 1995
Date of Patent: December 9, 1997
Assignee: The United States of America as represented by the Department of Health and Human Services
Inventors: H. Clifford Lane, Joseph A. Kovacs, Anthony S. Fauci

Immunologic Enhancement with Intermittent Interleukin-2 Therapy
Patent number: 6548055
Abstract: A method for activating a mammalian immune system entails a series of IL-2 administrations that are effected intermittently over an extended period. Each administration of IL-2 is sufficient to allow spontaneous DNA synthesis in peripheral blood or lymph node cells of the patient to increase and peak, and each subsequent administration follows the preceding administration in the series by a period of time that is sufficient to allow IL-2 receptor expression in peripheral or lymph node blood of the patient to increase, peak and then decrease to 50% of peak value. This intermittent IL-2 therapy can be combined with another therapy which targets a specific disease state, such as an anti-retroviral therapy comprising, for example, the administration of AZT, ddI or interferon alpha. In addition, IL-2 administration can be employed to facilitate in situ transduction of T cells in the context of gene therapy.
Type: Grant
Filed: August 9, 2000
Date of Patent: April 15, 2003
Assignee: The United States of America as represented by the Department of Health and Human Services
Inventors: H. Clifford Lane, Joseph A. Kovacs, Anthony S. Fauci

Immunologic Enhancement with Intermittent Interleukin-2 Therapy
Patent number: 6190656
Abstract: A method for activating a mammalian immune system entails a series of IL-2 administrations that are effected intermittently over an extended period. Each administration

of IL-2 is sufficient to allow spontaneous DNA synthesis in peripheral blood or lymph node cells of the patient to increase and peak, and each subsequent administration follows the preceding administration in the series by a period of time that is sufficient to allow IL-2 receptor expression in peripheral or lymph node blood of the patient to increase, peak and then decrease to 50% of peak value. This intermittent IL-2 therapy can be combined with another therapy which targets a specific disease state, such as an anti-retroviral therapy comprising, for example, the administration of AZT, ddI or interferon alpha. In addition, IL-2 administration can be employed to facilitate in situ transduction of T cells in the context of gene therapy.
Type: Grant
Filed: September 2, 1997
Date of Patent: February 20, 2001
Assignee: The United States of America as represented by the Department of Health and Human Services
Inventors: H. Clifford Lane, Joseph A. Kovacs, Anthony S. Fauci

Source: Justia Patents. "Patents by Inventor Anthony S. Fauci." https://patents.justia.com/inventor/anthony-s-fauci.

Afterword

During the book's editing, we witnessed the cold-blooded murder of Brian Thompson, CEO of UnitedHealthcare, on December 4, 2024. His murder is not justifiable but may be explainable when more details come to be known.

Medicine is a high-risk profession in ways many of you may have never considered.

Healthcare workers are at 16 times greater risk of suffering workplace violence than workers in other sectors, and around 50 percent experience workplace violence during their careers. Exposure to workplace violence is higher in healthcare workers than it is in prison guards and police officers.

Though a somewhat rare occurrence, doctors are murdered. An Italian study found that, in cases of the murder of physicians, 71 percent of the killers were patients of the doctor, and in 29 percent of the cases, the killer was a patient's family member. Revenge was the motivation in two-thirds of the cases. In 57 percent of the cases, the killer did not have a mental health disorder.

CEOs are accountable to their shareholders and boards of directors, not patients. Shareholders expect to see maximum profits. However, attempts to optimize profits are not always in the best interest of patients when they lead to the denial of care or involve a treatment that delivers more harm than good. CEOs must balance the drive for profits with the realization that their decisions affect the well-being of patients. At the moment, that realization has probably not been given due consideration.

As stated earlier, we have created a healthcare system liked by few, and many find it increasingly frustrating to deal with. That frustration, in some cases, is translating into anger.

Though Mr. Thompson's murder is unlikely to become a black swan event, it may serve as the first in a series of events that ultimately lead to the building of a healthcare system that is far more patient-centered than the one we currently have.

Endnotes

1 Kennedy, John F. "Commencement Address at Yale University." Goodreads.com. June 11, 1962. https://www.goodreads.com/quotes/14892-the-great-enemy-of-truth-is-very-often-not-the.
2 Merriam-Webster, s.v. "medicine (n.)," accessed April 3, 2025. https:/www.merriam-webster.com/dictionary/medicine.
3 Merriam-Webster, s.v. "scam (n.)," accessed April 3, 2025. https://www.merriam-webster.com/dictionary/scam.
4 Oxford Learners Dictionaries, s.v. "scam (n.)," accessed April 3, 2025. https://www.oxfordlearnersdictionaries.com/us/definition/english/scam_1?q=scam.
5 Horton, Richard. "Offline: What is Medicine's 5 Sigma?" *The Lancet,* 385, no. 9976 (2015). https://www.thelancet.com/journals/lancet/article/PIIS0140-6736(15)60696-1/fulltext.
6 Horton, Richard.
7 Angell, Marcia. "Drug Companies and Doctors: A Story of Corruption." Review. *The New York Review.* January 15, 2009. https://www.nybooks.com/articles/2009/01/15/drug-companies-doctorsa-story-of-corruption/.
8 Relman, Arnold S., and Marcia Angell. "America's Other Drug Problem: How the Drug Industry Distorts Medicine and Politics." *The New Republic*, 227, no. 25 (2002): 27-41.
9 Ley Jr, Herbert L. "The FDA protects the big drug companies." In "Institutions Seem To Protect You But Do The Exact Opposite." *Consumers' Association of Penang.* Accessed April 8, 2025. https://consumer.org.my/institutions-seem-to-protect-you-but-do-the-exact-opposite/#:~:text=The%20San%20Francisco%20

Chronicle%20immediately,threaten%20the%20big%20drug%20 companies.

10 Kennedy Jr, Robert F. *The Real Anthony Fauci: Bill Gates, Big Pharma, and and the Global War on Democracy and Public Health.* New York: Skyhorse Publishing, 2021.

11 Transparency International. "What is Corruption?" Transparency International. Accessed 3-13-2025. https://www.transparency.org/en/what-is-corruption.

12 Statista. "U.S. National Health Expenditure as Percent of GDP from 1960 to 2022." Statista. https://www.statista.com/statistics/184968/us-health-expenditure-as-percent-of-gdp-since-1960/.

13 Cantlupe, Joe. "Expert Forum: The Rise and (Rise) of the Healthcare Administrator." Athena Health (blog). November 7, 2017. Accessed 3-3-2025. https://www.athenahealth.com/knowledge-hub/practice-management/expert-forum-rise-and-rise-healthcare-administrator.

14 Kennedy Jr; Nass, Meryl. "Covid-19 Has Turned Public Health Into a Lethal, Patient-Killing Experimental Endeavor." *Alliance for Human Research Protection*, June 20, 2020. https://ahrp.org/covid-19-has-turned-public-health-into-a-lethal-patient-killing-experimental-endeavor/.

15 Thomas, Stephen J., Moreira, Jr, Edson D. Moreira, Jr, Nicholas Kitchin, Judith Absalon, Alejandra Gurtman, Stephen Lockhart, and John L. Perez. "Safety and Efficacy of the BNT162b2 mRNA Covid-19 Vaccine through 6 Months." *The New England Journal of Medicine*, 385, no. November 4, (2021): 1761-1773. DOI: 10.1056/NEJMoa2110345.

16 Pratap, Aayushi. "Pfizer Expects $33.5 Billion in Vaccine Revenue in 2021." *Forbes*, July 28, 2021. https://www.forbes.com/sites/aayushipratap/2021/07/28/pfizer-expects-335-billion-in-vaccine-revenue-in-2021/; Liu, Angus. "Pfizer to Become $100B Behemoth Next Year Thanks to COVID-19 Drug and Vaccine: Analyst." *Fierce Pharma.* November 23, 2021. https://www.fiercepharma.com/pharma/pfizer-to-exceed-100b-revenue-2022-thanks-to-covid-19-drug-and-vaccine-analyst.

17 Wei, Pei-Fang. "Diagnosis and Treatment Protocol for Novel Coronavirus Pneumonia Trial Version 7)." *Chinese Medicine Journal*, March 3, 2020. DOI: 10.1097/CM9.0000000000000819.

18 Association of American Physicians and Surgeons. "More Evidence Presented for Why Hydroxychloroquine Should be

Made Available, in a New Court Filing by the Association of American Physicians & Surgeons (AAPS)." PR NewsWire. July 22, 2020. https://www.prnewswire.com/news-releases/more-evidence-presented-for-why-hydroxychloroquine-should-be-made-available-in-a-new-court-filing-by-the-association-of-american-physicians--surgeons-aaps-301098030.html; Hope, Justus R. "Ivermectin Obliterates 97 Percent of Delhi Cases." *The Desert Review.* June 1, 2021. https://www.thedesertreview.com/news/national/ivermectin-obliterates-97-percent-of-delhi-cases/article_6a3be6b2-c31f-11eb-836d-2722d2325a08.html.

19 WorldoMeter. "COVID-19 Coronavirus Statistics." Accessed March 14, 2025. https://www.worldometers.info/coronavirus/#countries.

20 McCullough, Colin. "Mark Zuckerberg Says *META was 'Pressured' by Biden Administration to Censor COVID 19 Related Content in 2021." CNN.* August 27, 2024. https://www.cnn.com/2024/08/27/business/mark-zuckerberg-meta-biden-censor-covid-2021/index.html

21 Kennedy Jr, Robert F.

22 Physician Side Gigs. "About Physician Side Gigs." https://www.physiciansidegigs.com/about.

23 Shyrock, Todd. "Report: Supermajority of US Physicians are Employed by Health Systems or Corporate Entities." *Medical Economics.* April 19, 2022. https://www.medicaleconomics.com/view/supermajority-of-u-s-physicians-work-for-health-systems-or-corporations.

24 Rivera, Heidi. "What Is the Average Medical School Debt?" Bankrate. May 13, 2024. https://www.bankrate.com/loans/student-loans/average-medical-school-debt/.

25 Ridker, Paul M. "The JUPITER Trial: Results, Controversies, and Implications for Prevention." *Circulation, Cardiovascular Quality and Outcomes* 2, no. 3 (2009). https://doi.org/101161/circoutcomes.109.868299.

26 Erlich, Deborah R. "Evolocumab (Repatha) for the Treatment of Hyperlipidemia." *American Family Physician* 94, no. 10 (2016): 843-846. https://www.aafp.org/pubs/afp/issues/2016/1115/p843.html; Arbel, Ronen, Ariel Hammerman, and Joseph Azuri. "Usefulness of Ezetimibe Versus Evolocumab as Add-On Therapy for Secondary Prevention of Cardiovascular Events

in Patients with Type 2 Diabetes Mellitus." *American Journal of Cardiology* 123, no 8 (2019): 1273-1276. DOI: 10.1016/j.amjcard.2019.01.021.

27 Bero, Lisa. "When Big Companies Fund Academic Research, the Truth Often Comes Last." The Conversation. October 2, 2019. https://theconversation.com/when-big-companies-fund-academic-research-the-truth-often-comes-last-119164.

28 Muraуma, Anju, Akihiko Ozaki, and Tetsuya Tanimoto. "Pharmaceutical Company Payments to Clinical Practice Guideline Authors." In Faintuch, J., Faintuch, S. (eds.) *Integrity of Scientific Research*. Cham, Switzerland: Springer International, 2022. https://doi.org/10.1007/978-3-030-99680-2_45; Norris, Susan L., Haley K. Holmer, Lauren A. Ogden, and Brittany U. Burda. "Conflict of Interest in Clinical Practice Guideline Development: a Systematic Review." *PLoS One* 6, no. 10 (2011): e25153. DOI: 10.1371/journal.pone.0025153.

29 Schott, Gisela, Claudia Dunnweber, Bernd Mühlbauer, Wilhelm Niebling, Henry Pachl, andWolf-Dieter Ludwig. "Does the Pharmaceutical Industry Influence Guidelines?: Two Examples from Germany." Deutches Arzteblatt International, 110, no. 35-36 (2013): 575-583. DOI: 10.3238/arztebl.2013.0575; Choudry, Niteesh K, Henry Thomas Stelfox, and Allan S. Detsky. "Relationships Between Authors of Clinical Practice Guidelines and the Pharmaceutical Industry." *Journal of the American Medical Association* 287, no. 5 (2002): 612-617. DOI: 10.1001/jama.287.5.612.

30 Milestone Documents. "President Dwight D. Eisenhower's Farewell Address (1961)." National Archives. https://www.archives.gov/milestone-documents/president-dwight-d-eisenhowers-farewell-address.

31 Gail, Elizabeth. "Pablo Escobar's Unmatched Generosity, And His Crazy Lifestyle." *Inquisitr*. October 23, 2016. https://www.inquisitr.com/3633297/pablo-escobars-unmatched-generosity-his-crazy-lifestyle.

32 Kennedy Jr, Robert F.; Merck. "Merck Statement on Ivermectin Use During COVID-19 Pandemic." Merck. February 4, 2021. https://www.merck.com/news/merck-statement-on-ivermectin-use-during-the-covid-19-pandemic/.

33 Reagan, Ronald. "Radio Address on Socialized Medicine." American Rhetoric Online Speech Bank. May 9, 1961. https://www.americanrhetoric.com/speeches/ronaldreagansocializedmedicine.htm.

34 Marcovitch, Harvey. "Editors, Publishers, Impact Factors, and Reprint Income." *PLoS Medicine* 7, no. 20 (2010): e1000355. DOI: 10.1371/journal.pmed.1000355.

35 Lafayette, Jon. "TV Ad Revenue to Grow to $74.9B by 2022." *Broadcasting+Cable.* June 5, 2018. https://www.nexttv.com/news/tv-ad-revenue-to-grow-to-74b-by-2022-pwc; Bulik, Beth Snyder. "Hey, Big Spender: Pharmas $6.6 B TV Ad Outlay Outranks Most Other Industries, Report Says." *Fierce Pharma.* May 15, 2019. https://www.fiercepharma.com/marketing/hey-big-spenders-pharma-ranks-top-five-industries-for-tv-media-spending-says-report; LaMattina, John. "Pharma TV Ads and R&D Funding." Forbes. May 30,2022. ndustries-for-tv-media-spending-says-report. https://www.forbes.com/sites/johnlamattina/2022/03/30/pharma-tv-ads-and-rd-funding/.

36 Godlee, Fiona and Tom Jefferson. "Peer Review in Health Sciences." *British Medical Journal* 320 (2000): 1546. https://www.bmj.com/content/320/7248/1546.1.

37 Gunja, Munira, Evan Gumas, and Reginald D. Williams II. "US Health Care from a Global Perspective, 2022: Accelerating Spending, Worsening Outcomes." The Commonwealth Fund. January 31, 2023. https://www.commonwealthfund.org/publications/issue-briefs/2023/jan/us-health-care-global-perspective-2022.

38 Zuby. "20 Things I Learned (Or Had Confirmed About Humanity) During the 'Pandemic' (THREAD)." X.com. July 5, 2021. https://x.com/ZubyMusic/status/1412012537986568193?lang=en.

39 Stout, Martha. *The Sociopath Next Door.* New York: Harmony Books, 2005.

40 Freeman, David. "Are Politicians Psychopaths?" *HuffPost* (blog). Updated October 27, 2012. https://www.huffpost.com/entry/are-politicians-psychopaths_b_1818648.

41 Whitehead, John W. "From Democracy to Pathocracy: The Rise of the Political Psychopath." *HuffPost.* Updated April 1, 2017.

42 Bucksey, Colin, dir. Breaking Bad. Season 3, episode 8, "I See You." Aired May 9, 2010.
43 Statista. "Number of Mass Shootings in the United States between 1982 and September 2024." Statista. https://www.statista.com/statistics/811487/number-of-mass-shootings-in-the-us/.
44 Kennedy Jr, Robert F.
45 Jenkins, Rob. "America's Descent into Medical Fascism." *Townhall.* October 17, 2021. https://townhall.com/columnists/robjenkins/2021/10/17/americas-descent-into-medical-fascism-n2597550; Hague, Omar S. Julian De Freitas, Ivana Viani, Bradley Niederschulte, and Harold J. Bursztajn. "Why Did So Many German Doctors Join the Nazi Party Early?" *International Journal of Law and Psychiatry* 35, no. 5-6 (2012): 473-9. DOI: 10.1016/j.ijlp.2012.09.022.
46 "The Zyklon B Case: Trial of Bruno Tesch and Two Others." Law-Reports of Trials of War Criminals, The United Nations War Crimes Commission, Volume I, London, HMSO, 1947. https://phdn.org/archives/www.ess.uwe.ac.uk/WCC/zyklonb.htm#Dr.%20Tesch.
47 Kennedy Jr, Robert F.
48 Ortleb, Charles. *Fauci: The Bernie Madoff of Science and the HIV Ponzi Scheme that Concealed the Chronic Fatigue Syndrome Epidemic.* Independent. 2021.
49 Andrzejewski, Adam. "Rand Paul is Doing the Right Thing by Asking for Transparency in the NIH." Opinion. *Courier Journal.* June 20, 2022. https://www.courier-journal.com/story/opinion/2022/06/20/rand-pauls-questioning-dr-faucis-nih-royalty-payments-right/7622469001/.
50 Committee on Oversight and Government Reform. "COVID Select Subcommittee Releases Dr. Fauci's Transcript, Highlights Key Takeaways in New Memo." Press Release. May 31, 2024. https://oversight.house.gov/release/covid-select-subcommittee-releases-dr-faucis-transcript-highlights-key-takeaways-in-new-memo/.
51 Knudsen, Hannah. "Exclusive—Andrew Huff: Preemptive Pardon of Anthony Fauci, if Accepted, 'Incriminates Everyone'." *Breitbart.* January 8, 2025. https://www.breitbart.com/politics/2025/01/08/exclusive-andrew-huff-preemptive-pardon-anthony-fauci.

52 Long, Colleen and Zeke Miller. "Biden pardons Fauci, Milley and the Jan. 6 panel. It's a guard against potential 'revenge' by Trump." Associated Press. January 20, 2025. https://apnews.com/article/biden-trump-fauci-milley-pardons-january-6-3cba287f89051513fb48d7ae700ae747.
53 Maher, Bill. "Anti-Pharma Rant." YouTube.com. September 28, 2007. https://www.youtube.com/watch?v=rHXXTCc-IVg.
54 Mikhail, Alexa. "Healthspan May Be More Integral to Your Well-Being Than Lifespan. Here is How to Lengthen It." *Fortune Well.* April 15, 2023. https://fortune.com/well/2023/04/15/healthspan-may-be-more-integral-to-your-well-being-than-lifespan-how-to-lengthen-it/.
55 Duchaharme, Jamie. "Why 'Healthspan' May Be More Important Than Lifespan." *Time.* November 30, 2023. https://time.com/6341027/what-is-healthspan-vs-lifespan/.
56 Kitsis, Elizabeth A. "The Pharmaceutical Industry's Role in Defining Illness." *Virtual Mentor* 13, no. 12 (2011): 906-911. DOI: 10.1001/virtualmentor.2011.13.12.oped1-1112.
57 Schott, Gisela, et al.; Choudry, Niteesh K. et al.
58 LePan, Nicholas. "A Visual History of Pandemics." *World Economic Forum.* May 15, 2020. https://www.weforum.org/agenda/2020/03/a-visual-history-of-pandemics/.
59 Schuerger, Caroline, Steph Batalis, Katherine Quinn, Ronnie Kinoshita, Owen Daniels, and Anna Puglisi. "Understanding the Global Gain-of-Function Research Landscape." *Center for Security and Technology.* August 2023. https://cset.georgetown.edu/publication/understanding-the-global-gain-of-function-research-landscape/.
60 Field, Matt. "Gain-of-Function Pathogen Research Is Controversial and Widespread. Can It Be Regulated?" *Bulletin of the Atomic Scientists.* September 25, 2023. https://thebulletin.org/2023/09/gain-of-function-pathogen-research-is-controversial-and-widespread-can-it-be-regulated/.
61 Kanekoa. "Pfizer's History of Fraud, Corruption, and Using Nigerian Children as 'Human Guinea Pigs'." Kanekoa. December 14,2021. https://www.kanekoa.news/p/pfizers-history-of-fraud-corruption.
62 Lovelace Jr, Berkeley. "Pfizer CEO Says People Who Spread Misinformation on COVID Vaccines are 'Criminals'." CNBC. Updated November 9, 2021. https://www.cnbc.com/2021/11/09/

covid-vaccines-pfizer-ceo-says-people-who-spread-misinformation-on-shots-are-criminals.html.

63 Abramson, John. "Big Pharma is Hijacking the Information Doctors Need Most." *Time*. April 28, 2022. https://time.com/6171999/big-pharma-clinical-data-doctors/; Bero, Lisa. "When Big Companies Fund Academic Research, the Truth Often Comes Last."

64 Facher, Lev. "More Than Two-Thirds of Congress Cashed a Pharma Campaign Check in 2020, New STAT Analysis Shows." STAT News. June 9, 2021. https://www.statnews.com/feature/prescription-politics/federal-full-data-set/.

65 Wouters, Olivia J. "Lobbying Expenditures and Campaign Contributions by the Pharmaceutical and Health Product Industry in the United States, 1999-2018." *JAMA Internal Medicine* 180, no. 5 (2020): 1-10. DOI: 10.1001/jamainternmed.2020.0146.

66 Wouters, Olivia J.; Knight, Victoria, Rachana Pradhan, and Elizabeth Lucas. "Pharma Campaign Cash Delivered to Key Lawmakers with Surgical Precision. *KFF Health News*. October 27, 2021. https://kffhealthnews.org/news/article/pharma-campaign-cash-delivered-to-key-lawmakers-with-surgical-precision/.

67 Facher, Lev. "First of its Kind Examination Shows How Widely Pharma Showers Campaign Cash as the State Level." STAT News. October 15, 2020. https://www.statnews.com/feature/prescription-politics/state-level-examination/.

68 Facher, Lev. ""More Than Two-Thirds of Congress Cashed a Pharma Campaign Check in 2020, New STAT Analysis Shows."

69 US Food and Drug Administration. "FY4 2024 FDA Budget Summary." https://www.fda.gov/media/166050/download?attachment.

70 Department of Health and Human Services. "Food and Drug Administration Fiscal Year 2024." Figure 3, p. 15. https://www.fda.gov/media/166182/download?attachment.

71 Pradhan, Rachana, and McKenzie Beard. "Millions of Dollars Flow from Pharma to Patient Advocacy Groups." *The Washington Post*. December 15, 2023. https://www.washingtonpost.com/politics/2023/12/15/millions-dollars-flow-pharma-patient-advocacy-groups/.

72 McCoy, Matthew S., Michael Carniol, Katherine Chockley, John W. Urwin, Ezekiel J. Emanuel, and Harald Schmidt. "Conflicts of

Interest for Patient-Advocacy Organizations." *The New England Journal of Medicine* 376, no. 9 (2017): 880-885. https://www.nejm.org/doi/full/10.1056/NEJMsr1610625.

73 Almashat, Sammy; Sidney Wolfe, and Michael Carome. "Twenty-Five Years of Pharmaceutical Industry Criminal and Civil Penalties: 1991 Through 2017." Public Citizen. March 14, 2018. https://www.citizen.org/article/twenty-seven-years-of-pharmaceutical-industry-criminal-and-civil-penalties-1991-through-2017/.

74 Tanglis, Mike. "Mapping the PhRMA Grant Universe: An Analysis of the $6 Billion in Grants Distributed by PhRMA and its Member Companies." Public Citizen. December 14, 2023. https://www.citizen.org/article/mapping-the-phrma-grant-universe/.

75 Sismondo, Sergio. *Ghost-Managed Medicine: Big Pharma's Invisible Hands*. Manchester: Mattering Press, 2018.

76 Fabbri, Alice, Alexandra Lai, Quinn Grundy, and Lisa Anne Bero. "The Influence of Industry Sponsorship on the Research Agenda: A Scoping Review." *American Journal of Public Health* 10, no. 8 (2018): e9-e16. DOI: 10.2105/AJPH.2018.304677; Bero, Lisa. "When Big Companies Fund Academic Research, the Truth Often Comes Last." *The Conversation*. October 2, 2019. https://theconversation.com/when-big-companies-fund-academic-research-the-truth-often-comes-last-119164.

77 Ehrhardt, Stephen, Lawrence Appel, and Curtis Meinert. "Trends in National Institutes of Health Funding for Clinical Trials Registered in Clinicaltrials.gov." *Journal of the American Medical Association* 314, no. 23 (2015): 2566-2567. DOI:10.1001/jama.2015.12206.

78 Mello, Michelle M., Lindsey Murtagh, Steven Joffe, Patrick L. Taylor, Yelena Greenberg, and Eric G. Campbell. "Beyond Financial Conflicts of Interest: Institutional Oversight of Faculty Agreements at Schools of Medicine and Public Health." *PloS One*. October 29, 2018. https://doi.org/10.1371/journal.pone.0203179.

79 Lexchin, Joe, Lisa A. Bero, Benjamin Djulbegovic, Otavio Clark. "Pharmaceutical Industry Sponsorship and Research Outcome and Quality: Systematic Review." *British Medical Journal* 326, no. 7400 (2003): 1167. DOI: 10.1136/bmj.326.7400.1167.

80 Turner, Erick H., Annette M. Matthews, Efthiha Linardatos, Robert A. Tell, and Robert Rosenthal. "Selective Publication of

Antidepressant Trials and Its Influence on Apparent Efficacy." *The New England Journal of Medicine* 348 (2008): 252-260. DOI: 10.1056/NEJMsa065779.

81 Whoriskey, Peter. "As Drug Industry's Influence Over Research Grows, So Does the Potential for Bias." *The Washington Post.* November 24, 2012. https://www.washingtonpost.com/business/economy/as-drug-industrys-influence-over-researc h-grows-so-does-the-potential-for-bias/2012/11/24/bb64d596-1264-11e2-be82-c3411b7680a9_story.html.

82 Ehrhardt, Stephen, et al.

83 Helfand, Carly. "JAMA: Med-School Officials Risk Conflicts by Serving on Pharma Boards." *Fierce Pharma.* April 2, 2014. https://www.fiercepharma.com/pharma/jama-med-school-officials-risk-conflicts-by-serving-on-pharma-boards; Anderson, Timothy S., Shravan Dave, and Chester B. Good. "Academic Medical Center Leadership on Pharmaceutical Company Board of Directors." *JAMA Research Letter* 311, no. 13 (2014): 1353-1355. DOI: 10.1001/jama.2013.284925.

84 Elliott, Carl. Relationships Between Physicians and Pharma: Why Physicians Should Not Accept Money from the Pharmaceutical Industry." *Neurology Clinical Practice* 4, no. 2 (2014): 164-167. DOI: 10.1212/CPJ.0000000000000012.

85 Marcovitch, Harvey.

86 MacDonald, Fiona. "This Is the Sickening Amount Pharmaceutical Companies Pay Top Journal Editors." *Science Alert.* April 12, 2018. https://www.sciencealert.com/how-much-top-journal-editors-get-paid-by-big-pharma-corrupt; Liu, Jessica J., Chaim M. Bell, John J. Matelski, Allan S. Detsky, and Peter Cram. "Payments by US Pharmaceutical and Medical Device Manufacturers to US Medical Journal Editors: Retrospective Observational Study." *British Medical Journal* 349 (2017): j4619. DOI: 10.1136/bmj.j4619.

87 Redshaw, Megan. "US Physicians Received Billions From Pharmaceutical and Medical Device Industry, New Research Finds." *The Epoch Times.* April 1, 2024. https://www.theepochtimes.com/health/us-physicians-received-billions-from-pharmaceutical-and-medical-device-industry-new-research-finds-5619143; Sayed, Ahmed, Joseph S. Ross, John Mandrola, Lisa Soleymani Lehmann, and Andrew J. Foy. "Industry Payments to

US Physicians by Specialty and Product Type, Research Letter." *Journal of the American Medical Association* 331, no. 15 (2024): 1325-1327. DOI: 10.1001/jama.2024.1989.
88 Wright, Kristin, Daniel Meyers, Timothy Chisamore, Matthew D. F. McInnes, Sergio Sismondo, Bishal Gyawali, Vinay Prasad, et al. "Industry Relationships with Medical Oncologists: Who are the High-Payment Physicians?" *Journal of Oncology Practice* 18, no. 7 (2022): e1164-e1169. DOI: 10.1200/OP.21.00756.
89 Sood, Neeraj. "Should the Government Restrict Direct to Consumer Prescription Advertising? Six Takeaways on Their Effects." University of Southern California Leonard D.Schaeffer Institute for Public Policy and Government Service. March 23, 2023. https://schaeffer.usc.edu/research/should-the-government-restrict-direct-to-consumer-prescription-drug-advertising-six-takeaways-from-research-on-the-effects-of-prescription-drug-advertising/.
90 LaFayette, Jon.
91 Bulik, Beth Snyder.
92 LaMattina, John.
93 Light, David and Joel R. Lexchin. "Pharmaceutical Research and Development: What Do We Get for All That Money?" *British Medical Journal* 345 (2012): 34e4348. DOI: 10.1136/bmj.e4348.
94 Seeds Scientific Research & Performance Institute. https://ssrpinstitute.org/.
95 *Big Pharma's Business Model: Corporate Greed: United States Senate Hearing on Health, Education, Labor, and Pensions, February 6, 2024.* 108th Cong. (2024) (Majority Staff Report, Bernard Sanders, Chair). https://www.help.senate.gov/imo/media/doc/big_pharmas_business_model_report.pdf.
96 Elliott, Carl. Relationships Between Physicians and Pharma: Why Physicians Should Not Accept Money from the Pharmaceutical Industry." *Neurology Clinical Practice* 4, no. 2 (2014): 164-167. DOI: 10.1212/CPJ.0000000000000012.
97 Almashat, Sammy; Sidney Wolfe, and Michael Carome. "Twenty-Five Years of Pharmaceutical Industry Criminal and Civil Penalties: 1991 Through 2017." *Public Citizen*. March 14, 2018. https://www.citizen.org/article/twenty-seven-years-of-pharmaceutical-industry-criminal-and-civil-penalties-1991-through-2017/.

98 Grand View Research. "US Medical Device Manufacturers Market Size, Share & Trends Analysis Report By Application (Orthopedic Devices, Cardiovascular Devices, Neurology Devices, Drug Delivery Devices, Ophthalmic Devices, Nephrology & Urology Devices), And Segment Forecasts, 2025 - 2030." GVR Market Analysis Report. https://www.grandviewresearch.com/industry-analysis/us-medical-device-manufacturers-market.

99 Case Study. "GlaxoSmithKline Tried to Silence the Scientist Who Exposed the Dangers of Avandia." Union of Concerned Scientists. October 12, 2017. https://www.ucs.org/resources/glaxosmithkline-tried-silence-scientist-who-expose d-dangers-its-drug-avandia#:~:text=Multimedia%20%2F%20Case%20Study-,GlaxoSmithKline%20Tried%20to%20Silence%20the%20Scientist%20Who,Dangers%20of%20its%20Drug%20Avandia&text=When%20Dr.,threatened%20his%20integrity%20and%20career.

100 Wood, Shelley. "US Senate Committee Releases Report on GSK's 'Intimidation' of John Buse Over Rosiglitazone." *Medscape*. November 20, 2007. https://www.medscape.com/viewarticle/566298?form=fpf.

101 Jureidini, Jon, and Leemon B. McHenry. "The Illusion of Evidence Based Medicine." Opinion. *British Medical Journal*, 376 (2022). https://www.bmj.com/content/376/bmj.o702.

102 Jureidini, Jon, and Leemon B. McHenry; Goldacre, Ben. *Bad Pharma: How Drug Companies Mislead Doctors and Harm Patients.* Reprint ed. New York: Farrar, Straus and Giroux, 2013.

103 Noetel, Micheal, Taren Sanders, Daniel Gallardo-Gómez, .Paul Taylor, Borja del Pozo Cruz, Daniel van den Hoek, Jordan J Smith, et al. "Effect of Exercise for Depression: Systematic Review and Network Meta-Analysis of Randomised Controlled Trials." *British Medical Journal* 384 (2024): e075847. https://www.bmj.com/content/384/bmj-2023-075847.

104 Jureidini, Jon, and Leemon B. McHenry; Fugh-Berman, Adriane J. "The Haunting of Medical Journal: How Ghostwriting Sold 'HRT'." *PLoS Medicine* 7, no. 9 (2010): e1000335. https://journals.plos.org/plosmedicine/article?id=10.1371/journal.pmed.1000335

105 Fung, Jason. "The Corruption of Evidence Based Medicine—Killing for Profit." *The Fasting Method*. Accessed March 14, 2025. https://blog.thefastingmethod.com/the-corruption-of-evidence-based-medicine-killing-for-profit/.

106 Jureidini, Jon, and Leemon B. McHenry. "The Illusion of Evidence Based Medicine."
107 Sackett, David L. William M. C. Rosenberg, J. A. Muir Gray, and R. Brian Haynes, W. Scott Richardson. "Evidence Based Medicine: What It Is and What It Isn't." *British Medical Journal* 312 (1996): 71. https://www.bmj.com/content/312/7023/71.
108 Freddi, Goffredo and José Luis Romàn-Pumar. "Evidence-Based Medicine: What it Can and Cannot Do." *Annali dell'Istituto Superiore di Sanita* 47, no. 1 (2011): 22-5. DOI: 10.4415/ANN_11_01_06; Ioannidis, John P.A. "Evidence-Based Medicine Has Been Hijacked: A Report to David Sackett." *Journal of Clinical Epidemiology* 73, (2016): 82-6. DOI: 10.1016/j.jclinepi.2016.02.012; Fava, Giovanni A. "Evidence-Based Medicine Was Bound to Fail: A Report to Alvan Feinstein." *Journal of Clinical Epidemiology* 84 (2017): 3-7. DOI: 10.1016/j.jclinepi.2017.01.012.
109 Smith, Richard. "Medical Journals Are an Extension of the Marketing Arm of Pharmaceutical Companies." *PLoS Medicine* 2, no. 5 (2005): e138. DOI: 10.1371/journal.pmed.0020138.
110 Quraishi, Sadeq A., Edward A Bittner, Livnat Blum, Mathew M Hutter, and Carlos A. Camargo Jr. "Association Between Preoperative 25-Hydroxyvitamin D Level and Hospital-Acquired Infections Following Roux-en-Y Gastric Bypass Surgery." *JAMA Surgery* 149, no. 2 (2014): 112-8. https://jamanetwork.com/journals/jamasurgery/fullarticle/1782085.
111 The RECOVERY Collaborative Group. "Effect of Hydroxychloroquine in Hospitalized Patients with Covid-19." *The New England Journal of Medicine* 383, no. 21 (2020): 2030-40. DOI: 10.1056/NEJMoa2022926.
112 Kaplan, Robert M. and Veronica L. Irvin. "Likelihood of Null Effects of Large NHLBI Clinical Trials Has Increased over Time." *PloS One*. August 5, 2015. https://doi.org/10.1371/journal.pone.0132382.
113 Thacker, Paul D. "COVID-19: Researcher Blows the Whistle on Data Integrity Issues in Pfizer's Vaccine Trial." *British Medical Journal* 375 (2021): n2635. DOI: https://doi.org/10.1136/bmj.n2635.
114 Marcatto, Francesco, Jonathan J. Rolison, and Donatella Ferrante. "Communicating Clinical Trial Outcomes: Effects of Presentation Method on Physicians' Evaluations of New Treatments."

Judgment and Decision Making 8, no. 1 (2013): 29–33. https://doi.org/10.1017/S1930297500004472.

115 Sever, Peter S., Björn Dahlöf, Neil R Poulter, Hans Wedel, Gareth Beevers, Mark Caulfield, Rory Collins, et al. "Prevention of Coronary and Stroke Events with Atorvastatin in Hypertensive Patients Who Have Average or Lower-Than-Average Cholesterol Concentrations, in the Anglo-Scandinavian Cardiac Outcomes Trial—Lipid Lowering Arm (ASCOT-LLA): a Multicentre Randomized Controlled Trial." *The Lancet* 361, no. 9363 (2003): 1149-58. DOI: 10.1016/S0140-6736(03)12948-0.

116 Goldacre, Ben.

117 Goldacre, Ben.

118 Jureidini, Jon and McHenry Leemon B. *The Illusion of Evidence-Based Medicine.* Adelaide: Wakefield Press, 2020.

119 Heathers, James. "The Lancet Has Made One of the Biggest Retractions in Modern History. How Could this Happen?" *The Guardian.* June 5, 2020. https://www.theguardian.com/commentisfree/2020/jun/05/lancet-had-to-do-one-of-the-biggest-retractions-in-modern-history-how-could-this-happen; Piller, Charles. "Who's to Blame? These Three Scientists Are at the Heart of the Surgisphere COVID-19 Scandal." *ScienceInsider.* June 8, 2020. https://www.science.org/content/article/whos-blame-these-three-scientists-are-heart-surgisphere-covid-19-scandal; Offord, Catherine. "The Surgisphere Scandal: What Went Wrong?" *The Scientist.* September 30, 2020. https://www.the-scientist.com/the-surgisphere-scandal-what-went-wrong--67955; Mehra, Mandeep, Sapan Desai, SreyRam Kuy, Timothy D. Henry, and Amit N. Patel. "Retraction: Cardiovascular Disease, Drug Therapy, and Mortality in COVID-19." *The New England Journal of Medicine* 382, no. 2582 (2020). DOI:10:1056/NEJMc2021225; Mehra, Mandeep, Sapan S. Desai, Frank Rushchitzka, and Amit N. Patel. "RETRACTED: Hydroxychloroquine or Chloroquine With or Without a Macrolide for Treatment of COVID-19: a Multinational Registry Analysis." *The Lancet.* May 22, 2020. https://www.thelancet.com/journals/lancet/article/PIIS0140-6736%2820%2931180-6/fulltext.

120 Van Noorden, Richard. "Medicine is Plagued by Untrustworthy Clinical Trials. How Many Studies Are Faked or Flawed?" *Nature.* July 18, 2023. https://www.nature.com/articles/

d41586-023-02299-w; Crandon, Saul. "Be Sceptical: The Reasons Why Most Healthcare Research May Be Wrong." Cochrane.org. https://s4be.cochrane.org/blog/2017/05/12/be-sceptical-the-reason-why-most-healthcare-research-may-be-wrong/.

121 Bouter, Lex. "Fake Academic Papers are on the Rise: Why They're a Danger and How to Stop Them." *The Conversation*. March 6, 2024. https://theconversation.com/fake-academic-papers-are-on-the-rise-why-theyre-a-danger-and-how-to-stop-them-224650; Brainard, Jeffrey. "Fake Scientific Papers Are Alarmingly Common." *Science*, May 9, 2023. https://doi.org/doi:10.1126/science.adi6523; Elmore, Susan A., and Eleanor H. Weston. "Predatory Journals: What They Are and How to Avoid Them." *Toxicologic Pathology* 48, no. 4 (2020): 607–610. https://doi.org/10.1177/0192623320920209.

122 Broughel, James. "Surge in Academic Retractions Should Put US Scholars on Notice." *Forbes.* February 1, 2024. https://www.forbes.com/sites/jamesbroughel/2024/02/01/surge-in-academic-retractions-should-put-us-scholars-on-notice/; Else, Holly. "Biomedical Paper Retractions Have Quadrupled in 20 Years—Why?" *Nature*. May 31, 2024. https://www.nature.com/articles/d41586-024-01609-0; Van Noorden, Richard. "More Than 10,000 Research Papers Were Retracted in 2023—A New Record." *Nature*. December 12, 2023. https://www.nature.com/articles/d41586-023-03974-8.

123 Godlee, Fiona and Tom Jefferson.

124 Heathers, James.

125 Christian, Alexander. "On the Suppression of Medical Evidence." *Journal for General Philosophy of Science* 48 (2017): 395-418. https://link.springer.com/article/10.1007/s10838-017-9377-9; Levy, Raphaël. "Scientific Research: Should Negative Results Be Published?" HEC Paris. September 20, 2019. https://www.hec.edu/en/scientific-research-should-negative-results-be-published.

126 Snyder, Robert J. "Lack of Transparency in Publishing Negative Clinical Trial Results." *Clinics in Podiatric Medical and Surgery* 37, no. 2 (2020): 385-389. DOI: 10.1016/j.cpm.2019.12.013; Levy, Raphaël.

127 Turner, Erick H., Annette M. Matthews, Efthiha Linardatos, Robert A. Tell, and Robert Rosenthal. "Selective Publication of Antidepressant Trials and Its Influence on Apparent Efficacy."

The New England Journal of Medicine 348 (2008): 252-260. DOI: 10.1056/NEJMsa065779.
128 Turner, Erick H., et al.
129 Condon, Alan. "Nearly 80% of physicians now employed by hospitals, corporations: 5 things to know." April 11, 2024. Becker Hospital Review. https://www.beckershospitalreview.com/hospital-physician-relationships/nearly-80-physicians-now-employed-by-hospitals-corporations-report-finds/#:~:text=The%20analysis%20shows%20that%20health%20systems%20and,COVID%2D19%20pandemic.%20Five%20things%20to%20know:%201.
130 Fred, Herbert L. "What Makes a Medical Journal Successful? Five Crucial Components." *The Texas Heart Institute Journal* 44, no.2 (2017): 91-93. doi: 10.14503/THIJ-17-6196.
131 Marcovitch, Harvey.
132 Abramson, John.
133 Lexchin, Joe, et al.
134 Bourgeois, Florence, Srinivas Murthy, and Kenneth D. Mandl. "Outcome Reporting Among Drug Trials Registered in ClinicalTrials.gov." *Annals of Internal Medicine* 153, no. 3 (2010): 158-66. DOI: 10.7326/0003-4819-153-3-201008030-00006.
135 Bero, Lisa, Fieke Oostvogel, Peter Bachetti, and Kirby Leel. "Factors Associated with Findings of Published Trials of Drug to Drug: Why Some Statins Appear More Efficacious Than Others." *PLoS Medicine* 4, no. 6 (2007): e184. DOI: 10.1371/journal.pmed.0040184.
136 Kelly, Robert E., Lisa J. Cohen, Randye J. Semple, Philip Bialer, Adam Lau, Alison Bodenheimer, Elana Neustadter, et al. "Relationship Between Drug Company Funding and Outcomes of Clinical Psychiatric Research." *Psychological Medicine* 36, no. 11 (2006):1647-56. DOI: 10.1017/S0033291706008567.
137 Fugh-Berman, Adriane.
138 Fugh-Berman, Adriane.
139 Dinerstein, Chuck. "The True Cost of End-of-Life Medical Care." *American Council on Science of Health*. September 28, 2018. https://www.acsh.org/news/2018/09/28/true-cost-end-life-medical-care-13454.
140 National Center for Health Statistics. "Mortality Trends in the United States, 1900–2018." US Centers for Disease Control

and Prevention. https://www.cdc.gov/nchs/data-visualization/mortality-trends/index.htm.

141 Gurven, Michael and Hillard Kaplan: "Longevity Among Hunter-Gatherers: A Cross-Cultural Examination." *Population and Development Review* 33, no. 2 (2007): 321-65. https://gurven.anth.ucsb.edu/sites/secure.lsit.ucsb.edu.anth.d7_gurven/files/sitefiles/papers/GurvenKaplan2007pdr.pdf.

142 Schierling, Russell. "Live Long and Prosper: Why Modern Medicine Deserves Little Credit for Today's Lifespan." Dr. Schierling (blog). May 5, 2019. https://doctorschierling.com/blog/live-long-and-prosper-why-modern-medicine-deserves-little-credit-for-todays-lifespan.

143 Schierling, Russell; Rodrigues, Charlene M. C., and Stanley A. Plotkin. "Impact of Vaccines; Heath, Economic and Social Perspectives." *Frontiers in Microbiology* 11 (2020): 1526. DOI: 10.3389/fmicb.2020.01526.

144 Hinman, Alan R. "Vaccine-Preventable Diseases, Immunizations, and MMWR—1961–2021." Task Force Global Health. US Centers for Disease Control and Prevention. October 7, 2011. https://www.cdc.gov/mmwr/preview/mmwrhtml/su6004a9.htm.

145 Cutler, David, and Grant Miller. "The Role of Public Health Improvements in Health Advances: The Twentieth Century United States." *Journal of Demography* 42, no. 1 (2005): 1-22. DOI: 10.1353/dem.2005.0002; Scommegna, Paola. "Clean Water's Historic Effect on US Mortality Rates Provides Hope for Developing Countries." *PRB*. May 1, 2005. https://www.prb.org/resources/clean-waters-historic-effect-on-u-s-mortality-rates-provides-hope-for-developing-countries/.

146 Armstrong, Gregory L., et al.

147 Armstrong, Gregory L., et al.

148 Neilsberg Research. "United States Population by Age." Neilsberg. Updated February22, 2025. https://www.neilsberg.com/insights/united-states-population-by-age/.

149 Hinman, Alan R.

150 Bystrianik, Roman and Suzanne Humphries. *Dissolving Illusions: Disease, Vaccines, and the Forgotten History*. Independent. 2013; Humphries, Suzanne. "Dr. Suzanne Humphries Lectures on Vaccines and Health." YouTube.com https://www.youtube.com/watch?v=SFQQOv-Oi6U.

151 Schroeder, Steven A. "We Can Do Better—Improving the Health of the American People." *The New England Journal of Medicine* 357 (2007): 1221-28. https://www.nejm.org/doi/full/10.1056/NEJMsa073350.
152 Mokdad, Ali H., James S. Marks, Donna F. Stroup, and Julie L. Gerberding. "Actual Causes of Death in the United States, 2000." *Journal of the American Medical Association* 293, no. 3 (2005): 298. DOI: 10.1001/jama.291.10.1238.
153 Li, Yanping, An Pan, Dong D. Wang, Xiaoran Liu, Klodian Dhana, Oscar H. Franco, and Stephen Kaptoge, et al. "Impact of Healthy Lifestyle Factors on Life Expectancies in the US Population." *Circulation* 138, no. 4 (2018): 345-355. https://doi.org/10.1161/CIRCULATIONAHA.117.032047.
154 Li, Yanping, et al.
155 Li, Yanping, et al.
156 Dinerstein, Chuck.
157 Makary, Martin A., and Michael Daniel. "Medical Error—The Third Leading Cause of Death in the US." *British Medical Journal* 353 (2016): i2139. DOI: 10.1136/bmj.i2139.
158 Gasmi, Armin, Geir Bjørklund, Pavan Kumar Mujasdiya, Yuliya Semenova, Salva Piscopo, and Massimiliano Peana. "Coenzyme Q10 in Aging and Disease." *Critical Review in Food Science and Nutrition* 64, no. 12 (2024): 3907-19. DOI: 10.1080/10408398.2022.2137724; Sinatra, Stephen. "Medications that Interact with CoQ10." *Health Directions*. Accessed March 15, 2025. https://www.healthydirections.com/articles/heart-health/medications-that-deplete-coq10-and-the-coq10-dosage-you-need; "Drugs that Deplete: Coenzyme Q10." Lima Memorial Health System. https://www.limamemorial.org/health-library/Complementary%20and%20Alternative%20Medicine/33/000706.
159 Poulain, Michael. "Longevity Blue Zones: A Scientific Research Website." https://longevitybluezone.com/concept-and-history/.
160 Buettner, Dan. *The Blue Zones: 9 Lessons for Living Longer from the People Who've Lived the Longest*, second ed. Washington, DC: National Geographic, 2012.
161 Gladwell, Malcolm. *Outliers: The Story of Success*. New York: Little, Brown, and Company, 2008.
162 Mark. "How Long Do Amish People Live?" *AmishPedia*. February 5, 2024. https://amishpedia.com/?s=How+long+to+Amish+people+live; Kluger, Jeffrey.

"Amish People Stay Healthy in Old Age. Here's Their Secret." *Time*. February 15, 2018. https://time.com/5159857/amish-people-stay-healthy-in-old-age-heres-their-secret/.

163 LaBotz, Michele. "Anabolic-Androgenic Steroid Use in Sports, Health, and Society: A New Consensus Statement from ACSM." American College of Sports Medicine. August 31, 2021. https://acsm.org/anabolic-androgenic-steroid-use-consensus-statement/.

164 Wallinga, David and Kar, Avinash. New Data: Animal vs. Human Antibiotic Use Remains Lopsided. Keep Antibiotics Working. Blog. June 15, 2020. https://www.keepantibioticsworking.org/blog/2020/6/15/new-data-animal-vs-human-antibiotic-use-remains-lopsided.

165 Wallinga, David and Kar, Avinash. New Data: Animal vs. Human Antibiotic Use Remains Lopsided. Keep Antibiotics Working. Blog. June 15, 2020. https://www.keepantibioticsworking.org/blog/2020/6/15/new-data-animal-vs-human-antibiotic-use-remains-lopsided.

166 Aleci, Cristina, and Aaron Smith. "Cleveland Clinic Boots McDonald's From its Food Court." *CNN Money*. August 19, 2015. https://money.cnn.com/2015/08/19/news/companies/cleveland-clinic-mcdonalds/index.html.

167 "Dr. Jordan Vaughn Congressional Testimony." WeRockTV. July 13, 2024. Video, https://www.youtube.com/watch?v=qbr62DQR5PU&t=5s.

168 Fabbri, Alice, Alexandra Lai, Quinn Grundy, and Lisa Anne Bero. "The Influence of Industry Sponsorship on the Research Agenda: A Scoping Review." *American Journal of Public Health* 108, no. 11 (). https://doi.org/10.2105/ajph.2018.304677; Bero, Lisa. "When Big Companies Fund Academic Research, the Truth Often Comes Last." *The Conversation.* October 2, 2019. https://theconversation.com/when-big-companies-fund-academic-research-the-truth-often-comes-last-119164.

169 Sadow, Bernard. 1972. Rolling luggage. United States. US3653474A, filed 1970 and issued April 4, 1972; Wendorf, Marcia. "Who Actually Invented the Wheeled Suitcase?" *Interesting Engineering*, February 18, 2020. https://interestingengineering.com/innovation/who-actually-invented-the-wheeled-suitcase.

170 Lynch, James. "Dr. Fauci Could Not Recall Evidence for Child Masking, Admitted Six-Foot Distancing Came from Nothing, Transcripts Show." MSN. May 2024. https://www.msn.com/en-us/health/medical/dr-fauci-could-not-recall-evidence-for-child-masking-admitted-six-foot-distancing-came-from-nothing-transcripts-show/ar-BB1npVwl; Feiner, Laureen and Berkeley Lovelace Jr. "Fauci Tells Congress: 'There's No Guarantee That The Vaccine Is Actually Going to Be Effective.'" CNBC. May 12, 2020. https://www.cnbc.com/2020/05/12/fauci-tells-congress-no-guarentee-the-coronavirus-vaccine-will-be-effective.html; Dangor, Graison. "CDC's Six-Foot Social Distancing Rule Was 'Arbitrary', Says Former FDA Commissioner" *Forbes*. September 19, 2021. https://www.forbes/com/sites/graisondangor/2021/09/19/cdcs-six-foot-social-distancing-rule-was-arbitrary-says-former-fda-commissioner/; McNeil, Donald G." How Much Herd Immunity Is Enough?" *New York Times*. December 24, 2020. https://www.nytimes.com/2020/12/24/health/herd-immunity-covid-coronavirus.html.

171 Bouter, Lex. "Fake Academic Papers Are on the Rise: Why They're a Danger and How to Stop Them." *The Conversation*. March 6, 2024. https://theconversation.com/fake-academic-papers-are-on-the-rise-why-theyre-a-danger-and-how-to-stop-them-224650; Brainard, Jeffrey. "Fake Scientific Papers Are Alarmingly Common." *Science*. May 9, 2023. https://www.science.org/content/article/fake-scientific-papers-are-alarmingly-common; Elmore, Susan A., and Eleanor H. Weston. "Predatory Journals: What They Are and How to Avoid Them." *Toxicologic Pathology* 48, no. 4 (2020): 607-610. DOI: 10.1177/0192623320920209.

172 Woods, James. "The History of Estrogen." University of Rochester Medical Center. February 2016. https://www.urmc.rochester.edu/ob-yn/ur-medicine-menopause-and-womens-health/menopause-blog/february-2016/the-historyy-of-estrogen.

173 "Fluid Intake, Dehydration, and Exercise: Part I." *The Science of Sport*. Updated October 17, 2007. https://sportsscientists.com/2007/10/fluid-intake-dehydration-and-exercise-part-i-history-of-fluid-intake-and-a-conflict-of-interest/.

174 Murphy, Robert J. "Heat Illness in the Athlete." *American Journal of Sports Medicine* 12, no. 4 (1984). https://doi.org/10.1177/036354658401200404.
175 Makary, Martin A., and Michael Daniel; Starfield, Barbara. "Is US Health Really the Best in the World?" *Journal of the American Medical Association* 28, no. 4 (2000): 483-485. DOI: 10.1001/jama.284.4.483.
176 Britannica. "Prescription Drug Costs." Britannica ProCon. January 1, 2021. https://prescriptiondrugs.procon.org/fda-approved-prescription-drugs-later-pulled-from-the-market/.
177 Koutsos, Athanasios, Samantha Riccadonna, Maria M Ulaszewska, Pietro Franceschi, Kajetan Trošt, Amanda Galvin, Tanya Braune, et al. "Two Apples a Day Lower Serum Cholesterol and Improve Cardiometabolic Biomarkers in Mildly Hypercholesterolemic Adults: A Randomized, Controlled, Crossover Trial." *The American Journal of Clinical Nutrition* 111, no. 2 (2020): 307–18. https://doi.org/10.1093/ajcn/nqz282.
178 Brewer, Sarah. "Brazil Nuts Have Miraculous Effects on Cholesterol Balance." *Nutritional Health*. https://drsarahbrewer.com/brazil-nuts-have-miraculous-effects-on-cholesterol-balance; Ferrari, Carlos K.B. "Anti-Atherosclerotic and Cardiovascular Protective Benefits of Brazilian Nuts." *Frontiers in Bioscience* 12, no. 1 (2020): 38-56. https://doi.org/10.2741/s539.
179 Santos, Heitor O., Wilson M.A.M. de Moraes, Guilherme A.R. da Silva, Jonato Prestes, and Brad J. Schoenfeld. "Vinegar (Acetic Acid) Intake on Glucose Metabolism: A Narrative Review." *Clinical Nutrition ESPEN* 32 (August 2019): 1–7. https://doi.org/10.1016/j.clnesp.2019.05.008; Hadi, Amir, Makan Pourmasoumi, Ameneh Najafgholizadeh, Cain C. Clark, and Ahmad Esmaillzadeh. "The Effect of Apple Cider Vinegar on Lipid Profiles and Glycemic Parameters: A Systematic Review and Meta-Analysis of Randomized Clinical Trials." *BMC Complementary Medicine and Therapies 21*, no. 1 (2021). https://doi.org/10.1186/s12906-021-03351-w.
180 Ridker, Paul M.
181 Sackett, David L., et al.
182 Carr, Teresa. "Too Many Meds? America's Love Affair with Prescription Medication." *Consumer Reports*. August 3, 2017. https://www.consumerreports.org/

prescription-drugs/too-many-meds-americas-love-affai r-with-prescription-medication/.
183 "Flying High: The Real Odds of Experiencing a Plane Crash." Fly Fright. 2023. https://flyfright.com/plane-crash-statistics/.
184 Atkinson, Nancy. "Terrible Luck: The Only Person Ever Killed by a Meterorite- Back in 1888. *Universe Today*. April 30, 2020. https://www.universetoday.com/articles/terrible-luck-the-only-person-ever-killed-by-a-meteorite-back-in-1888#:~:text=%E2%80%9CStar%2Dshaped%E2%80%9D%20sign%20at,just%20waiting%20to%20be%20discovered.
185 National Weather Service. "How Dangerous is Lightning?" https://www.weather.gov/safety/lightning-odds.
186 International Shark Attack File. "Risk of Death: 18 Things More Likely to Kill You Than Sharks." Florida Museum. https://www.floridamuseum.ufl.edu/shark-attacks/odds/compare-risk/death/.
187 US Centers for Disease Control and Prevention. "Shingles Facts and Stats." US Centers for Disease Control and Prevention. Accessed March 18, 2025. https://www.cdc.gov/shingles/data-research/.
188 CDC. "Shingles."
189 Kennedy Jr, Robert F.
190 Starfield, Barbara.
191 Makary, Martin A., and Michael Daniel.
192 Hallahan, Gráinne. "The Alarming Link Between Poor Vocabulary and Behavior." *TES Magazine*. July 21, 2021. https://www.tes.com/magazine/teaching-learning/general/alarming-link-between-poor-vocabulary-and-behaviour; Peterson, Isaac T., Brian M D'Onofrio, Claire A. Coyne, Jennifer E.Lansford, Kenneth A. Dodge, Gregory S Pettit, and Carol A Van Hulle. "Language Ability Predicts the Development of Behavior Problems in Children." *Journal of Abnormal Psychology* 122, no. 2 (2013): 542-57. https://doi.org/10.1037/a0031963.
193 American Heart Association. "Understand Your Risks to Prevent a Heart Attack." American Heart Association. Accessed April 8, 2025. https://www.heart.org/en/health-topics/heart-attack/understand-your-risks-to-prevent-a-heart-attack.
194 DeVries, J. H. "Intensified Glucose Lowering in Type 2 Diabetes: Don't Throw the Baby Out with the Bathwater." *Diabetologia*, 53, no 3 (2010): 705-6. https://doi.org/10.1007/s00125-010-1991-6.

195 Reedy-Cooper, Alexi, Leesha Helm, and David Lee. "Metformin to Prevent Diabetes in Patients at Increased Risk." *American Family Physician* 102, no. 9 (2020): 531-32. https://www.aafp.org/pubs/afp/issues/2020/1101/p531.html; Madsen, Kasper, Yuan Chi, Maria-Inti Metzendorf, Bernd Richter, and Bianca Hemmingsen. "Metformin for Prevention or Delay of Type 2 Diabetes Mellitus and Its Associated Complications in Persons at Increased Risk for the Development of Type 2 Diabetes Mellitus." *The Cochrane Database of Systematic Reviews* 12, no. 12 (2019). DOI: 10.1002/14651858.CD008558.pub2.

196 The NNT. "SGLT-2 Inhibitors and GLP-1 Receptor Agonists for Type 2 Diabetes." Accessed April 8, 2025. https://thennt.com/nnt/sglt-2-inhibitors-and-glp-1-receptor-agonists-for-type-2-diabetes/.

197 Kokkinos, Peter, Charles Faselis, Immanuel Babu Henry Samuel, Andreas Pittaras, Michael Doumas, Rayelynn Murphy, et al. "Cardiorespiratory Fitness and Mortality Risk Across the Spectra of Age, Race, and Sex." *Journal of the American College of Cardiology* 80, no. 6 (2022). DOI: 10.1016/j.jacc.2022.05.031.

198 Thompson, Wade; Lucas Morin, Dorte Ejg Jarbøl, Jacob Harbo Andersen, Martin Thomsen Ernst, Jesper Bo Nielsen, Peter Haastrup, et al. "Statin Continuation and Cardiovascular Events Among Older People in Denmark." *JAMA Network Open* 4, no. 12 (2021): e2136802. DOI: 10.1001/jamanetworkopen.2021.36802.

199 National Institutes of Health. "According to a New Government Survey, 38 Percent of Adults and 12 Percent of Children Use Complementary and Alternative Medicine." Press release. December 10, 2008. https://www.nih.gov/news-events/news-releases/according-new-government-survey-38-percent-adults-12-percent-children-use-complementary-alternative-medicine.

200 US Food and Drug Administration. "FY4 2024 FDA Budget Summary."

201 Lietzen, Erika."User Fees Imposed by Federal Agencies." *The Regulatory Review*. July 3, 2024. https://www.theregreview.org/2024/07/03/lietzan-user-fees-imposed-by-federal-agencies/.

202 Depledge Strategic Wealth Management. "The US Printed More Than $3 Trillion in 2020 Alone. Here's Why it Matters Today." DePledge Straegic Wealth Management. June 17, 2022. https://www.depledgeswm.com/depledge/the-us-printed-more-than-

3-trillion-in-2020-alone-heres-why-it-matters-today/; Parlapiano, Alicia, Deborah Solomon, Madeline Ngo, and Stacy Cowley. "Where $5 Trillion in Pandemic Stimulus Money Went." *The New York Times*. March 11, 2022. https://www.nytimes.com/interactive/2022/03/11/us/how-covid-stimulus-money-was-spent.html.

203 Wolf, Zachary B. "$113 Billion: Where the US Investment in Ukraine Aid Has Gone." CNN, September 21, 2023. https://www.cnn.com/2023/09/21/politics/war-funding-ukraine-what-matters/index.html.

204 Christenson, John. "Migrant Crisis Has US Taxpayers on the Hook for Up to $451B, House GOP Report Says." *The New York Post*. November 13, 2023. https://nypost.com/2023/11/13/news/house-gop-report-cites-historic-451-billion-cost-of-migrant-crisis/; Ngo, Emily. "NYC Mayor Puts $12 Billion Cost On Migrant Crisis, Blames 'Broken National Immigration System'." *Politico*. August 9, 2023. https://www.politico.com/news/2023/08/09/eric-adams-new-york-migrants-cost-00110472.

205 Foley, Katherine Ellen. "Trust Issues Deepen as Yet Another FDA Commissioner Joins the Pharmaceutical Industry." *Quartz*. July 1, 2019. https://qz.com/1656529/yet-another-fda-commissioner-joins-the-pharmaceutical-industry.

206 Derep, Maxine. "What's the Average Time to Bring a Drug to Market in 2022?" *N-Side*. Blog. November 5, 2022. https://lifesciences.n-side.com/blog/what-is-the-average-time-to-bring-a-drug-to-market-in-2022.

207 Sever, Peter S., et al.

208 Pavlovic, Jelena, Philip Greenland, Oscar H. Franco, Maryam Kavousi, M. Kamran Ikram, Jaap W. Deckers, M. Arfan Ikram, et al. "Recommendations and Associated Levels of Evidence for Statin Use in Primary Prevention of Cardiovascular Disease: A Comparison at Population Level of the American Heart Association/American College of Cardiology/Multisociety, US Preventive Services Task Forces Department of Veterans Affairs/Department of Defense, Canadian Cardiovascular Society, and European Society of Cardiology/European Atherosclerosis Society Clinical Practice Guidelines." *Circulation: Cardiovascular Quality and Outcomes* 14, no. 9 (2021): e007183. DOI: 10.1161/CIRCOUTCOMES.120.007183.

209 Ridker, Paul M.

210 Rossignol, Michel, Michel Labrecque, Michel Cauchon, Marie-Claude Breton, and Paul Poirier. "Number of Patients Needed to Prescribe Statins in Primary Cardiovascular Prevention: Mirage and Reality." *Family Practice* 35, no. 4 (2018): 376-382. https://doi.org/10.1093/fampra/cmx124.

211 Carey, John. "Do Cholesterol Drugs Do Any Good?" *Businessweek*. January 2008. https://www.bloomberg.com/news/articles/2008-01-16/do-cholesterol-drugs-do-any-good.

212 Duke, Jon, Jeff Friedlin, and Patrick Ryan. "A Quantitative Analysis of Adverse Effects and 'Overwarning' in Drug Labelling." *Archives of Internal Medicine* 171, no. 10 (2011): 941-954. DOI: 10.1001/archinternmed.2011.182.

213 Sheikh, Hassan Z. "Drug Compounding: FDA Authority and Possible Issues for Congress." Congressional Research Service, R45069. Updated January 5, 2018. https://crsreports.congress.gov.

214 Fernandez, Maria Luz, Minu Sara Thomas, Bruno S. Lemos, Diana M. DiMarco, Amanda Missimer, Melissa Melough, Ock K. Chun, et al. "TA-65, A Telomerase Activator Improves Cardiovascular Markers in Patients with Metabolic Syndrome." *Current Pharmaceutical Design* 24, no. 17 (2018): 1905-1911. DOI: 10.2174/1381612824666180316114832; Bawamia, Bilal, Luke Spray, Vincent K. Wangsaputra, Karim Bennaceur, Sharareh Vahabi, Konstantinos Stellos, Ehsan Kharatikoopaei, et al. "Activation of Telomerease by TA-65 Enhances Immunity and Reduces Inflammation Post Myocardial Infarction." *Geroscience* 45, no. 4 (2023): 2689-705. DOI: 10.1007/s11357-023-00794-6; Salvador, Laura, Gunasekaran Singaravelu, Calvin B. Harley, Peter Flom, Anitha Suram, and Joseph M Raffaele. "A Natural Product Telomerase Activator Lengthens Telomeres in Humans: A Randomized, Double Blind, and Placebo Controlled Study." *Rejuvenation Research* 19, no. 6 (2016): 478-484. DOI: 10.1089/rej.2015.1793; Harley, Calvin B., Weimin Liu, and Joseph M Raffaele. "A Natural Product Telomerase Activator as Part of a Health Maintenance Program: Metabolic and Cardiovascular Response." *Rejuvenation Research* 16, no. 5 (2013): 386-95. DOI: 10.1089/rej.2013.1430.

215 Code of Federal Regulations. "§ 600.3; Biologic Products." https://www.ecfr.gov/current/title-21/chapter-I/subchapter-F/part-600/subpart-A/section-600.3.

216 Crump, Andy. "Ivermectin: Enigmatic Multifaceted 'Wonder Drug' Continues to Surprise and Exceed Expectations." *The Journal of Antibiotics* 70, no. 5 (2017): 495–505. https://doi.org/10.1038/ja.2017.11.

217 Henderson, David R., and Charles L. Hooper. "Why is the FDA Attacking a Safe, Effective Drug?" Opinion. *The Wall Street Journal.* July 28, 2021. https://www.wsj.com/articles/fda-ivermectin-covid-19-coronavirus-masks-anti-science-11627482393.

218 Lou Dobbs Staff. "Caught on Camera: DOJ Attorney Who Defended FDA in Court Admits Agency's Anti-Ivermectin Campaign Was a 'Mistake' and 'Abuse of Authority'." Lou Dobbs.com. August 27, 2024, https://loudobbs.com/news/caught-on-camera-doj-attorney-who-defended-fda-in-court-admits-agencys-anti-ivermectin-campaign-was-a-mistake-and-an-abuse-of-authority/.

219 Baletti, Brenda. "Whistleblower Case Against Merck Over MMR Vaccine Dismissed." *Advocatz*. August 14, 2024. https://advocatz.com/2024/08/14/whistleblower-case-against-merck-over-mmr-vaccine-dismissed/.

220 Gross, Terry. "How Drug Companies Helped Shape a Shifting, Biological View of Mental Illness." National Public Radio. May 2, 2019. https://www.npr.org/sections/health-shots/2019/05/02/718744068/how-drug-companies-helped-shape-a-shifting-biological-view-of-mental-illness; Kitsis, Elizabeth; Lacasse, Jeffrey R. and Jonathan Leo. "Serotonin and Depression: A Disconnect Between the Advertisements and the Scientific Literature." *PLoS Medicine* 2, no. 12 (2005): e392. https://journals.plos.org/plosmedicine/article?id=10.1371/journal.pmed.0020392; Moncrieff, Joanna; Ruth E. Cooper, Tom Stockmann, Simone Amendola, Michael P. Hengartner, and Mark Horowitz. "The Serotonin Theory of Depression: a Systematic Umbrella Review of the Evidence." *Molecular Psychiatry* 28, no. 8 (2022): 3243-56. DOI: 10.1038/s41380-022-01661-0.

221 Lidber, L., J. R. Tuck, M. Asberg, G. P. Scalia-Tomba, and L. Bertilsson. "Homicide, Suicide and CSF 5-HIAA." *Acta Pyschiatrica Scandinavica* 71, no. 3 (1985): 230-6. DOI: 10.1111/j.1600-0447.1985.tb01279.x. Asellus, P., P. Nordström, and J, Jokinen. "Cholesterol and CSF 5-HIAA in Attempted Suicide."

Journal of Affective Disorders 125, no. 1-3 (2010): 388-92. DOI: 10.1016/j.jad.2010.02.111.

222 Strand, Daniel S., Daejin Kim, and David A. Peura. "25 Years of Proton Pump Inhibitors: A Comprehensive Review." *Gut and Liver* 11, no. 1 (2017): 27-37. DOI: 10.5009/gnl15502.

223 Duke, Jon, Jeff Friedlin, and Patrick Ryan. "A Quantitative Analysis of Adverse Effects and 'Overwarning' in Drug Labelling." *Archives of Internal Medicine* 171, no. 10 (2011): 941-954. DOI: 10.1001/archinternmed.2011.182.

224 Rossouw, Jacques E., Garnet L. Anderson, Ross L. Prentice, Andrea Z. LaCroix, Charles Kooperberg, Marcia L. Stefanick, Rebecca D. Jackson, et al. "Risks and Benefits of Estrogen Plus Progestin in Healthy Postmenopausal Women: Principal Results From the Women's Health Initiative Randomized Controlled Trial." *Journal of the American Medical Association* 288, no. 3 (2002): 321-33. DOI: 10.1001/jama.288.3.321.

225 Miyagawa, Shinichi, Tomomi Sato, and Taison Iguchi. "Endocrine Disruptors." In *Handbook of Hormones: Comparative Endocrinology for Basic and Clinical Research*. Edited by Yoshio Takei, Yoshio, Kazuyoshi Tsutsui, Kazuyoshi, and Hironori Ando, 571-90. Oxford: Academic Press, 2015.

226 3M Careers. "3M's 15% Culture." 3M. Accessed April 8, 2025. https://www.3m.co.uk/3M/en_GB/careers/culture/15-percent-culture/.

227 Legal Information Institute. "15 U.S. §3710c - Distribution of Royalties Received by Federal Agencies." Cornell Law School. https://www.law.cornell.edu/uscode/text/15/3710c.

228 Kennedy Jr.

229 Cleary, Ekaterina Galkina, Jennifer M. Beirliein, Navleen Surjit Khanuja, Laura M. McNamee, and Fred D. Ledley. "Contribution of NIH Funding to New Drug Approvals 2010-2016." *Proceedings of National Academy of Sciences* 115, no. 10 (2018): 2329-2334. DOI: 10.1073/pnas.1715368115.

230 Andrzejewski, Adam. "Rand Paul is Doing the Right Thing by Asking for Transparency in the NIH"; Open the Books Investigation. "NIH Royalty Disclosures FY2010-FY2014." Open the Books. https://perma.cc/TDP3-Y7MD.

231 Gore, D'Angelo. "Some Posts About NIH Royalties Omit Fauci Statement That He Donates His Payments." FactCheck.org. May 20,2022. https://www.factcheck.org/2022/05/

scicheck-some-posts-about-nih-royalties-omit-that-fauci-said-he-donates-his-payments/.

232 *United States Sentencing Commission: Public Hearing. April 12, 2005.* 109th Cong. (2005). https://www.ussc.gov/sites/default/files/pdf/amendment-process/public-hearings-and-meetings/20050412-13/hearing_transcript.pdf.

233 Collins, Rick. *Legal Muscle: Anabolics in America*. East Meadow, NY: Legal Muscle Publishing, 2002.

234 LaBotz, Michele.

235 LaBotz, Michele.

236 Justia Patents. "Patents assigned to Centers for Disease Control and Prevention." Justia. https://patents.justia.com/assignee/centers-for-disease-control-and-prevention.

237 "IS CANCER A PARASITIC DISEASE?" *Journal of the American Medical Association* XVI, no. 13 (1891):452–453. DOI:10.1001/jama.1891.02410650020004.

238 Van Tong, Hoang, Paul J. Brindley, Christian G. Meyera, and Thirumalaisamy P. Velavana. "Parasite Infection, Carcinogenesis and Human Malignancy." *eBioMedicine* 15 (2016) :12-23. https://www.thelancet.com/article/S2352-3964(16)30551-5/fulltext; Wang, Fei, Wenbo Meng, Bingyuan Wang, and Liang Qiao. "Heliobacter pylori-induced Gastric Inflammation and Gastric Cancer." *Cancer Letters* 345, no. 2 (2014): 196-202. DOI: 10.1016/j.canlet.2013.08.016; Hosseininasab-Nodoushan, Seyed Albolfazi; Ghazvini, Kiarash; Jamialahmadi, Tannaz; et.al: Association of Chlamydia and Mycoplasma Infections with Susceptibility to Ovarian Cancer: A Systematic Review and Meta-Analysis." *Seminars in Cancer Biology* 86 (Pt 2) (2022): 923-928. DOI: 10.1016/j.semcancer.2021.07.016.

239 Keyarts, Els, Leen Vijgen, Piet Maes, Johan Neyts, and Marc Van Ranst. "In Vitro Inhibition of Severe Acute Respiratory Syndrome Coronavirus by Chloroquine." *Biochemistry and Biophysical Research Communications* 323, no. 1 (2004): 264-8. DOI: 10.1016/j.bbrc.2004.08.085.

240 Association of American Physicians and Surgeons. "More Evidence Presented for Why Hydroxychloroquine Should be Made Available, in a New Court Filing by the Association of American Physicians & Surgeons (AAPS)."

241 Mitchell, Aaron P., Stacie B. Dusetizine, and Akriti Mishra Meza, Niti U Trivedi, Peter B. Bach, and Aaron N. Winn.

"Pharmaceutical Industry Payments and Delivery of Non-Recommend and Low Value Cancer Drugs: Population Based Cohort Study." *British Medical Journal* 383 (2003): e075512. DOI: 10.1136/bmj-2023-075512.

242 Moss, Ralph. *Doctored Results: The Suppression of Laetrile at Sloan-Kettering Institute for Cancer Research.* Sheffield, England: Equinox, 2014.

243 Kirsch, Steve. "ABIM: Follow the Consensus, Not the Science. Saving Lives is Not a Priorty." *Steve Kirsch's Newsletter.* Substack. August 14, 2024. https://kirschsubstack.com/p/abim-follow-the-consensus-not-the; Weber, Lauren, and McKenzie Beard. "Doctors Accused of Spreading Misinformation Lose Certifications." *Washington Post.* May 13, 2024. https://www.washingtonpost.com/politics/2024/08/13/doctors-accused-spreading-misinformation-lose-certifications/.

244 Işık, H. Nazan. "SECOND OPINION: Laetrile at Sloan-Kettering—Uncovering a Cover-Up." NKENDiken. August 29, 2014. https://www.nkendiken.com/2014/08/29/second-opinion-laetrile-at-sloan-kettering-uncovering-a-cover-up/.

245 Saleem, Mohammed, Jawaria Asif, Muhammad Asif, and Uzma Saleem. "Amygdalin from Apricot Kernels Induces Apoptosis and Causes Cell Cycle Arrest in Cancer Cells; An Updated Review." *AntiCancer Agents in Medicinal Chemistry* 18, no. 12 (2018): 1650-55. DOI: 10.2174/18715206186661801051611 36; Barakat, Hassan, Thamer Aljutaily, Mona S. Almujaydil, Reham M. Algheshairy, Raghad M. Alhomaid, Abdulkarim S. Almutairi, Saleh I. Alshimali, et al. "Amygdalin: A Review on its Characteristics, Antioxidant Potential, Gastrointestinal Microbioata Intervention, Anticancer Therapeutic and Mechanisms, Toxicity, and Encapsulation." *Biomolecules* 12, no. 10 (2022): 1514. DOI: 10.3390/biom12101514; Spanoudaki, Maria, Sofia Stoumpou, Sousana K Papadopoulou, Dimitra Karafyllaki, Evangelos Solovos, Konstantinos Papadopoulos, Anastasia Giannakoula, Constantinos Giaginis, et al. "Amygdalin as a Promising Anticancer Agent: Molecular Mechanisms and Future Perspectives for the Development of New Nanoformulations for Its Delivery." *International Journal of Molecular Sciences* 24, no. 18 (2023): 14270. DOI: 10.3390/ijms241814270; Mani, Jens, Jens Neuschäfer, Christian Resch, Jochen Rutz, Sebastian

Maxeiner, Frederik Roos, Felix K-H Chun,et al. "Amygdalin Modulates Prostate Cancer Cell Adhesion and Migration in Vitro." *Nutrition and Cancer* 72, no. 3 (2020): 528-37. DOI: 10.1080/01635581.2019.1637442.

246 Cancer Trends Progress Report. "Financial Burden of Cancer Care." National Cancer Institute. Accessed March 16, 2025. https://progressreport.cancer.gov/after/economic_burden.

247 Mariotto, Angela B., Lindsey Enewold, Jingxuan Zhao, Christopher A. Zeruto, and K. Robin Yabroff. "Medical Care Costs Associated with Cancer Survivorship in the United States." *Cancer Epidemiology, Biomarkers & Prevention* 29, no. 7 (2020), 1304–1312. https://doi.org/10.1158/1055-9965.EPI-19-1534.

248 Tang, Mingyang, Xiaodong Hu, Yi Wang, Xin Yao, Wei Zhang, Chenying Yu, Fuying Cheng, et al. "Ivermectin, A Potential Anticancer Drug Derived from An Antiparasitic Drug." *Pharmacology Research* 163, no. 105207 (2021). DOI: 10.1016/j.phrs.2020.105207.

249 Makis, William. "FENBENDAZOLE and CANCER - at least 12 Anti-Cancer mechanisms of action. Not approved by FDA. Cheap. Safe. Kills aggressive cancers. Why no Clinical Trials? Nine research papers reviewed." COVID INT. Substack. October 3, 2023. https://makismd.substack.com/p/fenbendazole-and-cancer-at-least?ref=slightlyoffensive.com.

250 Nygren, Peter, Mårten Fryknäs, Bengt Agerup, and Rolf Larsson. "Repositioning of the Anthelmintic Drug Mebendazole for the Treatment for Colon Cancer." *Journal of Cancer Research and Clinical Oncology* 39, no. 12 (2013): 2133-2140. DOI: 10.1007/s00432-013-1539-5; DeWitt, Michelle, Alexander Gamble, Derek Hanson, Daniel Markowitz, Caitlin Powell, Saleh Al Dimassi, Mark Atlas, et. al. "Repurposing Mebendazole as a Replacement for Vincristine for the Treatment of Brain Tumors." *Molecular Medicine* 23 (2017): 50-56. DOI: 10.2119/molmed.2017.00011; Joe, Natalie S., Yuanfeng Wang, Harsh H. Oza, Inês Godet, Nubaira Milki, Gregory J. Riggins, and Daniele M. Gilkes. "Mebendazole Treatment Disrupts the Transcriptional Activity of Hypoxia-Inducible Factors 1 and 2 in Breast Cancer Cells." *Cancers* 15, no. 4 (2023):1330. doi: 10.3390/cancers15041330.

251 Sanare Lab. "Premium Fenbendazole Products." Sanare Lab. https://sanarelab.com/collections/

all?srsltid=AfmBOooUqNneBwrepLZD9Ly8GItVLM_VaTHjHwFG_b7oF2N0uEvGqin2.
252 GoodRx. "Emverm." GoodRx.com. https://www.goodrx.com/emverm/what-is.
253 Hanqing Xue et al., "Review of Drug Repositioning Approaches and Resources," International Journal of Biological Sciences 14, no. 10 (July 13, 2018): 1232–44, https://doi.org/10.7150/ijbs.24612.
254 Sudeep Pushpakom et al., "Drug Repurposing: Progress, Challenges and Recommendations," Nature Reviews Drug Discovery 18, no. 1 (October 12, 2018): 41–58, https://doi.org/10.1038/nrd.2018.168.
255 Willnat, Lars, David H. Weaver, and Cleve Wilhoit. "The American Journalist Under Attack: Media, Trust, & Democracy: Key Findings 2022." S.I. Newhouse School of Public Communication. Syracuse University, 2022.
256 O'Hare, Claire. "Latest Data Shows Astonishing Number of Journalists Align with Democrat Party." *State of the Union*. January 2, 2024. https://www.stateofunion.org/2024/01/02/latest-data-shows-astonishing-number-of-journalists-align-with-democrat-party/.
257 Bergman, Jerry. "Ratio of Liberal to Conservative Professors Has Profoundly Changed." Letter to the editor. KPCNews.com. October 10, 2019. https://www.kpcnews.com/opinions/article_72a36307-576f-517e-8a43-64eb7f024e27.html.
258 Gallup. "Party Affiliation." Gallup. Accessed March 14, 2025. https://news.gallup.com/poll/15370/party-affiliation.aspx.
259 Rothwell, Jonathan, and Dan Witters. "US Adults' Estimates of COVID-19 Hospitalization Risk." Gallup. September 27, 2021. https://news.gallup.com/opinion/gallup/354938/adults-estimates-covid-hospitalization-risk.aspx; Marken, Stephanie. "Roundup of Recent Gallup Data on Vaccines." Gallup Blog. November 13, 2020. https://news.gallup.com/opinion/gallup/324527/roundup-recent-gallup-data-vaccines.aspx.
260 Rothwell, Jonathan, and Dan Witters.
261 Moline, Heidi, Michael Whitaker, Li Deng, Julia C. Rhodes, Jennifer Milucky, Huong Pham, Kadam Patel, et al. "Effectiveness of COVID-19 Vaccines in Preventing Hospitalization Among Adults Aged > 65 Years – COVID-NET, 13 States, February-April, 2021." *CDC Morbidity and Mortality Report.*

August 13, 2021. https://www.cdc.gov/mmwr/volumes/70/wr/mm7032e3.htm.
262 Rothwell, Jonathan.
263 Glassner, Barry. *The Culture of Fear: Why Americans Are Afraid of the Wrong Things.* New York: Basic Books, 2018.
264 Takoff, Emma, and Ashley Fetters Malloy. "The Anti-Vax Wellness Influencers." *The Washington Post*. October 1, 2021. https://www.washingtonpost.com/podcasts/post-reports/the-antivax-wellness-influencers/.
265 Bezos, Jeff. "Opinion: The Hard Truth: Americans Don't Trust the News Media." *The Washington Post*, October 28, 2024.
266 Kurtzman, Daniel. "Baghdad Bob Quotes." May 9, 2019. https://www.liveabout.com/baghdad-bob-quotes-4068522.
267 Guo, Ming, Xiaoxiao Liu, Xiangmei Chen, and Qinggang Li. "Insights into New-Onset Autoimmune Diseases After COVID-19 Vaccination." *Autoimmune Review* 22, no. 7 (2023). DOI: 10.1016/j.autrev.2023.103340; Chen, Yue, Zhiwei Xu, Peng Wang, Xiao-Mei Li, Zong-Wen Shuai, Dong-Qing Ye, and Hai-Feng Pan. "New-Onset Autoimmune Phenomena Post COVID-19 Vaccination." *Immunology* 165, no. 4 (2022): 386-401.
268 Canadian COVID Care Alliance. "The Pfizer Inoculations for COVID-19: More Harm than Good." December 21, 2021. https://www.canadiancovidcarealliance.org/wp-content/uploads/2021/12/The-COVID-19-Inoculations-More-Harm-Than-Good-REV-Dec-16-2021.pdf.
269 Insurance Forums Staff. "OneAmerica CEO Says Death Rates Among Working-Age People Up 40%." Insurance Forums. January 3, 2022. https://www.insurance-forums.com/life-insurance/oneamerica-ceo-says-death-rates-among-working-age-people-up-40/.
270 National Institutes of Health. "According to a New Government Survey, 38 Percent of Adults and 12 Percent of Children Use Complementary and Alternative Medicine."
271 Kennedy Jr, Robert F. "Full, Controversial Speech at 'Defeat the Mandates'." YouTube.com. January 23, 2022. https://www.youtube.com/watch?v=joiLT2IT2qQ.
272 Now This. "Dr. Fauci Predicted a Pandemic Under Trump in 2017." YouTube.com. May 18, 2020. https://www.youtube.com/watch?v=puqaaeLnEww&t=95s.

273 "Redefining Philanthropic Drug Discovery." Milken Institute Future of Health Summit. November 26, 2019. https://www.youtube.com/watch?v=-kFJijSgXnQ&list=PLwJK8JzK8C_dEtHeihV0ut3akPfo488Jr&index=7.
274 Chan, Alina. "Why the Pandemic Probably Started in a Labs, in 5 Key Points." *The New York Times.* June 3, 2024. https://www.nytimes.com/interactive/2024/06/03/opinion/covid-lab-leak.html; Alwine, James, Felicia Goodrum, Bruce Banfield, David Bloom, William J. Britt, Andrew J. Broadbent, Samuel K. Campos, et al. "The Harms of Promoting the Lab Leak Hypothesis for SARS-CoV-2 Origins Without Evidence." *Journal of Virology* 98, no. 9 (2024): e0124024. DOI: 10.1128/jvi.01240-24.
275 Akpan, Nsikan, and Victoria Jaggard. "Fauci: No Scientific Evidence the Coronavirus Was Made in a Chinese Lab." N*ational Geographic.* May 4, 2020. https://www.nationalgeographic.com/science/article/anthony-fauci-no-scientific-evidence-the-coronavirus-was-made-in-a-chinese-lab-cvd.
276 McNeil Jr, Donald J.
277 Porterfield, Carlie. "Dr. Fauci on GOP Criticism." June 9, 2021. *Forbes.com.* https://www.forbes.com/sites/carlieporterfield/2021/06/09/fauci-on-gop-criticism-attacks-on-me-quite-frankly-are-attacks-on-science/.
278 Statista. "Number of Coronavirus Disease 2019 (COVID-19) Deaths in the US as of June 14, 2023, by Age." Statista. https://www.statista.com/statistics/1191568/reported-deaths-from-covid-by-age-us/.
279 McNicholas, Celine and Margaret Poydock. "Who Are Essential Workers?" *Economic Policy Institute.* May 19, 2020. https://www.epi.org/blog/who-are-essential-workers-a-comprehensive-look-at-their-wages-demographics-and-unionization-rates/.
280 World Health Organization. "Coronavirus Disease (COVID-19) : Herd Immunity, Lockdowns, and COVID-19." World Health Organization. December 31, 2020. https://www.who.int/news-room/questions-and-answers/item/herd-immunity-lockdowns-and-covid-19.
281 Parlapiano, Alicia, et al.
282 Dangor, Graison.
283 Kampf, G. A., et al.; Abraham, Jonathan, Cohen; Marc. "Turning up the Heat on COVID-19: Heat as a Therapeutic Intervention." *F1000 Research* 9, no. 292 (2020). DOI: 10.12688/

f1000research.23299.2; Liikkanen, Lassi A., and Jari A. Laukkanen. "Sauna Bathing Frequency in Finland and the Impact of COVID-19." *Complementary Therapies in Medicine* 56, no. 102594 (2021). DOI: 10.1016/j.ctim.2020.102594.

284 Statista. "Number of Households in the U.S. from 1960 to 2023." Statista. (2025). https://www.statista.com/statistics/183635/number-of-households-in-the-us/.

285 Mehra, Mandeep, Sapan S. Desai, Frank Rushchitzka, and Amit N. Patel.

286 Kennedy Jr., Robert F.

287 Crump, Andy.

288 World Health Organization. "WHO Model Lists of Essential Medicines." Accessed March 17, 2025. https://www.who.int/groups/expert-committee-on-selection-and-use-of-essential-medicines/essential-medicines-lists.

289 Heidary, Fatemeh and Reza Gharebaghi. "Ivermectin: A Systematic Review from Antiviral Effects to COVID-19 Complementary Regimen." *Journal of Antibiotics* 73, no. 9 (2020): 593-692. https://doi.org/10.1038/s41429-020-0336-z.

290 Monash University. "Lab Experiments Show Anti-Parasitic Drug, Ivermectin, Eliminates SARS-CoV-2 in Cells in 48 Hours." April 4, 2020. https://www.monash.edu/news/articles/coronavirus-fight-possible-covid-19-drug-identified-by-scientists.

291 Santin, A.D., D. E. Scheim, P. A. McCullough, M. Yagisawa, and T. J. Borody. "Ivermectin: A Multifaceted Drug of Nobel Prize-Honoured Distinction with Indicated Efficacy Against a New Global Scourge, COVID-19." *New Microbes New Infections* 43, no. 100924 (2021). DOI: 10.1016/j.nmni.2021.100924.

292 Carvallo, Hector, Roberto Raul Hirsh, Alkis Psaltis, and Veronica Contreras. "Study of the Efficacy and Safety of Topical Ivermectin + Iota- Carrageenan in the Prophylaxis." *Journal of Biomedical Research and Clinical Investigation* 2 (2020). DOI: 10.31546/2633-8653.1007.

293 Keyarts, Els, et al.

294 Wei, Pei-Fang.

295 Risch, Harvey A. "Early Outpatient Treatment of Symptomatic, High Risk COVID-19 Patients That Should Be Ramped Up Immediately as Key to Pandemic Crisis." *American Journal of Epidemiology* 189, no. 11 (2020): 1218-1226. DOI: 10.1093/aje/kwaa093.

296 Risch, Havery A. "The Key to Defeating COVID-19 Already Exists. We Need to Start Using It." Opinion. *Newsweek.* Updated July 28, 2020. https://www.newsweek.com/key-defeating-covid-19-already-exists-we-need-start-using-it-opinion-1519535.

297 Nass, Meryl. "Covid-19 Has Turned Public Health Into a Lethal, Patient-Killing Experimental Endeavor." *Alliance for Human Research Protection.* June 20, 2020. https://ahrp.org/covid-19-has-turned-public-health-into-a-lethal-patient-killing-experimental-endeavor/.

298 Kennedy Jr, Robert F.

299 Canadian COVID Care Alliance.

300 Varney, James. "Leprosy, Polio, Malaria, TB, Measles…, and Massive Unscreened Illegal Immigration." *Real Clear Investigations.* Updated March 2024. https://www.realclearinvestigations.com/articles/2023/12/27/leprosy_polio_malaria_tb_measles__and_massive_unscreened_illegal_immigration_1000817.html; McCaughey, Betsy. "Biden's Open Borders Are Bringing Contagious Diseases to Your Neighborhood." *The New York Post.* April 18, 2023. https://nypost.com/2023/04/18/bidens-open-borders-are-bringing-contagious-diseases-to-your-neighborhood/.

301 Clark County. "Active Tuberculosis Disease in Clark County, 2013-2023." Clark County Combined Health District. https://ccchd.com/wp-content/uploads/2024/01/TB-Incidence-Rates-and-Counts_1.4.24.pdf.

302 Camero, Katie. "Why Did CDC Change Its Definition for 'Vaccine'? Agency Explains Move as Skeptics Lurk." *The Charlotte Observer.* Updated September 27, 2021. https://www.charlotteobserver.com/news/coronavirus/article254111268.html.

303 Paul, Rand. "The Great COVID Cover-Up: Shocking Truth About Wuhan and 15 Federal Agencies." Opinion. Fox News. April 9, 2024. https://www.foxnews.com/opinion/great-covid-cover-up-shocking-truth-about-wuhan-15-federal-agencies.

304 Reynolds, Alan. "How One Model Simulated 2.2 Million U.S. Deaths from COVID-19." Cato Institute. April 21, 2020. https://www.cato.org/blog/how-one-model-simulated-22-million-us-deaths-covid-19; Ryan, Chatelain. "US COVID-19 Deaths in 2021 Surpass 2020 Total." *Spectrum News NY*! October 6, 2021.

https://ny1.com/nyc/all-boroughs/health/2021/10/06/u-s--covid-deaths-in-2021-top-2020-total.

305 Feiner, Laureen and Berkeley Lovelace Jr.

306 Thomas, Stephen J., et al.

307 Gorkhali, Ritesh, Prashanna Koirala, Sadikshya Rijal, Ashmita Mainali, Adesh Baral, Hitesh Kumar Bhattarai. "Structure and Function of Major SARS-CoV-2 and SARS-CoV Proteins." *Bioinformatics and Biology Insights.* June 2022. DOI: 10.1177/11779322211025876.

308 Patel, Rikin, Mohamad Kaki, Venkat S. Potluri, Payal Kahar, and Deepesh Khannal. "A Comprehensive Review of SARS-CoV-2 Vaccines: Pfizer, Moderna & Johnson & Johnson." *Human Vaccines & Immunotherapeutics* 18, no. 1 (2022): 2002083. DOI: 10.1080/21645515.2021.2002083.

309 Parry, Peter, Astrid Lefringhausen, Conny Turni, Christopher J. Neil, Robyn Cosford, Nicholas J, Hudson, and Julian Gillespie. "'Spikeopathy': COVID-19 Spike Protein Is Pathogenic, from Both Virus and Vaccine and RNA." *Biomedicine* 11, no. 8 (2023): 2287. DOI: 10.3390/biomedicines11082287.

310 McCullough, Peter A. "McCullough Protocol Base Spike Detoxification." *Focal Points.* September 30, 2024. https://www.thefocalpoints.com/p/mccullough-protocol-base-spike-detoxification.

311 Alexander, Paul Elias. "160 Plus Research Studies Affirm Naturally Acquired Immunity to COVID-19: Documented, Linked, and Quoted." Brownstone Institute. October 17, 2021. https://brownstone.org/search-results/?_keywords=160+Plus+Research+Studies+Affirm+Naturally+Acquired+Immunity+to+COVID-19%3A+Documented%2C+Linked%2C+and+Quoted.

312 "Redefining Philanthropic Drug Discovery." Milken Institute Future of Health Summit. November 26, 2019. https://www.youtube.com/watch?v=-kFJijSgXnQ&list=PLwJK8JzK8C_dEtHeihV0ut3akPfo488Jr&index=7.

313 Le Bert, Nina, Anthony T. Tan, Kamini Kunasegaran, Christine Y. L. Tham, Morteza Hafezi, Adeline Chia, Melissa Hui Yen Chng, et al. "SARS-CoV-2 Specific T-Cell Immunity Cases of COVID-19 and SARRS, and Uninfected Controls." *Nature* 584, no. 7821 (2020): 457-62. DOI: 10.1038/s41586-020-2550-z.

314 Hope, Justus R.

315 Parry, Peter, et al.

316 Berenson, Alex. "URGENT: Yale researchers have found Covid spike protein in the blood of people never infected with Covid—years after they got mRNA jabs." *Unreported Truths* (blog). December 19, 2024. https://www.thefocalpoints.com/p/mccullough-protocol-base-spike-detoxification.
317 Mullis, Kary. "Dr. Kary Mullis Explains the PCR Test." YouTube.com. https://www.youtube.com/watch?v=ZmZft4fXhQQ&t=144s.
318 Racaniello, Vincet and Rich Condit. "COVID-19 with Dr. Anthony Fauci." TWiV (This Week in Virology) (podcast) Episode 641. July 16, 2020. https://www.youtube.com/watch?v=a_Vy6fgaBPE.
319 Trusdell, Brian. "Harvard Medical Professor to Newsmax: Vax Mandates Create Distrust." August 13, 2021. https://www.newsmax.com/newsmax-tv/covid-vaccine-mandates-harvard/2021/08/13/id/1032333/.
320 Dutta, Sinjari Sutta. "No Point Vaccinating Those Who've Had COVID-19: Cleveland Clinic Study Suggests." June 8, 2021. https://www.news-medical.net/news/20210608/No-point-vaccinating-those-whoe28099ve-had-COVID-19-Findings-of-Cleveland-Clinic-study.aspx; Emory University News Center. "COVID-19 Survivors May Possess Wide-Ranging Resistance to the Disease." Emory University. July 22, 2021. http://news.emory.edu/stories/2021/07/covid_survivors_resistance/index.html; Bhandari, Tamara. "Good News: Mild COVID-19 Induces Lasting Antibody Protection." WashU Medicine Press Release. May 24, 2021. https://medicine.wustl.edu/news/good-news-mild-covid-19-induces-lasting-antibody-protection/; Cho, Alice, Frauke Muecksch, Dennis Schaefer-Babajew, Zijun Wang, Shlomo Finkin, Christian Gaebler, Victor Ramos, et al. "Antibody Evolution after SARS-CoV-2 mRNA Vaccination." *BioRxiv*. July 29, 2021. https://www.biorxiv.org/content/10.1101/2021.07.29.454333v1.
321 Le Bert, Nina, et al.
322 Li, Steven. "Most COVID-19 Patients at Israel Hospital Fully Vaccinated, Doctor Calls Mandates 'Diabolic'." *Vision Times*. August 8, 2021. https://www.visiontimes.com/2021/08/08/israel-hospital-vaccinated.html.
323 Aravindan, Aradhana and Chen Lin. "Vaccinated People Make Up 75% of Recent COVID-19 Cases in Singapore, but Few Fall Ill." *Vision Times*. July 23, 2021. https://www.reuters.com/world/

asia-pacific/vaccinated-people-singapore-make-up-three-quarters-recent-covid-19-cases-2021-07-23/.

324 Li, Steven. "Higher Death, Hospitalization Rates Among Vaccinated Individuals: UK COVID-19 Data." *Vision Times*. July 4, 2021. https://www.visiontimes.com/2021/07/04/deaths-hospital-vaccinated-uk.html.

325 "27 People Aboard Carnival Cruise Test Positive for COVID-19." Associated Press. August 13, 2021. https://apnews.com/article/lifestyle-business-health-travel-caribbean-4dd34f14b6a6365f48b3375c57ba4fb4.

326 Aygun, Hatice. "Vitamin D Can Prevent COVID-19 Infection-Induced Multiple Organ Damage." *Naunyn-Schmiedeberg's Archives of Pharmacology* 393, no. 7 (2020): 1157–60. DOI: 10.1007/s00210-020-01911-4; Daneshkhah, Ali, Adam Eshein, Hariharan Subramanian, Hemant K. Roy, and Vadim Backman. "The Role of Vitamin D in Suppressing Cytokine Storm in COVID-19 Patients and Associated Mortality." *medRxiv*. April 10, 2020. https://www.medrxiv.org/content/medrxiv/early/2020/04/10/2020.04.08.20058578.full.pdf?mod=article_inline; Parpia, Rishman. "Open-Air Treatment During the "Spanish Flu" Pandemic." *The Vaccine Report*. April 12, 2020. https://thevaccinereaction.org/2020/04/open-air-treatment-during-the-spanish-flu-pandemic/.

327 Hobday, Richard. "Coronavirus and the Sun: A Lesson from the 1918 Influenza Pandemic." Medium. March 10, 2020. https://medium.com/@ra.hobday/coronavirus-and-the-sun-a-lesson-from-the-1918-influenza-pandemic-509151dc8065.

328 Sun Online Desk. "Mass vaccination during COVID-19 pandemic historic blunder, says French Nobel laureate and virologist Luc Montagnier." *Daily Sun*. May 25, 2021. https://www.daily-sun.com/post/554588.

329 Canadian COVID Care Alliance.

330 Thomas, Stephen J., et al.

331 Bar-On, Yinon M., Yair Goldberg, Micha Mandel, Omri Bodenheimer, Ofra Amir, Laurence Freedman, Sharon Alroy-Preis, et al. "Protection by a Fourth Dose of BNT162b2 against Omicron in Israel." *The New England Journal of Medicine* 386 (2022): 1712-20. https://www.nejm.org/doi/full/10.1056/NEJMoa2201570.

332 Le Bert, Nina, et al.

333 Miltimore, Jon. "Athletes Who Had COVID Will Be Considered 'Fully Vaccinated,' NCAA Says in New Guidelines." *Foundation for Economic Freedom*. January 10, 2022. https://fee.org/articles/athletes-who-had-covid-will-be-considered-fully-vaccinated-ncaa-says-in-new-guidelines/.
334 VAERS Weekly Summary. "VAERS Summary for COVID-19 Vaccines through 10/29/2021." VAERS Analysis. November 5, 2021. https://vaersanalysis.info/2021/11/05/vaers-summary-for-covid-19-vaccines-through-10-29-2021//.
335 Wire Editor. "OneAmerica Insurance CEO: Deaths Increase 40% Among People Ages 18-64." *Headline USA*. January 3, 2022. https://headlineusa.com/oneamerica-insurance-ceo-deaths-increase-40-among-people-ages-18-64/; Conradson, Julian. "It's Not Just the US: Excess Deaths Skyrocket Worldwide in 2021 Following Rollout of the Experimental Covid Vaccine." *The Gateway Pundit*. April 2, 2022. https://www.thegatewaypundit.com/2022/04/not-just-us-excess-deaths-skyrocket-worldwide-2021-following-rollout-experimental-covid-vaccine/.
336 Jureidini, Jon, and Leemon B. McHenry. "The Illusion of Evidence Based Medicine."
337 Kanekoa. 'Pfizer's History of Fraud, Corruption, and Using Nigerian Children as 'Human Guinea Pigs'." *Kanekoa News* Substack. December 5, 2021.https://kanekoa.substack.com/p/pfizers-history-of-fraud-corruption?s=.
338 CDC. "Shingles."
339 Canadian COVID Care Alliance.
340 United States Holocaust Memorial Museum. "Medical Ethics." The Nuremberg Code. Accessed April 9, 2025. https://encyclopedia.ushmm.org/content/en/article/the-nuremberg-code.
341 Committee on Oversight and Government Reform. "COVID Select Subcommittee Releases Dr. Fauci's Transcript, Highlights Key Takeaways in New Memo." Press Release. May 31, 2024. https://oversight.house.gov/release/covid-select-subcommittee-releases-dr-faucis-transcript-highlights-key-takeaways-in-new-memo/.
342 Bergman, Frank. "Official Data Shows Kidney Failure Deaths Surging Among Covid-Vaxxed." *Slay*. October 17, 2024. https://slaynews.com/news/official-data-shows-kidney-failure-deaths-surging-among-covid-vaxxed/.

343 Lovelace Jr, Berkeley. "Pfizer CEO Says People Who Spread Misinformation on COVID Vaccines are "Criminals." CNBC. November 9, 2021. https://www.cnbc.com/2021/11/09/covid-vaccines-pfizer-ceo-says-people-who-spread-misinformation-on-shots-are-criminals.html.
344 Thomas, Stephen J., et al.
345 Canadian COVID Care Alliance; Pratap, Aayushi.
346 Liu, Angus.
347 Polack, Fernando, Stephen J. Thomas, Nicholas Kitchin, Judith Absalon, Alejandra Gurtman, Stephen Lockhart, John L. Perez, et al. "Safety and Efficacy of the BNT162b 2mRNA Covid-19 Vaccine." *The New England Journal of Medicine,* 383 (2020): 2603-26. https://www.nejm.org/doi/full/10.1056/NEJMoa2034577.
348 Thomas, Stephen J., et al.
349 Canadian COVID Care Alliance. "The Pfizer Inoculations For COVID-19 – More Harm Than Good – PDF." Accessed April 9, 2025. https://www.canadiancovidcarealliance.org/media/the-pfizer-inoculations-for-covid-19-more-harm-than-good/
350 Levin, Einav; Yaniv Lustig, Carmit Cohen, Ronen Fluss, Victoria Indenbaum, Sharon Amit, Ram Doolman, et al. "Waning Immune Humoral Response to BNT162b2 Covid-19 Vaccine Over 6 Months." *The New England Journal of Medicine* 385, no. 24 (2021): e84. DOI: 10.1056/NEJMoa2114583; Chemaitelly, Hiram, Patrick Tang, Mohammad R. Hasan, Sawsan AlMukdad, Hadi M. Yassine, Fatiha M. Benslimane, Hebah A. Al Khatib, et al. "Waning of BNT162b2 Vaccine Protection Against SARS-CoV-2 Infection in Qatar." *The New England Journal of Medicine* 385, no. 24 (2021): e83. DOI: 10.1056/NEJMoa2114114.
351 Statista. "Resident Population of the United States by Sex and Age as of July 1, 2023." Statista. https://www.statista.com/statistics/241488/population-of-the-us-by-sex-and-age/.
352 Thacker, Paul D. "COVID-19: Researcher Blows the Whistle on Data Integrity Issues in Pfizer's Vaccine Trial." *British Medical Journal* 375 (2021): n2635. DOI: https://doi.org/10.1136/bmj.n2635.
353 Mercola, Joseph. "How CDC Manipulated Data to Create 'Pandemic of the Unvaxxed' Narrative." *The Defender*. August 16, 2021. https://childrenshealthdefense.org/defender/cdc-manipulated-data-create-pandemic-unvaxxed-narrative/;

Our World in Data. "US: Total COVID-19 Vaccination Doses Administered per 100 People." Our World in Data. https://ourworldindata.org/grapher/us-state-covid-vaccines-per-100.
354 Langmaid, Virgina. "Data on Hospitalizations and Deaths in the Unvaccinated Do Not Reflect Delta Variant, CDC Director Says." CNN. August 5, 2021. https://www.cnn.com/us/live-news/coronavirus-pandemic-vaccine-updates-08-05-21/h_82f976bb0f238323e3e0482af5d2d563.
355 "The CDC licences vaccine technology, but isn't a vaccine company; the CDC doesn't sell vaccines, it buys and distributes vaccines free of charge." Sophie Fessl, ed. Science Feedback. March 4, 2021. https://science.feedback.org/review/the-cdc-licences-vaccine-technology-but-isnt-a-vaccine-company-the-cdc-doesnt-sell-vaccines-it-buys-and-distributes-vaccines-free-of-charge/.
356 VAERS Adverse Event Reporting Systems. "About Us." https://vaers.hhs.gov/about.html.
357 VAERS Analysis. "VAERS Summary for COVID-19 Vaccines through 11/05/2021." https://vaersanalysis.info/2021/11/12/vaers-summary-for-covid-19-vaccines-through-11-05-2021/.
358 Delépine, Gérard. "High Recorded Mortality in Countries Categorized as 'Covid-19 Vaccine Champions'. Increased Hospitalization." *Freedom of Speech*. October 1, 2021. https://childrenshealthdefense.org/citation/1e-42-gerard-delepine-high-recorded-mortality-in-countries-categorized-as-covid-19-vaccine-champions-increased-hospitalization-freedom-of-speech-oct-1-2021/.
359 Chung, Frank. "Pfizer CEO Says Vaccine Offers 'Very Limited Protection, If Any' Against 0micron." News.com.au. January 12, 2022. https://www.news.com.au/technology/science/human-body/pfizer-boss-says-two-doses-provides-limited-protection-if-any-against-omicron/news-story/9d76126d080e2010f05eb0b4ae5e0c45
360 Hu, Charlotte. "These Are the Most—and Least—Reputable Drug Companies in the US." *Business Insider*. June 19, 2018. https://www.businessinsider.com/pharmaceutical-company-reputation-rankings-2018-6#22-pfizer-reptrak-points-545-1

361 RepTrack. "2021 Global RepTrak 100." The RepTrak Company. (2021). https://ri.reptrak.com/hubfs/_2021%20GRT/2021%20Global%20RepTrak%20100%20-%20Report.pdf
362 UPI. "Court Approves Settlement in Shipley Heart-Valve Case." UPI Archives. August 19, 1992. https://www.upi.com/Archives/1992/08/19/Court-approves-settlement-in-Shiley-heart-valve-case/4515714196800/.
363 Meier, Barry. "Pfizer Unit to Settle Charges of Lying About Heart Valve." *New York Times.* July 2, 1994. https://www.nytimes.com/1994/07/02/business/pfizer-unit-to-settle-charges-of-lying-about-heart-valve.html.
364 Smith, David. "Pfizer Pays Out to Nigerian Families of Meningitis Drug Trial Victims." *The Guardian.* August 12, 2011. https://www.theguardian.com/world/2011/aug/11/pfizer-nigeria-meningitis-drug-compensation.
365 Reuters. "Pfizer to Pay $49 Million in Fraud Case." *New York Times.* October 29, 2002. https://www.nytimes.com/2002/10/29/business/pfizer-to-pay-49-million-in-fraud-case.html.
366 Harris, Gardiner. "Pfizer to Pay $430 Million Over Promoting Drug to Doctors." *New York Times.* May 14, 2004. https://www.nytimes.com/2004/05/14/business/pfizer-to-pay-430-million-over-promoting-drug-to-doctors.html.
367 Saul, Stephanie. "Experts Conclude Pfizer Manipulated Studies." *New York Times.* October 8, 2008. https://www.nytimes.com/2008/10/08/health/research/08drug.html.
368 Office of Public Affairs. "Justice Department Announces Largest Health Care Fraud Settlement in Its History." Press release. US Department of Justice. September 2, 2009.
369 Girion, Lisa, Myron Levin, and David Willman. "Pfizer Agrees to Settle Suit Over Diabetes Drug Rezulin." *Los Angeles Times.* December 22, 2001. https://www.latimes.com/archives/la-xpm-2001-dec-22-mn-17267-story.html.
370 Feeley, Jef and Janelle Lawrence. "Pfizer to Pay $142.1 Million Over Neurontin Marketing." January 28, 2011. https://www.bloomberg.com/news/articles/2011-01-28/pfizer-ordered-to-pay-142-1-million-in-damages-over-neurontin-marketing.
371 Wilson, Duff. "Pfizer Gives Details on Payments to Doctors." *New York Times.* March 31, 2010.

372 Edwards, Jim. "Blue Cross Names and Shames Pfizer Execs Linked to Massages-for-Prescription Push." CBS Money Watch. June 10, 2010. https://www.cbsnews.com/news/blue-cross-names-and-shames-pfizer-execs-linked-to-massages-for-prescriptions-push/.
373 Boseley, Sarah. "WikiLeaks Cables: Pfizer 'Used Dirty Tricks to Avoid Clinical Trial Payout'." *The Guardian.* December 9, 2010. https://www.theguardian.com/business/2010/dec/09/wikileaks-cables-pfizer-nigeria.
374 Newsroom. "SEC Charges Pfizer with FCPA Violations." Press release. US Securities and Exchange Commission. August 7, 2012. https://www.sec.gov/newsroom/press-releases/2012-2012-152htm.
375 Feeley, Jef. "Pfizer Paid $896 Million in Prempro Settlement." *Bloomberg.* June 19, 2012. https://www.bloomberg.com/news/articles/2012-06-19/pfizer-paid-896-million-in-prempro-accords-filing-shows-1-.
376 Turner, Terry. "Proton Pump Inhibitor (PPI) Lawsuits." DrugWatch. Updated April 1, 2025. https://www.drugwatch.com/proton-pump-inhibitors/lawsuits/.
377 Staton, Tracy. "Pfizer Settles 2000-Plus Chantix Suits, Takes $273 M Charge." *Fierce Pharma.* March 4, 2013. https://www.fiercepharma.com/sales-and-marketing/pfizer-settles-2-000-plus-chantix-suits-takes-273m-charge.
378 Palmer, Eric. "Pfizer Settles More Off-Label Marketing Cases Tied to Rapamune." *Fierce Pharma.* August 7, 2014. https://www.fiercepharma.com/regulatory/pfizer-settles-more-off-label-marketing-cases-tied-to-rapamune.
379 Espiner, Tom. "Pfizer Fined Record £84.2 M for Overcharging NHS." BBC News. December 7, 2016. https://www.bbc.com/news/business-38233852#:~:text=Drugs%20giant%20Pfizer%20has%20been,drugs%20industry%2C%20the%20CMA%20said.
380 Weber, Lauren, and McKenzie Beard.
381 Kirsch, Steve.
382 Kirsch, Steve.
383 Nevradakis, Michael. "'Medical Warfare': Doctors Who Questioned COVID Shots, Promoted Ivermectin Lose Certification." *The Defender*. August 14, 2024.

About the Author

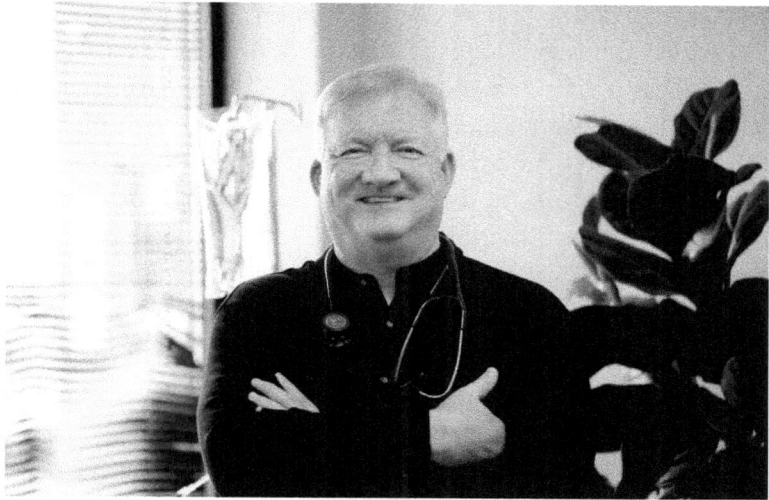

Dr. Joseph Jacko is a thought leader in the medical field. His selective contrarian mindset allows him to abandon conventional beliefs that become stale over time, recognizing that breakthroughs in any field occur when there is a breakthrough in thought.

The author has more than 39 years of experience in the medical field. He was one of the first internists in the country to complete a formal primary care sports medicine fellowship at the Hughston Orthopaedic Clinic (now the

Hughston Clinic). From there, he went to the Cooper Clinic and Institute for Aerobics Research in Dallas, founded by Kenneth Cooper, MD, PhD. He spent most of his career with Southwest Orthopedic Institute (since merged with the Texas Orthopaedic Association) in Dallas, Texas, where he treated some of the best high school athletes in the Dallas Independent School District. Later, he joined the Steadman-Hawkins Clinic of the Carolinas, the Cenegenics Medical Institute, and now has a concierge practice in Columbus, Ohio.

Along the way, Dr. Jacko practiced under and with some of the best physicians and surgeons in the country, many of whom have been pioneers in their fields. He completed a fellowship in regenerative medicine and has certifications in the use of peptides and as a personal trainer. The author's current practice provides patients with a wide selection of treatment options, including access to dieticians, exercise physiologists, personal trainers, massage therapists, athletic coaches, and three fitness centers with the latest technology in sports performance recovery.

Connect with Dr. Jacko at www.jackomd180.com.

Interested in Finding Out More About Preventive Medicine?

Dr. Jacko has given numerous talks on sports medicine, exercise, nutrition, and hormones. Reach out today to have him speak at your next event!

KEYNOTE SPEAKER

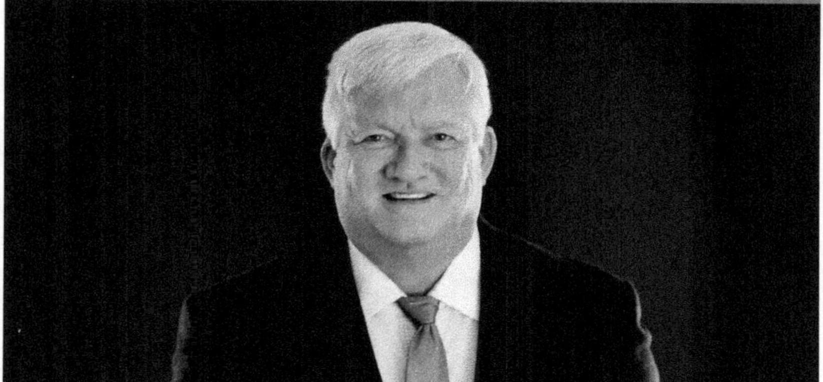

START THE CONVERSATION TODAY

JackoMD180.com

Living Life

THROUGH HEALTHY AGING

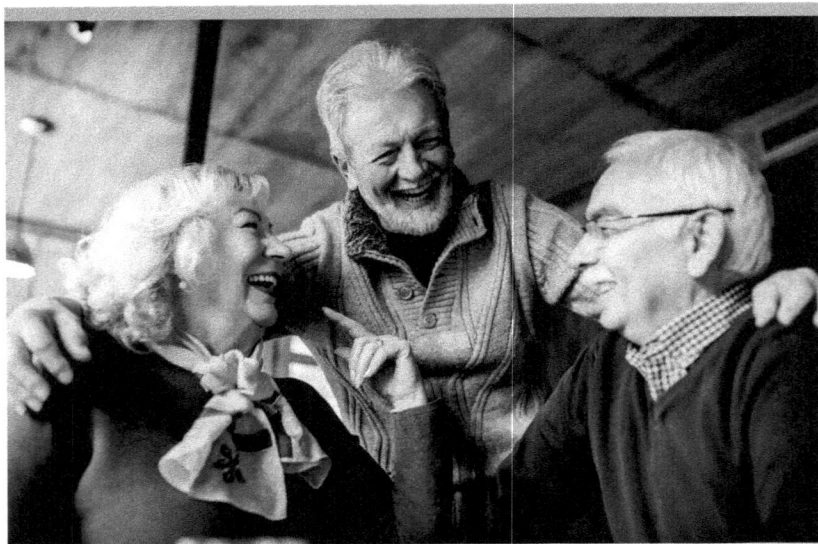

Take The First Step To Better Health Today!

JackoMD180.com